T0227125

Rabies

Clinical Considerations and Exposure Evaluations

Rabies

Clinical Considerations and Exposure Evaluations

PAMELA J. WILSON, MEd, LVT, MCHES
Texas Department of State Health Services
Zoonosis Control Branch
Austin, TX, United States

RODNEY E. ROHDE, PhD, MS, SM(ASCP)^{CM}, SV^{CM},
MB^{CM}, FACSc
College of Health Professions
Clinical Laboratory Science Program
Texas State University
San Marcos, TX, United States

ERNEST H. OERTLI, DVM, PhD, Diplomate, ACVPM
Private Consultant
Bertram, TX, United States

RODNEY E. WILLOUGHBY, Jr., MD
Professor of Pediatrics
Medical College of Wisconsin
Milwaukee, WI, United States

ELSEVIER

RABIES: CLINICAL CONSIDERATIONS AND EXPOSURE EVALUATIONS   ISBN: 978-0-323-63979-8
Copyright © 2019 Elsevier, Inc. All rights reserved.

No part of this publication may be reproduced or transmitted in any form or by any means, electronic
or mechanical, including photocopying, recording, or any information storage and retrieval system,
without permission in writing from the publisher. Details on how to seek permission, further information about the Publisher's permissions policies and our arrangements with organizations such
as the Copyright Clearance Center and the Copyright Licensing Agency, can be found at our website:
www.elsevier.com/permissions.

This book and the individual contributions contained in it are protected under copyright by the Publisher
(other than as may be noted herein).

Notices

Practitioners and researchers must always rely on their own experience and knowledge in evaluating
and using any information, methods, compounds or experiments described herein. Because of rapid
advances in the medical sciences, in particular, independent verification of diagnoses and drug dos-
ages should be made. To the fullest extent of the law, no responsibility is assumed by Elsevier, authors,
editors or contributors for any injury and/or damage to persons or property as a matter of products
liability, negligence or otherwise, or from any use or operation of any methods, products, instructions,
or ideas contained in the material herein.

Publisher: Dolores Meloni
Acquisition Editor: Sarah Barth
Editorial Project Manager: Megan Ashdown
Project Manager: Kiruthika Govindaraju
Cover Designer: Alan Studholme

ELSEVIER

3251 Riverport Lane
St. Louis, Missouri 63043

Working together
to grow libraries in
developing countries

www.elsevier.com • www.bookaid.org

List of Contributors

Ernest H. Oertli, DVM, PhD, Diplomate, ACVPM
Private Consultant
Bertram, TX, United States

Rodney E. Rohde, PhD, MS, SM(ASCP)^{CM}, SV^{CM}, MB^{CM}, FACSc
College of Health Professions
Clinical Laboratory Science Program
Texas State University
San Marcos, TX, United States

Rodney E. Willoughby, Jr., MD
Professor of Pediatrics
Medical College of Wisconsin
Milwaukee, WI, United States

Pamela J. Wilson, MEd, LVT, MCHES
Texas Department of State Health Services
Zoonosis Control Branch
Austin, TX, United States

Preface

Anyone seriously working in the field of rabies has been fascinated by its complexity and frustrated by its mysteries.

From Rupprecht CE, Hanlon CA, Hemachudha T. Rabies Re-Examined. *Lancet Infect Dis.* 2002;2:327–343.

With over 50 combined years working with rabies, we are in full agreement with this insightful quote and feel fortunate that we have been able to delve deeply into these complexities and mysteries together, accompanied by our remarkably distinguished collaborators, Drs. Skip Oertli and Rodney E. Willoughby. Our journey into the realms of rabies began under the guidance of one of the legendary leaders of this disease, Dr. Keith Clark, and allowed us to thankfully and exuberantly meet more respected, renowned rabies experts than we ever could have imagined, including Dr. Charles Rupprecht, who we obviously continue to quote today. Although our careers eventually took diverse pathways, we have maintained a fervor for rabies accompanied with a focus on education.

The original title for this book was *Rabid Revelations: The Fallacies and Realities of Rabies*, which in ways is more descriptive of its original intent. The purpose of this book is not to provide a comprehensive review and inclusion of all the literature, history, and theories of rabies or a detailed description of the causative virus and its pathogenesis; for readers with an interest for in-depth elements of the disease, more extensive information is provided in other books, such as Jackson's *Rabies: Scientific Basis of the Disease and Its Management* by Elsevier. Rather, as described in Chapter 1, this book is designed to provide approachable, compact information for physicians, veterinarians, veterinary technicians, public health and health department professionals, and academic faculty in health care on pertinent aspects pertaining to means of transmission and clinical signs and symptoms of rabies (Chapter 2) and the prevalence and epidemiology of rabies in geographic areas (Chapter 3), plus routes of exposure, what constitutes an exposure, and when rabies postexposure prophylaxis (PEP) is warranted (Chapter 6).

Additionally, although some global perspectives will be presented pertaining to prevalence and epidemiology (which are decisively relevant when determining if PEP administration is warranted, especially for people who may have been exposed abroad), the focus of the book will be rabies and administration of PEP in the United States. Pertinent information pertaining to specimen submission and laboratory testing for humans and animals will also be covered (Chapter 4). The need for a book with this quick-reference design became evident after we formed a positive team with Dr. Alison Bert, then Editor-in-Chief of Elsevier Connect, to prepare two articles, *8 Things You May Not Know About Rabies - But Should* and *The Many Faces of Rabies*. Upon publication, the first article in particular went viral (as a disease such as rabies inherently does) and subsequently received about 400,000 views and 200 comments in the 3 years since, with no sign of slowing down. We continue to receive and reply to questions from people throughout the world. Upon seeing the response to these articles and realizing the need for more education on rabies, Dr. Bert astutely proposed that we write a book for Elsevier that would include some of these real-life scenarios, which are presented in Chapter 7. Many of the website inquiries were generated through misunderstandings related to rabies, partially created by folklore; therefore, common myths and legends of the disease are clarified in Chapter 5. In sync with these issues is the apparent need for education concerning the prevention of rabies not only for health professionals but also for the public at large, which is covered in Chapter 8. We hope that our passion for rabies education is contagious.

Wishing you well—Pam and Rodney R.

Biographies

Pamela J. Wilson is a Licensed Veterinary Technician and a Master Certified Health Education Specialist. For more than 25 years, she has worked in Zoonosis Control at the Texas Department of State Health Services (DSHS) in Austin subsequent to working at Hyde Park Animal Clinic for multiple years. Additionally, Wilson was an adjunct instructor for 16 years teaching veterinary medical terminology with a focus on anatomy and physiology at Austin Community College and has done veterinary assistant training programs with the Texas Veterinary Medical Association.

She has published multiple articles on rabies in the peer-reviewed *Journal of the American Veterinary Medical Association*, plus articles on various topics in *Texas Veterinarian* and *Best Friends Magazine*. Wilson wrote the chapter on rabies for the seventh edition of *Robinson's Current Therapy in Equine Medicine*, published by Elsevier. She is also the author of three books about animals, including *Puppy Pal Pointers: From the True Tails of Ripple and Jessie*, which contains helpful care tips for dogs (and cats) of all ages, plus *Tales From Tubblewood* and *Tales From Tubblewood Too*, which includes guidance on responsible pet ownership— www.tubblewoodtales.com or www.authorhouse.com.

Wilson graduated with honors while earning a Bachelor of Science degree in zoology from Southern Illinois University Carbondale and a Master of Education degree in health education with a focus on zoonotic diseases from the University of Texas at Austin. Her awards include the Charles L. Foote Achievement Award in Zoology (SIU Carbondale), Humane Educator (Texas Animal Control Association), Veterinary Technician of the Year (Texas Veterinary Medical Association), Alumni Achievement Award (Spoon River College), and the Honors for Excellence in Achievement, Leadership, and Teamwork in Health (HEALTH) Award from the Texas DSHS. She has a deep passion and compassion for animals. Her heart and home have been shared with many beloved dogs and cats.

Dr. Rodney E. Rohde is Professor and Chair of the Clinical Laboratory Science Program (CLS), as well as Research Dean, in the College of Health Professions at Texas State University. He has been recognized for numerous awards, including Fellow of the Association of Clinical Scientists, Global Citizenship Alliance Global Fellow, Everette Swinney Faculty Senate Teaching Award, Texas State Alumni Association Teaching Award of Honor, and Mariel M. Muir Mentoring Award. Dr. Rohde continues to enjoy being an adjunct associate professor of biology in the biology department for Austin Community College where he received the Teaching Excellence Award and John and Suanne Roueche Excellence Award for Teaching. He holds certifications as a Specialist in Virology, Specialist in Microbiology, and Molecular Biologist from the American Society for Clinical Pathology.

Prior to his academic career, Rodney spent a decade as a public health microbiologist and molecular epidemiologist with the Texas Department of State Health Services (DSHS) Bureau of Laboratories and Zoonosis Control Division, including two terms as a CDC Visiting Scientist. Dr. Rohde helped establish the DSHS laboratory as an internationally recognized regional reference laboratory for rabies typing. He was an inaugural and founding member with the internationally successful Oral Rabies Vaccination Program that helped eliminate canine rabies from parts of Texas. Rodney received the prestigious J.V. Irons Award for Scientific Excellence from the DSHS Bureau of Laboratories for his efforts in rabies control and prevention.

He has published more than 50 research articles and abstracts and presented at over 100 international, national, and state conferences. As recipient of the 2015 urEssential Award from Cardinal Health, the Rodney E. Rohde endowed scholarship was established for Texas State's CLS Program for students seeking careers in laboratory science. He has been recognized multiple times as the Distinguished Author by ASCLS and was awarded by the same organization the 2016, 2015, 2014, and 2007 ASCLS Scientific Research Award for his work with rabies and MRSA. A TEDx speaker, he is one of the global "Top 20 Professors of Clinical Laboratory Science You Should Know."

Dr. Rohde's background is in public health and clinical microbiology. His research focuses on adult education and public health microbiology with respect to rabies virology, oral rabies wildlife vaccination, antibiotic resistant bacteria, and molecular diagnostics/biotechnology. He is a Past President of the Texas Association for Clinical Laboratory Science. For more information about Dr. Rohde, see http://rodneyerohde.wp.txstate.edu/ and follow on Twitter @RodneyRohde & @TXST_CLS, as well as Facebook and Linkedin.

Dr. Ernest "Skip" Oertli, married 50 years, a father of 3, and a grandfather of 8 grandchildren/6 step grandchildren, is now retired and works part time as a Consultant. Upon graduation from high school, Dr. Oertli entered Texas A&M University, where he completed the first of his three degrees, a BS in 1969. He later returned to complete a second degree, a DVM, in 1976. The interlude was spent as a Combat Engineer in the Marine Corps. The utilization of his veterinary medicine training was deployed as a veterinarian in the Air Force. Leaving the Air Force active duty forces upon deciding to pursue a specialized education, Dr. Oertli graduated from Texas A&M University a third time with a Ph.D. in Toxicology in 1985. He then practiced veterinary medicine for 2 years, starting the Hwy 29 Veterinary Clinic in Bertram, Texas. Having stayed in the Air Force Reserves, he sold his solo mixed animal practice and reentered active duty. Completing a military career, Dr. Oertli retired from the Air Force as a Colonel in 1997. To date, he is associated with the following professional organizations: Diplomate American College of Veterinary Preventive Medicine; Society of Forensic Toxicologists; Southwest Association of Toxicologists; and Midwest Association for Toxicology and Therapeutic Drug Monitoring. Dr. Oertli's work experience includes working as Chief, Bureau of Epidemiology, Texas Department of Health, and the Texas Department of State Health Services' Director of the Oral Rabies Vaccination Program (retired on August 31, 2013).

Dr. Rodney E. Willoughby, Jr., is a Professor of Pediatrics (Infectious Diseases) at the Medical College of Wisconsin and Children's Hospital of Wisconsin. He is the originator of the Milwaukee Protocol for treatment of human rabies, counting 18 survivors of this previously untreatable encephalitis. The current version of the protocol is available online at www.mcw.edu/rabies.

Dr. Willoughby survived many wild animal and conventional warm-blooded pet zoonoses during his childhood in Spain, California, and Peru (opossum, spider monkey, parrot, parakeets, duck, cats, dogs, horse, lamb, kid, outside rabbits, guinea pigs). He graduated with a BA in Biology from Princeton University (2007) and a MD from Johns Hopkins University (JHU, 1982), including a year working in Switzerland and Cameroon. He underwent further training in pediatrics (University of California at San Diego and JHU), infectious diseases (JHU), biochemistry (JHU), and clinical investigation (JHU). He was Clinical and Fellowship Director, Pediatric Infectious Diseases, at Johns Hopkins Hospital and moved to Wisconsin (2004) where the Milwaukee Protocol was improvised during his second week on call. He is a past member of the Committee on Infectious Diseases of the American Academy of Pediatrics and has served on diverse working groups at the Centers for Disease Control and Prevention. He has lectured on rabies in Brazil, Chile, China, Colombia, and Japan. His research interests include brain infections, including rabies, NMR metabolomics, and bacterial pathogenesis by hydrogen sulfide as a toxicant. He is married to a Brazilian ceramicist/sculptor, with three children and three dogs. Coyotes, raccoons, foxes, opossums, deer, flying squirrels, rabbits, chipmunks, voles, mice, and wild turkey share the author's ecosystem.

Acknowledgments

Sincere appreciation is extended to the Zach Jones Memorial Fund for their unwavering efforts to assist with educational awareness, early detection, and ultimately the cure for rabies—www.zachjonesmemorial.org/.

Gratitude is given to Drs. Tom Sidwa, James Alexander, James Wright, Eric Fonken, and David Florin for lending their considerable expertise to insightfully assess the content of various chapters; Dr. Ryan Wallace for patiently responding to numerous technical questions; David McLellan for efficiently assisting with literature searches; Elizabeth Wilson and Deborah Speicher for graciously reviewing chosen chapters; Dr. Laura Robinson for being a fountain of information and advice on rabies issues; Patrick Hunt for kindly providing database assistance; Zoonosis Control colleagues past and present for sharing thought-provoking case investigations; Dr. Keith Clark for being an encouraging rabies mentor; William D. Wilson for inspiring a passion for science and education; and Mary A. Wilson for being an endless source of unconditional support in every element of life.

Pamela J. Wilson

I would like to acknowledge all of the amazing public health, academic, medical/clinical laboratory professionals, and friends who have mentored and supported me during my life. You know who you are, and I thank God every day you entered my life!

I would like to thank my dear wife Bonnie for being my best friend and the foundation of our beautiful family, daughter Haley and son Landry; my parents, David and Nelda Rohde, for raising me as a child of God and instilling in me the work ethic to be successful; and my siblings, Winchel and Wendy, and my wife's entire family. I love you all so much!

I am passionate about teaching and mentoring students toward productive and exciting careers and life experiences. I would like to thank all of my current and former Texas State and ACC students who have helped shape my life and career. I hope I have helped you all with advocacy, leadership, research, and integrity in your educational experience and challenged you to strive for lifelong learning. #WeSaveLivesEveryday #TXST #Lab4Life

Rodney E. Rohde

Contents

CHAPTER 1

Introduction

PAMELA J. WILSON, MEd, LVT, MCHES

PERPLEXITIES OF RABIES

An animal infected with this disease may show any one or all of these signs or none of them.

From Center for Disease Control (now the Centers for Disease Control and Prevention), Public Health Services, Viral Diseases Division, Bureau of Epidemiology. *Clinical Rabies in Animals.* Video (discontinued).[1] https://www.cdc.gov/.

This quote is taken from a rabies educational film that has been used in classroom and training settings for decades as the video gives a concise, precise overview of the more common clinical signs of rabies in animals. The message that is relayed embodies the perplexity and elusiveness of rabies that holds true not only for its diverse clinical signs and symptoms but also for its problematic routes of exposure and varying incubation period. It is, indeed, amazing that with all the advances in science and health care, a disease that was noted in legal documents in Mesopotamia as early as 2300 BC in which owners were held responsible for deaths resulting from bites from their "mad" or "vicious" dogs and described as a disease that drives the animal mad by Aristotle in the 4th century BC[2,3] is still, with a few exceptions, fatal by the time clinical signs and symptoms develop. If rabies postexposure prophylaxis (PEP) is administered before the virus enters the nervous system and prior to the onset of clinical features, the disease can be prevented,[4] but this mode of prevention requires that the person exposed to the virus knows to seek medical attention and the attending physician knows to prescribe the proper rabies biologics. Throughout this length of history, Pasteur's development of an effective rabies vaccine in the 1880s was a landmark advancement in preventing rabies[3,5] and made rabies one of the frontrunners among vaccine-preventable diseases.[6] However, elements of the pathogenesis and core etiology of rabies, as well as a reliably effective cure, remain

an enigma after centuries of awareness of this disease and how it manifests (see Fig. 1.1).

NEEDS OF HEALTH PROFESSIONALS

Pertaining to salve applied to a bite wound of a potentially rabid dog, remove it and feed it to a hen.

If the bird eats it and does not die, the victim was not bitten by a rabid dog.

Oribasius (AD 325–399).[7]

Antiquated practices such as this might have been limited in the catacombs of history, but PEP recommendations are much more complex. (Note: for up-to-date testing techniques, refer to Chapter 4; don't use the "feeding salve to a hen" approach.) While dealing with multiple clients on a daily basis or an endless stream of emergencies, most health professionals for both humans and animals do not have time to read extensive history, research descriptions, and experimental designs to locate the basic information they require to effectively evaluate a potential rabies exposure to determine if administration of PEP is warranted. The intent of this book is to aid them in the goal of quickly accessing this information, which includes common modes of transmission, fundamental pathogenesis, clinical signs and symptoms, and modes of prevention. Critical concerns specific to possible exposure to rabid bats and details on potential exposure scenarios are also outlined.

When conducting a literature search on rabies, one can develop an appreciation for the frustration a health professional might experience when trying to find basic information to address a case involving a potential exposure to rabies. On many of the disease topics, such as the incubation period, disease stages, and clinical signs and symptoms, volumes may have to be read on studies with varying, sometimes opposing, outcomes with

Rabies. https://doi.org/10.1016/B978-0-323-63979-8.00001-5
Copyright © 2019 Elsevier Inc. All rights reserved.

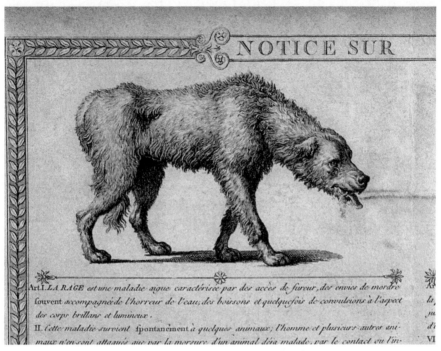

FIG. 1.1 Vintage Rabies Notice—French Line Engraving—1785 (Wellcome Library, London). Precautions on rabies, describing an acute disease characterized by fits of rage, the desire to bite, often accompanied by a fear of water and drinks, and sometimes convulsions of the body. (Translation courtesy of Steve Rogers, Austin, Texas.)

the potential result of still lacking clarity on the topic or a concrete answer to an issue in question. Such is the elusive nature of this disease as there sometimes are no clear resolves or concrete answers. Thus, these observations should not be construed as criticisms, as that is not the intent, but rather as rabies realities. Even within the confines of this book, research had to be directed toward trying to resolve discrepancies created by use of varying references and experiences. Another actuality made apparent was that narratives of the various aspects of the disease are lengthy. Concise, yet comprehensive, tables are difficult to design because of numerous qualifiers that need to be expressed to provide an accurate description and capture not only the more common elements of the disease but also outliers that may be of importance in a particular situation for implementing a proper PEP evaluation or considering differential diagnoses. Additionally, oftentimes experimental models are used when trying to describe the disease in animals. For example, it would be impossible to know when a rabid wild animal was actually exposed to the virus in nature and, hence, the range of the incubation period remains uncertain. Therefore, timeframes for different periods and stages of the disease in animals are frequently based

on experimental inoculation of animals with rabies virus, which may or may not reflect how the disease would progress in naturally infected animals.[6] There are even impending changes in the viral taxonomy, so the standard systematic classification is also in a state of evolution.[8] In essence, the more this disease is studied, the more exceptions are uncovered, which adds to the difficulty presented to physicians and veterinarians (in locales where PEP for animals is permitted) in determining when to prescribe and administer PEP. In the realm of rabies, one size certainly does not fit all. One goal of this book is to present some of these broad concepts and ranges in pertinent scientific findings while trying to provide need-to-know facts in a manageable format.

Another goal is to present real-life scenarios through website inquiries and rabies cases, plus anecdotal reports, to give examples of situations that might be presented to a practitioner. There is a quote from an undetermined source (it has been attributed by some to the astronomer, Carl Sagan) that "The plural of anecdote is not data." However, there are insights to be gained when considering reviews of such scenarios. They also provide memorable avenues for applying lessons learned by others in future similar circumstances.

PREVALENCE OF RABIES AND RABIES POSTEXPOSURE PROPHYLAXIS

Rabies is not a simple long-ago vestige, nightmarish myth, or literary allegory but rather a significant viral encephalitis with the highest case fatality of any conventional infectious disease.

From Rupprecht C, Kuzmin I, Meslin F. Lyssaviruses and rabies: current conundrums, concerns, contradictions and controversies. F1000Res. 2017;6(184):1–22.[8]

Despite the severity of the clinical course of rabies, awareness of the disease can be lacking. Rabies is relatively rare in humans in the United States with generally one to three cases reported annually,[9] so it is oftentimes a forgotten disease not only by the general public but also by health professionals when considering it as a differential in diagnoses, which could contribute to underreporting of rabies cases. The importance of detecting rabies is evident when considering cases in which recipients of transplants subsequently developed rabies and the case investigations led to confirmation that the donors had died of undiagnosed rabies.[10,11] Rabies in animals in the United States is not so unusual with thousands of reported cases yearly.[4,12]

Globally, rabies is not as rare as one may think and remains a disease of public health significance. Rabies (or rabies-related viruses) exists in every continent except Antarctica.[13] Australia is free of dog-associated rabies[14]; however, Australian bat lyssavirus (rabies is a lyssavirus[15]) is diagnosed with standard rabies diagnostic reagents and prevented with traditional rabies vaccine, plus it has resulted in fatal human disease that is indistinguishable from classic rabies.[16] The list of rabies-free countries fluctuates and is updated by and available through the Centers for Disease Control and Prevention (CDC).[17]

It is difficult to assess the annual number of human rabies deaths worldwide because of underreporting in developing countries, but the estimation is in the tens of thousands with approximations reaching 59,000 cases per year or higher, placing rabies among the deadliest of zoonotic diseases.[5,14,18] The estimation is that more than 99% of rabies case fatalities occur in developing countries,[14,19] particularly Africa and Asia, with India accounting for the most reported deaths in Asia.[14] The low number of cases in humans in the United States compared with that in many developing countries can be attributed partially to exposed individuals in the United States having expeditious access to medical care and rabies biologics, which are nearly 100% effective if administered promptly and properly.[20] Annually, an estimated 40,000 people in the United States[21,22] and 15 million people worldwide[5] receive PEP.

Rabies in humans and animals has been a notifiable condition in the United States since 1944.[4] From 1946 (the year the Communicable Disease Center, which was the forerunner of the CDC, established its national rabies control program) to 1965, there were 236 cases of rabies in humans reported in the United States. Most of these cases were attributed to exposures to rabid dogs.[21,23] Campaigns involving vaccination of dogs and control of stray animals during the 1940s and 1950s,[23,24] coupled with progressive animal control programs highlighting knowledgeable, dedicated animal control officers, enactment of leash laws and vaccination requirements, and an emphasis on sterilization of pets to reduce overpopulation issues,[25] have been credited with the reduction of rabies cases in dogs in the United States.[23] The most common rabies virus variants involved in indigenous rabies cases in humans in the United States then changed from dog variant to those associated with bats.[6,9,26]

Adding to the difficulties of assessing the need for PEP is the variety of animals considered to be high risk for transmitting rabies in different locales. This becomes a significant issue for health professionals being presented with a possible exposure that may have occurred in another country or even a different area of the United States. Some species have an increased possibility of being rabid in certain geographic locations compared with other areas. For example, PEP is recommended for patients bitten or otherwise potentially exposed to rabies by a nonhuman primate in countries where rabies is enzootic.[27,28] However, observation of the animal for a defined period may be all that is warranted if the biting nonhuman primate is a pet in the United States. In the United States, rabies in wildlife constitutes more than 90% of the cases of rabies in animals with the highest numbers usually being attributable to bats, raccoons, and skunks.[4,12] Conversely, on a worldwide basis, at least 99% of human rabies cases are caused by exposure to rabid dogs.[12,14,29]

Even though rabies is more common in wildlife than domestic animals in the United States, reports have indicated that people are more likely to be exposed to rabies through a domestic animal than a wild one.[30,31] The American Veterinary Medical Association estimated that 59.5% of all US households owned pets and that 64% of these pet-owning households owned more than one pet.[32] This provides ample opportunities for pets to bring rabies into the home environment after being exposed to rabid wildlife. They may also bring the actual rabid animal into the home, such as a cat carrying in a downed rabid bat.[33] Even a pet door can be an open invitation for a rabid animal, such as a skunk, to enter a house.[34] In the United States, an estimated

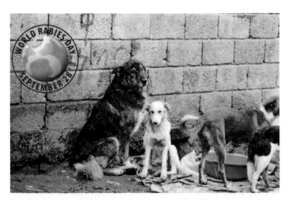

FIG. 1.2 **World Rabies Day: Share the Word; Save a Life.** (Courtesy of the Centers for Disease Control and Prevention, Atlanta, Georgia.)

4.5 million people are bitten by dogs annually[35]; all of these bite scenarios should be evaluated to determine if the administration of PEP is warranted.

Although the majority of rabies cases in the United States occur in wildlife, research showed that approximately 86% of humans who received PEP did so because of potential exposure through dogs and cats, which reflects the close association between people and dogs and cats.[31,36] It has been estimated that nearly half of pet owners in the United States consider their pets to be family members while the other half consider their pets to be pets/companions.[32] This strong human-animal bond illustrates the need for knowledgeable and appropriate implementation of PEP not only from a public health perspective, including both preventing rabies when administration of PEP is warranted and avoiding needless PEP in situations in which there has not been a valid exposure, but also to prevent unnecessary euthanatizing and testing of animals by allowing observation and quarantine or confinement when possible. Client education on rabies awareness and the importance of rabies vaccinations for animals is an essential component for proactively preventing challenging rabies exposure scenarios.

In addition to the tragic toll taken on human life due to this disease, there is an estimated economic cost worldwide of $8.6 billion annually, of which 6% is because of livestock losses.[14,18] In the United States alone, the expenditure on rabies prevention has been approximated at $500 million annually.[22]

Rabies is such a worldwide health problem that September 28 is dedicated annually toward educating the world about this disease (see Fig. 1.2). World Rabies Day uses a One Health approach, which encompasses the inextricable connections among human health, animal health, and the state of the environment. Given that rabies is a neglected disease even among neglected diseases,[6] this commemorative day is intended to raise awareness of rabies and encourage people to vaccinate their pets; the focus is on rabies-endemic countries with the goal of increasing community consciousness about the disease and its prevention.[24,37] These should be fundamental goals for all health professionals.

REFERENCES

1. Center for Disease Control (now the Centers for Disease Control and Prevention), Public Health Services, Viral Diseases Division, Bureau of Epidemiology. *Clinical Rabies in Animals.* Video (discontinued). https://www.cdc.gov/.
2. Baer GM, Neville J, Turner GS. *Epidemiology.* In: *Rabbis and Rabies: A Pictorial History of Rabies Through the Ages.* Mexico: Laboratorios Baer; 1996:13–26.
3. Wilkinson L. History. In: Jackson AC, Wunner WH, eds. *Rabies.* Academic Press-Elsevier Science; 2002:1–22.
4. Birhane MG, Cleaton JM, Monroe BP, et al. Rabies surveillance in the United States during 2015. *JAVMA.* 2017;250(10):1117–1130.
5. Singh R, Singh KP, Cherian S, et al. Rabies – epidemiology, pathogenesis, public health concerns and advances in diagnosis and control: a comprehensive review. *Vet Q.* 2017;37(1):212–251.
6. Willoughby RE. Rabies: rare human infection – common questions. *Infect Dis Clin N Am.* 2015;29:637–650.
7. Baer GM, Neville J, Turner GS. *Symptoms and diagnosis.* In: *Rabbis and Rabies: A Pictorial History of Rabies Through the Ages.* Mexico: Laboratorios Baer; 1996:29–45.
8. Rupprecht C, Kuzmin I, Meslin F. Lyssaviruses and rabies: current conundrums, concerns, contradictions and controversies. *F1000Res.* 2017;6(184):1–22.
9. Centers for Disease Control and Prevention. Rabies Surveillance in the U.S.: Human Rabies – Rabies. https://www.cdc.gov/rabies/location/usa/surveillance/human_rabies.html.
10. Centers for Disease Control and Prevention. Investigation of rabies infections in organ donor and transplant recipients – Alabama, Arkansas, Oklahoma, and Texas, 2004. *Morb Mortal Wkly Rep.* 2004;53:1–3.
11. Wallace RM, Stanek D, Griese S, et al. A large-scale, rapid public health response to rabies in an organ recipient and the previously undiagnosed organ donor. *Zoonoses Public Health.* 2014;61:560–570.
12. Ma X, Monroe BP, Cleaton JM, et al. Rabies surveillance in the United States during 2016. *JAVMA.* 2018;252(8):945–957.
13. Fooks AR, Banyard AC, Horton DL, et al. Current status of rabies and prospects for elimination. *Lancet.* 2014;384:1389–1399.

14. World Health Organization. *WHO Expert Consultation on Rabies*; 2018. WHO Technical Report Series No. 1012. Third report.

15. Wunner WH, Conzelmann KK. Rabies virus. In: Jackson AC, ed. *Rabies: Scientific Basis of the Disease and its Management*. San Diego: Academic Press, An Elsevier Science Imprint; 2013:17–60.

16. Hanlon CA, Childs JE. Epidemiology. In: Jackson AC, ed. *Rabies: Scientific Basis of the Disease and its Management*. San Diego: Academic Press, An Elsevier Science Imprint; 2013:61–121.

17. Centers for Disease Control and Prevention. Rabies-Free Countries and Political Units. https://www.cdc.gov/importation/rabies-free-countries.html.

18. Food and Agriculture Organization of the United Nations. The Food and Agriculture Organization and Rabies Prevention and Control. http://www.fao.org/3/a-i7873e.pdf.

19. Chacko K, Parakadavathu T, Al-Masiamani, et al. Diagnostic difficulties in human rabies: a case report and review of the literature. *Quar Med J*. 2016;(2):15. Published online 21.04.17 https://www.ncbi.nlm.nih.gov/articles/PMC5427514/.

20. Susilawathi NM, Darwinata AE, Dwija IB, et al. Epidemiological and clinical features of human rabies cases in Bali 2008-2010. *BMC Infect Dis*. 2012;12(81):1–8.

21. Gibbons RV. Cryptogenic rabies, bats, and the question of aerosol transmission. *Ann Emerg Med*. 2002;39(5):528–536.

22. Centers for Disease Control and Prevention. Take a Bite Out of Rabies. https://www.cdc.gov/features/rabies/index.html.

23. Childs JE. Epidemiology. In: Jackson AC, Wunner WH, eds. *Rabies*. Academic Press-Elsevier Science; 2002:113–162.

24. Petersen BW, Rupprecht CE. Human Rabies Epidemiology and Diagnosis. Intechopen; November 16, 2011. https://www.intechopen.com/books/non-flavivirus-encephalitis/human-rabies-epidemiology-and-diagnosis.

25. Rupprecht CE. A tale of two worlds: public health management decisions in human rabies prevention. *Clin Infect Dis*. 2004;39(2):281–283.

26. De Serres G, Dallaire F, Cote M, et al. Bat rabies in the United States and Canada from 1950 through 2007: human cases with and without bat contact. *Clin Infect Dis*. 2008;46:1329–1337.

27. Blaise A, Parola P, Brouqui P, et al. Rabies postexposure prophylaxis for travelers injured by nonhuman primates, Marseille, France, 2001–2014. *Emerg Infect Dis*. 2015;21(8).

28. Gautret P, Blanton J, Dacheux L, et al. Rabies in nonhuman primates and potential for transmission to humans: a literature review and examination of selected French national data. *PLoS Neg Trop Dis*. 2014;8(5):e2863.

29. Hergert M, Le Roux K, Nel LH. Characteristics of owned dogs in rabies endemic KwaZulu-Natal province, South Africa. *BMC Vet Res*. 2018;14(278):1–10.

30. Wilson PJ, Oertli EH, Hunt PR, et al. Evaluation of a postexposure rabies prophylaxis protocol for domestic animals in Texas: 2000-2009. *JAVMA*. 2010;237(12):1395–1401.

31. Murray KO, Holmes KC, Hanlon CA. Rabies in vaccinated dogs and cats in the United States, 1997–2001. *JAVMA*. 2009;235(6):691–696.

32. American Veterinary Medical Association. *Key Findings. U.S. Pet Ownership & Demographics Sourcebook*. Schaumburg: AVMA; 2007:1–6.

33. Mayes BC, Wilson PJ, Oertli EH, et al. Epidemiology of rabies in bats in Texas (2001-2010). *JAVMA*. 2013;243(8):1129–1137.

34. Oertli EH, Wilson PJ, Hunt PR, et al. Epidemiology of rabies in skunks in Texas. *JAVMA*. 2009;234(5):616–620.

35. American Veterinary Medical Association. Dog Bite Prevention. https://www.avma.org/public/Pages/Dog-Bite-Prevention.aspx.

36. Moran GJ, Talan DA, Mower W, et al. Appropriateness of rabies postexposure prophylaxis treatment for animal exposures. *JAMA*. 2000;284(8):1001–1007.

37. Global Alliance for Rabies Control. World Rabies Day. https://www.rabiesalliance.org/world-rabies-day/.

CHAPTER 2

Clinical Signs and Symptoms of Rabies

PAMELA J. WILSON, MEd, LVT, MCHES

SCENARIO

From an actual rabies case investigation: a man was checking on his son's cattle in a pasture. All the cattle were grazing except one that was lying down by itself. It got up and went to the water trough, but it did not drink. He called a veterinarian who suggested the cow might have "wooden tongue," a condition that renders the tongue stiff as a result of a bacterial infection. As the man tried to feel the cow's tongue, she slung her head and knocked him into the side of his pickup; he fell to the ground and broke his hip. Every time he moved, the cow head butted him. She finally lost interest and he crawled away and called for help. The first person to arrive on the scene started to make a call on his cell phone and while he was walking, the cow attacked him. In a struggle that ensued, the cow fell on this man, but the ambulance crew arrived in time to assist. The cow was killed, a specimen was submitted for rabies testing, and the result was positive. In retrospect, it was recalled that a dead skunk previously had been found near the water trough. A total of seven people had rabies postexposure prophylaxis (PEP) administered.[a]

Note: As can oftentimes be the case while considering different diagnoses, people put their hands in the mouths of rabid animals trying to determine why they are having difficulty eating, drinking, swallowing, or sounding like they are choking (all clinical signs of rabies, as are aggression, head butting, and a change in behavior). Unfortunately, they usually do not use precautions such as wearing gloves and, although saliva contact with intact skin does not constitute an exposure to rabies, if there is a chance that they had any type of nick, scratch, or other break in the skin, saliva contacting that break would constitute an exposure; the recommendation would be to err on the side of caution and administer PEP.

CHAPTER FORMAT

To aid in making need-to-know information readily accessible, this chapter is designed to present the fundamental facts in boxes on transmission and pathogenesis of rabies (see Overview of Rabies

Transmission and Pathogenesis section, Box 2.1); rabies in animals (see Rabies in Animals section, Box 2.2); and rabies in humans (see Rabies in Humans section, Box 2.3). Each box also contains guidance on where more detailed information on each fact is in the text, plus specific references. There are additional sections with special studies, reports, and cases for those interested.

OVERVIEW OF RABIES TRANSMISSION AND PATHOGENESIS

Description of the Rabies Virus

"Rabere" in Latin means "to be mad" or "to rage or rave."[1] Lyssaviruses are negative-sense, single-stranded, enveloped RNA viruses that contain a single-surface glycoprotein and a ribonucleoprotein core.[2] The rabies virus has a bullet-shaped morphology[3] and is highly neurotrophic[2,4]; it belongs to the family Rhabdoviridae ("rhabdos" is Greek for "rod"), genus *Lyssavirus*.[3]

"Lyssa" is Greek for "madness,"[1] "rage,"[3] or "violent" (from the root "lud").[5,6] "Lyssa" was also a deity in Greek mythology; she was the spirit of mad or blind rage, fury, raging madness, and rabies in animals.[7,8] Some have suggested that "lyssa" was derived from "lykos," meaning wolf, signifying that the madness stemmed from the absorption of a bestial nature; others have contended that its root was "lysis" implying the loosening or dissolving of one's rational faculties.[9] These Latin and Greek meanings and associations are descriptive of the nature of this elusive, behavior-changing disease.

Typical Transmission, Infectious Materials, and Basics of Pathogenesis

Rabies is a rapidly progressive infection of the central nervous system (CNS) and can affect any warm-blooded animal, although most concern about the disease centers around mammals. It usually is spread when saliva containing the virus enters a defect in the skin barrier. This is typically achieved through a bite from a rabid animal. Although rare, transmission could potentially occur with infected saliva contacting

Rabies. https://doi.org/10.1016/B978-0-323-63979-8.00002-7
Copyright © 2019 Elsevier Inc. All rights reserved.

7

BOX 2.1
Fundamental Facts: Transmission and
Pathogenesis of Rabies

The rabies virus belongs to the family Rhabdoviridae, genus *Lyssavirus* (see Description of the Rabies Virus section).

Rabies is caused by negative-sense, single-stranded, enveloped RNA viruses (see Description of the Rabies Virus section).

Rabies is a rapidly progressive encephalomyelitis that can affect any warm-blooded animal (see Typical Transmission, Infectious Materials, and Basics of Pathogenesis section).

Transmission is typically through the bite of a rabid animal. Although rare, transmission could occur by infectious materials, such as saliva and neural tissue (conceivably tears), contacting mucous membranes or a scratch or other break in the skin (see Typical Transmission, Infectious Materials, and Basics of Pathogenesis section).

Contact with intact skin does not constitute an exposure (see Typical Transmission, Infectious Materials, and Basics of Pathogenesis section).

Contact with feces, blood, or urine does not constitute an exposure nor does skunk spray (see Typical Transmission, Infectious Materials, and Basics of Pathogenesis and Human-to-Human Transmission sections).

On entry into the body, the rabies virus typically replicates in muscle tissue (or skin with some bat variants) for a variable length of time; the virus then enters the nervous system (see Typical Transmission, Infectious Materials, and Basics of Pathogenesis section).

Once the virus enters the nervous system, rabies is almost always fatal (see Typical Transmission, Infectious Materials, and Basics of Pathogenesis section).

Although other modes of transmission are theoretically possible, the only documented human-to-human transmission of rabies has been in recipients of transplants from donors who died of undiagnosed rabies (see Human-to-Human Transmission section).

Oral transmission could occur with the consumption of infected raw meat; cooking inactivates the virus. Transmission through unpasteurized milk is unlikely; pasteurization destroys the virus (see Oral Transmission section).

Airborne transmission may be possible under extreme conditions, for example, in a rabies laboratory or an unventilated cave with millions of bats (this route has been subject to debate) (see Airborne Transmission section).

No cases of rabies have been reported in association with transmission by fomites or environmental surfaces (see Fomite Transmission section).

Exposures to bats cause special concerns and customized recommendations for rabies postexposure prophylaxis; the bite marks from some species of bats are small enough to go unnoticed (see Exposures to Bats – Special Concerns section).

a mucous membrane or a scratch or other break in the skin,[10] including a wound inflicted by a saliva-contaminated claw of a rabid animal.[11] In a study conducted in India of 19 deaths in humans due to rabies, 5 were attributed to dog-related scratches/abrasions that created a break in the skin without any bleeding.[12] Virus contacting intact skin is not considered to be a mode of transmission.[7,13]

Contact with feces, blood, or urine does not constitute an exposure[2] nor does skunk spray.[14,15] There are some other potential modes of transmission, however, such as a mucous membrane or a break in the skin having contact with virus-laden neural tissue or conceivably tears.[16-20] Transplantation of corneas, organs, and tissue from an individual with rabies could transmit the virus.[4,7,18-20]

After the rabies virus is introduced into the body (see Fig. 2.1), it avoids immune detection (but is susceptible to neutralization if antibodies are present) and replicates in muscle tissue (may also occur in skin with some bat variants) for a variable length of time, leading to a wide range in the incubation period.[21-23] The virus ultimately binds to nicotinic acetylcholine receptors at the neuromuscular junction[23] (or possibly to unknown receptors in the skin with bat rabies[21]) and enters the nervous system. Once the virus enters the nervous system, rabies is, with few exceptions, fatal.[24] Centripetal propagation of the virus from the muscle is via the motor[22,23] (and perhaps sensory[23]) axons of peripheral nerves. The virus travels within axons in peripheral nerves via retrograde transport to the CNS[22,24,25] at a fairly constant rate of 8–20 mm/day[21]; the time this transport takes depends on the distance from the site of virus inoculation to the CNS.[21] The virus is propagated solely across synapses at the rate of approximately one synaptic network every 12 h.[2,22] Dorsal root ganglia become infected and contribute to the clinical syndrome but do not extend the infection.[2,22] The virus moves by centrifugal spread along peripheral nerves to the salivary glands and various organs of the body, including hair follicles in the skin.[23,25,26] Replication in most organs is limited to the nerves.

Human-To-Human Transmission

The only laboratory-confirmed rabies cases with human-to-human transmission have been through transplantation from a donor who succumbed to undiagnosed rabies.[4,18,19,27] It is theoretically possible to have human-to-human transmission via infectious material, notably saliva or neural tissue (potentially tears), from a person with rabies contacting a mucous membrane or break in the skin of another person.[16-20]

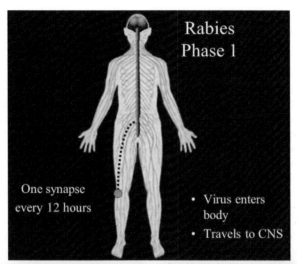

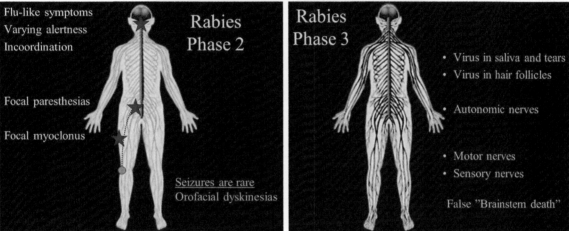

FIG. 2.1 **Pathogenesis of Rabies.** Slide 1 - rabies virus travels to the central nervous system at a rate of approximately one synaptic network every 12 h. Slide 2 - with the brain now completely full of rabies, the **peripheral** immune system finally notices this massive infection, causing flu-like symptoms. The motor cortex has been mapped, with focal myoclonus present in the bitten limb. The sensory system has been mapped, with local pain and paresthesias of the bitten limb. The cerebellum has been mapped, leading to incoordination. A notable feature of rabies, in addition to focal myoclonus and paresthesias, is that rabies patients are intermittently alert until just before death and can personally tell family and medical staff how horrible the disease is. Based on experience (REW), seizures are very rare unless there has been asphyxia or other complication. On the other hand, unusual movements of the face and mouth are common **and can be mistaken for seizures.** Slide 3 - rabies virus has to replicate to survive in nature. To do so, the virus moves in both directions, out as well as in. It populates every nerve in the body. This allows it to get to the salivary gland, to transmit by contaminated bite to the next victim. Rabies virus is found in small sensory nerves surrounding hair follicles in the skin, allowing easy diagnostic sampling of this highly innervated tissue by PCR or antigen detection. Saliva can also be sampled. Rabies virus in autonomic nervous system causes extreme dysautonomia that often causes death. Involvement of motor nerves leads to eventual paralysis. Involvement of the sensory nerves (including pain fibers) renders the patient unsuitable for a formal neurologic evaluation. Such a neurologic evaluation will make it appear as if the patient is brain dead, a false conclusion also seen in Miller-Fisher variants of Guillain-Barre syndrome and Bickerstaff encephalitis. Many patients are probably prematurely removed from critical care support because of this. (Courtesy of Dr. Rodney E. Willoughby, Medical College of Wisconsin, Milwaukee, Wisconsin.)

Similar contact with cerebrospinal fluid (CSF) being a potential source of exposure has been considered[11,17] and is under review (rabies antibodies have been found in CSF, but virus has not[b]).

Contact with urine from an infected person (or a rabid animal) is not considered to be an exposure.[2,20,28] In one study, rabies viral RNA (not infectious) was detected in urine[22] and in an investigation involving rabies in a recipient of a kidney from a donor who had died of undetected rabies, presumably rabies virus antigen (also not infectious) was found in high concentrations throughout kidney tissue[18]; however, these examples are atypical and urine is not recognized as an infectious material for rabies.

Congenital transmission is not considered to be a route of exposure nor is hematogenous transmission.[2] There has been at least one account of transplacental transmission mentioned in rabies literature[27] but with no defining mechanism[21] and no laboratory confirmation,[4] the evidence is insufficient to support congenital transmission as a route of exposure.

Oral Transmission

Oral transmission potentially could occur with the consumption of raw meat. This would be plausible with wild animals feeding on the carcasses of rabid animals[29] or humans eating raw meat, particularly in areas endemic for rabies in dogs where raw dog meat is consumed.[23,30] Although some references state that there have been no documented cases in humans transmitted via this route,[7] there have been reports of cases associated with the processes of slaughtering, preparing, and consuming street animals (dog and cat), including a study of 1839 rabies cases in humans in the Philippines, in which 21 were ascribed to eating raw dog meat.[30] Nonetheless, cooking will inactivate the rabies virus.[31] Contact with infected neural tissue could be a potential transmission concern during the process of butchering or skinning an infected carcass.[7,27,32] Ingestion of unpasteurized milk from a rabid cow has been considered to be a theoretical route of exposure.[11,27] The known pathology and progression of rabies virus makes it unlikely for rabies to be shed into milk[32]; additional study is warranted. Infectious rabies virus has not been isolated from the milk of rabid cows.[7] To avoid the dilemma of addressing a possible exposure via this route, the process of heat pasteurization destroys the rabies virus.[31-33]

Airborne Transmission

Airborne transmission has been reported in at least one laboratory worker.[34,35] Additionally, reports of two humans developing rabies by airborne transmission in a cave with a dense population of bats has been mentioned in rabies literature. Subsequent experiments in the same cave revealed airborne transmission to animals[34-37]; however, the oppressive conditions (kept in cages for 7–30 days in an environment in which the severe degree of heat, humidity, and ammonia-charged atmosphere apparently caused the death of some of the animals[36]) to which the animals in this experiment were subjected were not reflective of natural conditions.[34] It is thought that the presence of millions of bats and an unventilated area would be necessary for possible airborne transmission of the rabies virus.[23] There is also controversy as to the exact method of infection of the human cases in the cave; it is possible that they were caused by an undetected bat bite or other direct exposure.[34,37]

Fomite Transmission

Lyssaviruses replicate primarily in mammalian tissue and do not survive outside the host. The rabies virus can be destroyed by such elements as ultraviolet radiation, pH extremes, organic solvents, desiccation, excessive heat, and putrefaction. Therefore, transmission in the abiotic environment is unlikely[13] unless, for instance, the infected saliva was still moist and contacted a mucous membrane or a break in the skin. No cases of rabies have been reported in association with transmission by fomites or environmental surfaces[19,20]; bodies of water and inanimate objects do not have a role in rabies.[38]

Exposures to Bats—Special Concerns

When trying to diagnosis a possible case of rabies, one cannot rely on the patient to report a bite or other potential exposure. In close to 80% of US cases of a human with laboratory-confirmed bat rabies virus variant, there was no history of animal exposure.[2] Occasionally, the patient reported awakening to find a bat on the bed near the head and neck region or a family member reported that there were bats in the patient's home, but no bites or direct contact with a bat were noted. Bat teeth are very fine and a bite easily may go unnoticed (see Fig. 2.2); bat bites can be an undetectable pinpoint puncture mark less than or equal to 1 mm in diameter.[39] This led to the guidance that rabies postexposure prophylaxis (PEP) be considered for a person who was sleeping in the same room in which a bat was found or for an unattended child, a cognitively impaired person, or an intoxicated person in the same room in which a bat was found even if no noticeable bite wound is detected. This would be applicable when

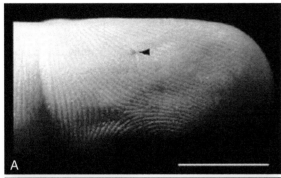

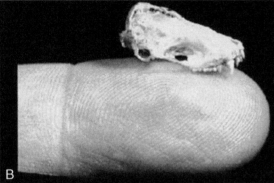

FIG. 2.2 Puncture wound (by *arrowhead*) of a bite from a canine tooth of a silver-haired bat **(A)** and skull of a silver-haired bat (17.1 mm in length and resting on a distal phalanx) **(B)**. (Reprinted with permission from Elsevier) (Reproduced from Jackson AC, Fenton MB. Human rabies and bat bites. *The Lancet.* 2001;357:1714.)[42]

circumstances were such that the bat could not be laboratory-confirmed negative for rabies.[2,40,41] Additionally, a person may know they were bitten by a bat but not be aware of the danger the exposure presented, particularly because bat bites are so small.

RABIES IN ANIMALS

For purposes of this discussion on rabies, the term "animal" refers to a nonhuman mammal.

Stages and Associated Clinical Signs of Rabies in Animals

Perhaps in no other major zoonosis does routine concentration upon the health of an individual animal determine a cascade of actions directly targeting Homo sapiens.

From Rupprecht CE. A tale of two worlds: public health management decisions in human rabies prevention. *Clin Infect Dis.* 2004;39(2):281–283.[43]

BOX 2.2
Fundamental Facts: Rabies in Animals*

Key clinical signs of rabies usually include unexplained paralysis and a change in behavior (see Stages and Associated Clinical Signs of Rabies in Animals section).

Traditional stages of rabies include an incubation period, prodromal period, acute neurologic period, coma, and death (see Stages and Associated Clinical Signs of Rabies in Animals section; Table 2.1).

A commonly cited incubation period is 3 weeks to 3 months; it could be days or years but rarely exceeds 6 months (see Length of incubation period in animals section; Table 2.1).

The prodromal period may last approximately 1–3 days; initial clinical signs (if present) during this period are nonspecific, such as anorexia, fever, lethargy, and vomiting. Behavior changes and paralysis may also start during this time (see Prodromal period in animals section; Table 2.1).

There are many potential additional clinical signs in the prodromal and/or acute neurologic periods. Some generally observed ones are aggression, agitation, ataxia, chewing at the bite site, dysphagia, hypersalivation, hypersensitivity to stimuli, paralysis, and altered phonation. Ataxia and head pressing/tilting are common clinical signs of diseases that cause encephalitis in horses (see Prodromal period in animals, Clinical signs in the acute neurologic period, and Differential diagnoses in horses sections; Table 2.1).

Death usually occurs within 7 days (with a range of 1–10 days) of development of clinical signs (see Coma and death in animals section; Table 2.1).

The animal can be infectious with virus being shed in the saliva before development of clinical signs (see Infectious period section).

A common differential diagnosis in dogs (plus raccoons and foxes) is canine distemper. In horses, some of the differential diagnoses include tetanus, plus eastern equine, western equine, and West Nile virus encephalitis (see Canine distemper as a differential diagnosis and Differential diagnoses in horses sections).

In the United States, customary high-risk animals for transmitting rabies are bats, foxes, raccoons, and skunks. Low-risk animals are rabbits, opossums, armadillos, and rodents (such as squirrels, rats, and mice) (see High-risk animals for transmitting rabies and Low-risk animals for transmitting rabies sections).

Dogs, cats, and domestic ferrets can be observed for rabies for 10 days after biting a person to determine if transmission of rabies could have occurred at the time of the bite (see Dogs, cats, and domestic ferrets section).

Rabies has been laboratory-confirmed in multiple other species (see Animals in the "other" category section).

*Refer to full text for detailed information, ranges of time periods, diversity of clinical signs, and associated outliers, plus specific references.

Traditionally, rabies has had a series of stages used to define the clinical course of the disease, including an incubation period (the interval between the exposure and the first clinical signs); prodromal period; acute neurologic period, which historically has been categorized into the furious or paralytic forms of rabies depending on the predominant clinical signs; coma; and death[13] (see Table 2.1). As with most elements of rabies, though, these stages can be somewhat nebulous. For instance, there is no absolute defining moment when the prodromal period ends and the acute neurologic period begins, but generally it is when clinical signs become more pronounced. In addition, it is possible to have furious signs first followed by paralytic signs or vice versa in any one case of rabies.[13] However, since they are frequently used as descriptors of rabies cases, the following sections will provide a general overview of these categorizations. Presenting the descriptions of what have been referred to as the furious and paralytic forms also brings awareness to the varied presentations that rabies can have, which will hopefully aid in considering this disease as a differential diagnosis.[4]

Clinical signs of rabies are not pathognomonic. The most typical signs of rabies in animals are unexplained paralysis and a change in behavior. There is a litany of other clinical signs that a rabid animal may or may not exhibit (see Table 2.1). The clinical course may be affected by the site(s) of the primary CNS lesion, the variant (strain or type) of rabies virus, the dose of virus, and the route of infection.[13] When a rabid animal is first presented to a veterinarian for evaluation because of exhibiting signs of illness, the thought of rabies as a diagnosis rarely occurs unless the owner reports a fight with a high-risk animal, such as a skunk or raccoon, or some other history that would alert the veterinarian to this disease.

Incubation period in animals

The only universal truth from all the numbers is that the rabies incubation period is highly variable. The more people look into it, the more "exceptions to the rule" we find.

Dr. Ryan M. Wallace, Centers for Disease Control and Prevention, Atlanta, Georgia[b]

TABLE 2.1
Traditional Stages of Rabies and Associated Clinical Signs in Animals[a]

Stage of Disease	Typical Duration	Examples of Clinical Signs
Incubation	3 weeks to 3 months; rarely exceeds 6 months; can be days or years	No clinical signs
Prodromal[b]	1–3 days	Nonspecific: anorexia, fever, lethargy, vomiting Clinical signs may not be present Behavior changes may begin May start to have chewing at the bite site, choking noises, dysphagia, hypersalivation, hypersensitivity, altered phonation, priapism, straining to defecate, stranguria, trismus Cranial nerve involvement may start (anisocoria; extension of nictitating membrane; facial, lingual, and laryngeal paralysis)
Acute neurologic[c]:	2–7 days	Aggressiveness, agitation, ataxia, behavior changes, biting, chewing at bite site (with possible self-mutilation), choking sounds, dysphagia, head tilt/head pressing/head butting, hyperactivity, hypersalivation, hypersensitivity to stimuli, altered phonation, paresis/paralysis, pica, priapism, weakness
Furious (classic or encephalitic)		Furious: Focus of clinical signs is on those associated with hyperactivity
Paralytic (dumb)		Paralytic: Focus of clinical signs is on paralysis, appearing early and throughout the clinical course
Coma		Respiratory and cardiac failure
Death	1–10 days, usually within 7 days after onset of clinical signs	Due to respiratory or cardiac arrest

[a]For more information on clinical signs and how they manifest and ranges in duration of stages, plus specific references, refer to the text.
[b]Clinical signs in the prodromal period can extend into the acute neurologic period.
[c]There can be a continuum of clinical signs between furious and paralytic.

Length of incubation period in animals. The variable length of time that the virus is replicating in muscle tissue or skin and the time that it takes for the virus to travel from the peripheral nerves to the CNS contribute to a significantly variable incubation period. In general, the incubation period for any mammal typically has been referred to as 3–8 weeks[15,44] or 3 weeks to 3 months[31,38,b] (see Fig. 2.3). This period in animals could be days to several months[13,45,46] to years[37,46]; it rarely exceeds 6 months.[31]

Reports and studies—incubation period in animals. The variation in the incubation period apparently can be dependent on multiple factors, such as the severity and the location of the bite, quantity of virus introduced, and variant of rabies virus involved.[45–47] Results of studies involving inoculating mice with a mouse-adapted stock rabies virus have suggested that the virus is capable of entering the peripheral nerves without replicating in the muscle first, which would cause the incubation period to be short.[25,48] The incubation period could potentially be years, but that is difficult to document in naturally infected animals,[46] particularly wild animals that are naturally exposed to rabies.[49] For instance, when an abnormally acting skunk is discovered by someone and subsequently tests positive for rabies, there is no way to know when it was exposed to rabies in the wild.

Results on animals experimentally infected with rabies may not necessarily reflect the true nature of the disease as manifested in naturally infected animals. The biology of wild-type rabies (also called street-rabies virus) varies from laboratory-adapted variants (also called fixed-rabies virus). In contrast to fixed-rabies virus, the street-rabies virus is highly neurotropic and replicates at low levels with a prolonged and highly variable incubation period while not causing pronounced cytopathic effects and not generating a significant immune response.[2] Natural exposure of wildlife in the field can vary with such factors as the species of the biting animal, rabies variant involved, amount of virus in the exposure, and location of the bite. With these caveats kept in mind, refer to the Appendix for studies on incubation periods for various species.

Prodromal period in animals

The prodromal period may progress for 1 to 3 days before clinical signs become more noticeable.[37] If clinical signs are present, they initially are nonspecific, such as **anorexia**,[38,45] **fever**,[37,38] **lethargy**,[13,45] and **vomiting**[13,45] (see Table 2.1).

The **change in behavior** may start during this period,[37,46,50] such as a friendly cat becoming very aggressive; a normally playful puppy being shy and withdrawn; a nocturnal animal appearing during the day; or a wild animal losing its fear of people or domestic animals, which leads to reports of finding, for example, a rabid skunk in a pen with dogs or a rabid fox in a stall with a horse. Note that sometimes a healthy nocturnal animal temporarily may be wandering in the daylight looking disoriented because it was displaced from its resting place (for instance, a plumber working under a home disturbs a nocturnal animal that was residing there) or it could be an easily confused juvenile animal that is still trying to get its bearings.

Cranial nerve involvement may begin to be reflected in **anisocoria**,[13] **extension of the nictitating membrane**,[13,29] **facial paralysis**,[13] **lingual paralysis**,[13] **laryngeal paralysis**, altered phonation (speculated to be the result of laryngeal paralysis),[46] and **dilated pupils**.[46,50]

Other clinical signs that may manifest during the prodromal period include **chewing at the bite site**,[37] **choking sounds**,[13] **dysphagia**,[13] **hypersalivation** and thick, **rope-like drool**,[13,46] **hypersensitivity**,[37] **priapism**,[37] **straining to defecate**,[13] **stranguria**,[13] and **trismus**.[13]

Chewing at the bite site is presumably stimulated by irritation or a tingling sensation (akin to **paresthesia**), is commonly reported, and may lead to self-mutilation to the extent of self-amputation of an appendage.[38,45,51] Keep in mind that nonrabid animals can have excessive chewing in response to allergies, thereby creating lick granulomas or hot spots.

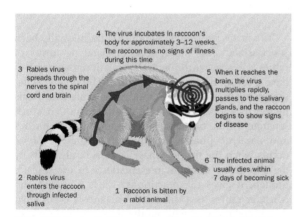

4 The virus incubates in raccoon's body for approximately 3–12 weeks. The raccoon has no signs of illness during this time

3 Rabies virus spreads through the nerves to the spinal cord and brain

5 When it reaches the brain, the virus multiplies rapidly, passes to the salivary glands, and the raccoon begins to show signs of disease

6 The infected animal usually dies within 7 days of becoming sick

2 Rabies virus enters the raccoon through infected saliva

1 Raccoon is bitten by a rabid animal

FIG. 2.3 Cycle of rabies—beginning with a bite transmitting infected saliva and leading to virus entry into peripheral nerves followed by movement to the central nervous system resulting in encephalitis and transit to salivary glands, facilitating infection of another host. (Reprinted with permission from Elsevier: Rupprecht CE, Hanlon CA, Hemachudha T. Rabies re-examined. *The Lancet - Infect Dis.* 2002;2:327–343.[38])

In a study of 21 experimentally infected horses, tremor of the muzzle was the most frequently reported and the most common initial clinical sign[15,52]; in a group of 21 naturally infected horses, clinical signs at the time of initial examination included ataxia and paresis of the hindquarters, lameness, recumbency, pharyngeal paralysis, and colic.[53]

Besides the conventional signs of rabies, hemorrhagic gastroenteritis with dark, slimy feces was noted in 18% of dogs in two studies 1–2 days after clinical signs were observed; the hemorrhagic gastroenteritis persisted until the animals died. At necropsy, no macroscopic changes were observed in the oral cavity, esophagus, or stomach; the pathologic changes were noted caudad to the pyloric sphincter; and the small and large intestines, including the rectum, were markedly affected.[46] It is not clear as to the cause of diarrhea in these study cases.

Acute neurologic period in animals

If you hear that the dog is wasted in body, dry, red in the eyes, tail hanging limp, drooling saliva, its tongue hanging out and discolored, bumping into people it meets, irrationally running and stopping, biting with furious rage people it has never met before, then you may be sure the dog is rabid.

Galen (AD 131–201)[54]

Clinical signs in acute neurologic period. Through ancient writings such as those of Galen, it is evident that the clinical signs of rabies have been acknowledged for eons. During the acute neurologic period, clinical signs become more pronounced. Some that may be evident are **ataxia**,[38,46] in which the animal is stumbling and may be described by an onlooker as appearing "intoxicated" (see Fig. 2.4), **chewing at the bite site**,[13,45] **dysphagia**,[45,46] and **hypersalivation**[37,45,46] (see Table 2.1). **Paresis** and **paralysis** occur at some point depending on how the disease has manifested[38] (see Fig. 2.5).

Hypersalivation is a commonly observed and distinctive clinical sign (see Fig. 2.6). The combination of excessive saliva and dysphagia, which makes it difficult for the animal to swallow anything, including its own saliva, can produce copious amounts of saliva; the drool can have a heavy, rope-like consistency.[13,45] This sizable volume of virus-laden saliva has the potential for transmitting rabies, so these clinical signs can aid in the continued propagation of the disease.[45] With dysphagia, which is created by spasms and paralysis of pharyngeal muscles,[37,45,46] the animal also will have difficulty drinking water, which can lead to dehydration.

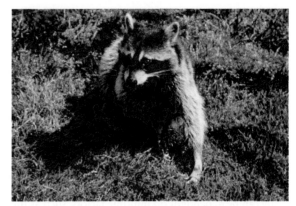

FIG. 2.4 Rabid raccoon exhibiting ataxia. (Courtesy of the Centers for Disease Control and Prevention, Atlanta, Georgia.)

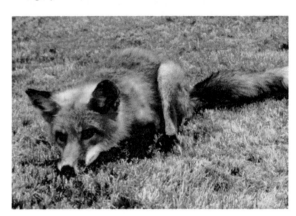

FIG. 2.5 Rabid fox with paresis. (Courtesy of the Centers for Disease Control and Prevention, Atlanta, Georgia.)

The acute neurologic period has traditionally been subclassified into the furious or paralytic forms of rabies. However, furious and paralytic rabies tend to have a continuum of clinical signs.[2] The different presentations of clinical signs during the acute neurologic period have been described by some as not so much separate forms, but as a progression between furious and paralytic phases, in which the paralytic phase occurs when the furious phase is short or absent.[46] By describing the different presentations of the disease, though, it gives the practitioner cause to pause and consider rabies as a differential diagnosis even when the animal presents without the classic clinical signs of rabies, which is one of the goals of this chapter.

Furious rabies is also referred to as classic or encephalitic rabies. In this version of clinical-sign presentation, the focus is on **hyperactivity**. The archetypal vision of the vicious mad dog may be encapsulated with

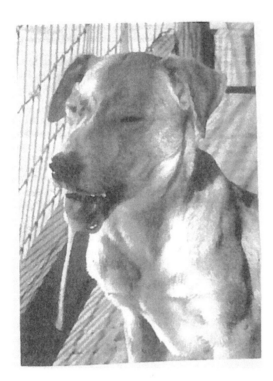

FIG. 2.6 Rabid dog with hypersalivation (thick, rope-like saliva). (Reprinted with permission from Elsevier: Niezgoda M, Hanlon CA, Rupprecht CE. Animal rabies. In: Jackson AC, Wunner WH, eds. *Rabies*. San Diego: Academic Press, An Elsevier Science Imprint; 2002:163–218.[13])

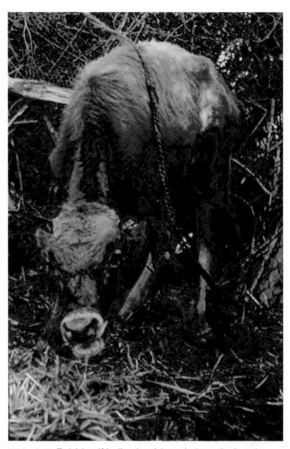

FIG. 2.7 Rabid calf bellowing (altered phonation) and exhibiting hypersalivation. (Courtesy of L. Mahin; Wikimedia Commons.)

the animal **snapping** and **biting** at real or imaginary objects (a rabid animal may look like it is "**snapping at flies**," which is akin to a rabid human experiencing hallucinations),[45] **running** for long distances, and **attacking** anything in its path.[37]

Clinical signs that might be evident in the furious form include **aggression**,[13,37,51] **agitation**,[13,37,46] **biting**,[51] **hypersensitivity to stimuli**, such as light, sound, and touch[13] (e.g., the animal will overreact and be agitated by a sound, such as a phone ringing, as typified in the legendary rabid-dog movie, *Cujo*[55]), **altered phonation** (high-pitched howling in dogs; bellowing in cattle)[46,51] (see Fig. 2.7), **pica**, in which the animal tries to eat nonfood items, such as wood or stones,[43,51,56] **priapism**,[37] and **seizures**[37,46] (or possibly movement disorders that resemble seizures).

Head tilting, **head pressing**, and/or **head butting**, plus **circling**, may also be evident[13]; particularly in horses, these clinical signs can lead to misdiagnosis with other more common encephalitic diseases.

Paralytic rabies is so named because in this form of the disease the main clinical sign is **paralysis**[13]; although paralysis can eventually occur in furious rabies, it is not the primary clinical sign throughout the duration of the disease (see Fig. 2.8). It has commonly been called dumb rabies, a name that is reflective of how the animal may exhibit clinical signs, such as **facial paralysis** creating a drooping mandible (dropped jaw) caused by paralysis of the masseter muscle[46] and **lingual paralysis** causing a lolling tongue.[13,37] The animal may make **choking sounds**, which can lead to human exposures when an attempt is made to determine the cause of the choking. These exposures occur particularly in horses when dental problems are suspected; multiple exposures have occurred with a rabid horse in which the owner, plus friends and neighbors, have had their hands in the mouth of the horse searching for dental complications before veterinary staff were called upon and

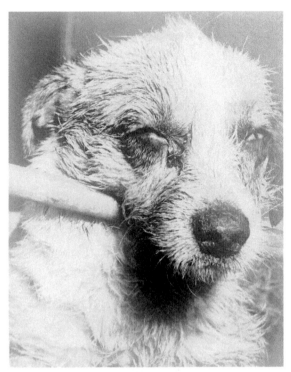

FIG. 2.8 Classic photo of a rabid dog that is frequently featured in books and articles on rabies. (Courtesy of the Centers for Disease Control and Prevention, Atlanta, Georgia.)

did the same. Similar exposures have occurred involving rabid dogs with the "bone in the throat" syndrome in which the animal gives the mistaken appearance of choking on a bone.[46] Cattle and sheep may also appear to be choking, leading to a person inserting a hand in the animal's mouth to try to locate a foreign object.[13] Motor neuropathy creates flaccid muscle **weakness in the hind limbs** and paresis.[13,51] **Recumbency** is oftentimes exhibited in horses[53] and cattle.[57]

Clinical signs in animals—reports and anecdotal scenarios

Bats. Signs of rabies in bats include being active during the day, disoriented, and clumsy, plus losing their ability to fly, resulting in fluttering on the ground; less commonly, they may become aggressive.[40,58] Virus isolation was noted in 0.5% of flying adults compared with 50% or higher in sick bats found fluttering on the ground in bat caves.[58] Of bats submitted for testing, usually 4%–15% are positive.[34,38]

Bobcats. There have been reports in case investigations of rabid bobcats threatening or stalking humans

for no apparent reason, chasing dogs and cats, attacking livestock, and jumping against a picture window or glass door.[a,c,d]

Coyotes. In South Texas, there have been reports of coyotes approaching people and being hand-fed by someone or even jumping into a truck and sitting on the seat while a person fed or petted it.[59,e] Each coyote in the various situations suddenly bit the person and frequently escaped or possibly got shot in the head, thereby destroying the brain and making it untestable. Note: In such scenarios, even if testing of the animal to confirm rabies is not possible, rabies PEP should be recommended given the unusually tame behavior of a wild animal with no fear of people; additionally, in that geographic location (Texas), coyotes are defined in law as high-risk species for transmitting rabies.[60] Although not always possible in emergency field conditions in which an animal is attacking a person, attempts should be made to avoid destroying the brain via gunshot, thereby preserving it for testing.

Coyotes play a valuable role in maintenance of the environment, including their scavenging and consuming of animals that have expired.[59] Unfortunately, urban spread has overrun their habitat and created conditions in which they are more frequently in contact with people and domestic animals.

Foxes. A behavioral tendency noted during reviews of case investigations of laboratory-confirmed rabid foxes in Texas was aggression, such as jumping on car or truck wheels or the legs of hunters and repeatedly biting them.[61]

Skunks. In a study conducted in Texas, the more commonly reported behaviors during case investigations of skunks that had exposed a human to rabies included attacking dogs, appearing outside during the day, attacking humans, entering a dog pen, approaching or entering a house, acting sick, attacking a cat or other animal, and entering a tent. Multiple behaviors could be exhibited by an individual skunk. In the same study, frequent behaviors in rabid skunks, regardless of human exposure, were similar and included entering a dog pen, appearing outside during the day, and attacking pets.[62] Rabid skunks have been reported to have entered houses through pet doors.[62] There are also situations in which a person unfortunately could be exposed just by being at the wrong place at the wrong moment, such as one in which someone was bitten in the buttocks by a rabid skunk while crawling under a mobile home.[61,62] As a reminder, the rabies virus is not transmitted through skunk spray.[14,15]

Rabid skunks are known to bite with tenacity, a characteristic that makes skunks particularly good vectors and effective in transmitting rabies.[13] In reviews of case investigations of laboratory-confirmed rabid skunks in Texas, the biting behavior exhibited by rabid skunks was noted to be quite insidious with multiple reports of rabid skunks attacking litters of puppies or kittens that regrettably were housed outside; the skunks in these cases were sometimes found chewing on the heads of the young animals.[61]

Coma and death in animals
The clinical course of rabies generally terminates with coma and respiratory or cardiac failure. Death usually ensues within 7 days[38,63] with a range of 1–10 days[13] after clinical signs begin. The physiologic mechanism resulting in death could result from autonomic dysfunction that leads to variations in respiration, body temperature, blood pressure, and cardiac rhythm.[45] Refer to the Appendix for studies and reports on the length of clinical illness in animals.

Infectious period
The infectious period is the span of time when it is possible that the rabid animal (or person) is shedding rabies virus in saliva. Studies conducted on cats, dogs, and domestic ferrets (see below) have shown that shedding begins within 10 days before first clinical signs and that a 10-day period should be used for investigations involving rabies exposure to these three animals. Because an asymptomatic shedding period has not been fully determined in other species, including humans, a conservative approach has been recommended by using 14 days before clinical signs (or symptoms) for PEP.[7,18]

Cats. Clinical signs develop within 10 days of starting to shed virus in the saliva.[45,64] In a study of 26 cats inoculated with street-rabies virus from four different species of animals (cat, dog, fox, and skunk), 23 cats excreted virus in saliva with initiation of viral excretion detected 1 day before onset of clinical illness to 3 days after onset.[65]

Dogs. Clinical signs develop within 10 days of starting to shed virus in the saliva.[45,64] In a study of 54 dogs inoculated with street-rabies virus from three different species of animals (dog, fox, and skunk), 26 excreted virus in the saliva with initiation of viral excretion detected 3 days before onset of clinical illness to 2 days after onset (a conclusion was offered by the researchers that, based on the findings of their study, consideration could be made for possibly reducing the observation period following an exposure incident to as short as 5 days and no longer than 7 days).[66] Other references

also have noted virus in saliva 3–6 days before clinical signs appeared.[46] In another experiment in which dogs were inoculated with various street-rabies viruses from dogs, the viral shedding period before development of clinical signs was 1–14 days.[46] However, virologic data from pathogenesis studies support the practice of a 10-day observation period for a dog that has bitten a person; if the dog is alive and well after 10 days, data support that there would not be risk of infection.[45]

Domestic ferrets. Clinical signs develop within 10 days of starting to shed virus in the saliva.[45,64] In a study of 19 domestic ferrets inoculated with raccoon rabies virus variant (9 of which shed virus in the saliva), virus excretion in the saliva ranged from 2 days before development to 6 days after onset of clinical signs.[67]

Differential Diagnoses in Animals
Importance of proper diagnosis of rabies
An effective treatment may be forthcoming at which time prompt diagnosis to initiate that treatment could save an animal's life. At present, it is still extremely important to make a proper diagnosis for the purpose of public health. By confirming that the animal was positive for rabies, a case investigation can ensue and proper evaluations made to enable informed decisions on the administration of PEP for potentially exposed humans and domestic animals (if PEP is allowed for animals in a particular locale). It may also be the case that a bite incident (or other exposure) to a human or domestic animal might be determined after the biting animal has expired and the body disposed, so it is no longer available for testing. If rabies was not considered as the cause of an animal's medical condition and rabies testing was not conducted, PEP would probably need to be administered even though the biting animal might have tested negative for rabies if it had been tested. Undue expense and mental anguish can be avoided if proper steps are taken to prove or disprove rabies as the causative disease if possible exposures to humans and domestic animals are involved.

Canine distemper as a differential diagnosis
Many of the clinical signs of rabies can mimic those of canine distemper in dogs, raccoons, and foxes.[13,68] Clinical signs of encephalitis in distemper (for example, chomping, agitation, and irritability) tend to be periodic in frequency and seizures occur intermittently throughout the disease.[46] Sporadically, there will be an outbreak of what appears to be rabies in raccoons or foxes; this disease outbreak may actually be due to canine distemper, especially in areas where rabies in

that species is not endemic. However, because you cannot determine the disease just by looking at the animal, laboratory testing is needed for confirmation and to eliminate rabies as a differential diagnosis. Vaccination against distemper in dogs can save animal lives and reduce costs by not having to test as many dogs for rabies because of the similarity of clinical signs.[f] Vaccination, along with laboratory testing for rabies when considered as a differential diagnosis, may also prevent the associated financial costs and mental stress humans experience as a result of having to be treated for exposure to what may have been a canine disease, which poses no threat to humans. See Miscellaneous differential diagnoses in animals section for an extensive list of other potential differential diagnoses.

Differential diagnoses in horses

As with other animals, the clinical signs of rabies in horses are diverse and vary in their expression. Several, including ataxia, circling, head tilt, and head pressing, are similar to those found in arboviral encephalopathy, such as West Nile virus, eastern equine, western equine, and Venezuelan equine encephalitis.[13,15] Whenever neurologic signs are involved, rabies should be considered as a differential diagnosis.

There have been reports of rabies infection in previously vaccinated horses (specifics on the vaccinations in these cases could not be definitely documented)[53]; protection by vaccination is not guaranteed, so even a currently vaccinated horse should be tested for rabies if it exhibits neurologic clinical signs. If testing for another disease in addition to rabies is being considered, priority should be given to submission for rabies testing because of its critical zoonotic potential.[15] Some of the other potential equine conditions that can have clinical signs similar to those of rabies may include tetanus (trismus is a clinical sign of rabies), equine herpes myeloencephalopathy, colic, botulism, lead poisoning, moldy feed poisoning, equine protozoal myeloencephalitis, or brain or spinal cord injury.[13,15]

Miscellaneous differential diagnoses in animals

Categories of other differential diagnoses for encephalitis compatible with rabies may include the following: viral (pseudorabies, feline infectious peritonitis, herpes myelitis, infectious canine hepatitis, porcine enteroviral encephalomyelitis, malignant catarrhal fever, Borna disease); bacterial (listeriosis, Rocky Mountain spotted fever, sporadic bovine encephalomyelitis); fungal (cryptococcosis, blastomycosis); parasitic (baylisascariasis, strongylosis, toxoplasmosis); neoplastic

(lymphosarcoma, osteosarcoma, fibrosarcoma, meningioma, metastatic neoplasia); traumatic (hit by car, gunshot, intervertebral disk disease, esophageal foreign body); toxic (heavy metals, chlorinated hydrocarbons, organophosphates, strychnine); metabolic (ketosis, hypocalcemia); and developmental (hydrocephalus, cerebellar hypoplasia).[13]

In a case involving the discovery of a single dead horse or cow with no other contributing history, consider rabies. There have been multiple cases in which, on necropsy and testing, such an animal was determined to be rabid, unfortunately after multiple humans already had been exposed, resulting in the need for PEP.[f]

Rabies Susceptibility in Different Species of Animals

All warm-blooded animals, particularly mammals, can acquire rabies, but some are more likely to transmit it than others. In the United States, typically more than 90% of reported rabies cases in animals occur in wildlife.[10,69]

High-risk animals for transmitting rabies

Some species are considered "reservoirs" for rabies and have a higher risk for transmitting the virus. Rabies reservoirs are animal species in which a species-associated rabies virus variant has evolved and circulates. Although the virus variant is adapted to that species, it can infect other species. Rabies infection in a species other than the reservoir species for a particular rabies virus variant is considered "spillover"[13] or cross-species transmission.[70] Random examples of spillover would be a raccoon infected with a fox variant of rabies virus, a skunk infected with a raccoon variant, or a cat infected with a skunk variant. For a more comprehensive overview of reservoir hosts worldwide, see Chapter 3.

Some species are more prevalently rabid in certain geographic locations than in other areas. In the United States, bats, raccoons, and skunks typically are the most commonly reported species for rabies,[10,69] and they, along with foxes, are customarily classified as high-risk animals for rabies. The prevalent species for transmitting rabies can vary from state to state. For instance, in Texas, coyotes were added to this list of high-risk animals[60] because of an epizootic of rabies in coyotes that occurred in the southern portion of the state.[71] In Puerto Rico, the mongoose is the primary reservoir for rabies[10,69]; in 2015, the first reported case in the United States or its territories of human rabies caused by a bite from a mongoose occurred in Puerto Rico.[72,73] The mongoose was introduced to the Caribbean from Asia for the purpose of snake and rodent control in sugarcane plantations.[38]

Low-risk animals for transmitting rabies

Examples of low-risk animals for transmitting rabies include rabbits, opossums, armadillos, shrews, and moles, plus rodents such as mice, rats, squirrels, nutria, prairie dogs, beavers, and gophers (if they are cage-raised animals, they are considered to be very low risk partially because of an unlikely potential for being exposed to rabies). Generally, bites from small rodents, such as squirrels, chipmunks, rats, and mice, plus hamsters, gerbils, and guinea pigs, do not constitute an exposure concern.[74] These animals have little chance of surviving an attack by a rabid animal, although larger rodents, such as beavers and groundhogs/woodchucks, may have more potential for survival.[51] There have been occasional reports of rabies in squirrels,[69,74] groundhogs, beavers, opossums, and rabbits.[69]

Opossums appear relatively resistant to experimental infection; additionally, the consistently low number of naturally occurring cases in opossums helps to support this finding.[13,23,47] One theory for this resistance is that the muscle content of an opossum has a low quantity of nicotinic acetylcholine receptors (to which the rabies virus binds at the neuromuscular junction) compared with, for example, a high-risk animal such as the fox.[23] Ironically, during the writing of this chapter, Texas had an unusual occurrence with two opossums that were laboratory-confirmed positive for rabies, both from the same county and with the south central skunk rabies virus variant. Even given this uncommon occurrence, opossums are still considered to be low-risk animals; since 1962 (over five decades), more than 5000 opossums were tested for rabies in Texas with only 8 positives (including the two previously mentioned cases).[8]

There have been rare cases in which a rabbit that was caged outside developed rabies. The supposition was that an aggressive rabid animal was able to bite the animal through the caging material, but the animal was protected enough in its housing to survive the attack.[61] An interesting article pertains to a pet guinea pig and seven rabbits in New York that developed rabies.[51] In the case of the rabid guinea pig, the owner remembered seeing a raccoon in the yard when the guinea pig was allowed outside and heard the guinea pig squeal followed by seeing the raccoon run and climb a tree. Three of the rabbits were exposed to raccoons (one was chased out of its cage by a raccoon, and the other two each had a raccoon found on top of its cage), one was exposed to a skunk (attacked while tethered outside), and three had unknown exposures; all the rabbits and the guinea pig were confirmed to have the raccoon variant of rabies virus. Closely supervising pet rabbits and rodents when they are allowed to be in the open and using double caging for these pets if housed outside will help to avert contact with wild animals.

The human-behavior element can compound problems pertaining to exposure concerns when there are interactions with low-risk animals, especially animals that have learned through positive reinforcement to interact with humans. It is not uncommon for some animals, such as squirrels and chipmunks, to appear tame and friendly because of people feeding them. They become trusting of people and get positive reinforcement for doing so via the reward of food, so friendliness and tameness could be considered normal behavior for these animals.[61,h] However, it could lead to the unnecessary demise of a healthy animal due to suspicion of rabies infection.

Dogs, cats, and domestic ferrets

Dogs, cats, and domestic ferrets have a special grouping in the world of rabies. If they bite or otherwise expose someone to rabies, they can be observed for 10 days rather than euthanatized and tested.[31,45,75] If they are healthy and alive 10 days after the bite incident, they could not have transmitted rabies in their saliva at the time of the bite.[20,45] Supportive in the 10-day observation option are results from studies of cats and dogs naturally infected with rabies, all of which died within 10 days of onset of clinical signs.[43,75] That does not mean that they could not have been incubating rabies; it just means that the disease would not have progressed to the point where the virus had traveled to the salivary glands and would not have been present at the time of the bite (See Infectious period section for details).

Animals in the "other" category

Rabies has been reported in a multitude of species in the United States that are not dogs, cats, or domestic ferrets and are not defined as being high or low risk for transmitting rabies. One such animal is a wolf-dog hybrid.[76] Domestic animals that usually have some yearly reported cases include cattle and equines, plus the occasional sheep, goats, and swine.[69] In addition to those already mentioned in this section, a few examples of the many other wildlife species reported with rabies include carnivores such as the otter and badger,[69,76] plus wolf, ringtail, coati, mink, weasel, fisher, puma, bear, and lesser panda (located in a national zoo and infected with the raccoon variant of rabies virus, which is another example of spillover).[76] In addition, rabies has been confirmed in species such as deer,[69] antelope,[10] nonhuman primate,[77] and bison.[78]

In Norway, rabies was confirmed in a ringed seal. The animal was found with a wound and in a state of confusion. It deteriorated during the next 4–5 days, had exudate from its eyes and mouth, and became aggressive. This case was presumed to be associated with an epizootic of rabies in arctic foxes, showing that even marine animals can be infected with the rabies virus. Rabid reindeer located in the same area were also thought to be associated with the rabies epizootic in arctic foxes.[79]

Because of nonhuman primates sometimes having a close association with humans leading to a higher possibility for being involved in bite incidents, it is prudent to keep in mind their potential for rabies transmission especially in areas where rabies is enzootic.[77,80,81] (When dealing with a bite incident involving a macaque monkey or another primate species with a history of being co-housed with macaques, in addition to evaluating the need for rabies PEP, prophylactic treatment should also be considered against herpes B virus.[81,i,j,k])

Although rabies typically affects mammals, there have been rare reports of rabies in birds,[82] including one in India in 2015 involving a domestic fowl that was attacked by a dog in an area endemic for canine rabies.[83] Birds, like smaller mammals, usually would not survive being attacked by a rabid animal. Additionally, the transmission potential of birds, including absence of teeth and limited development of salivary glands,[13] is questionable, although contact of neural tissue with mucous membranes or a break in the skin during butchering and handling of rabies-infected poultry could be a possible exposure risk.[83] Because this is a rarity, caution should be taken to not overly project concern about acquiring rabies through birds.[84]

RABIES IN HUMANS

Stages and Associated Clinical Signs and Symptoms in Humans

Rabies is an unpredictable disease—the only characteristic feature is that it is uncharacteristic in its presentation.

From Rupprecht CE, Hanlon CA, Hemachudha T. Rabies re-examined. *Lancet Infect Dis.* 2002;2: 327–343.[38]

Rabies in humans in the United States is rare with generally one to three cases per year.[85] The majority of indigenous rabies cases in the United States are due to bat variants of rabies virus. Often there was no known bite; in some of these cases, there was not even any known contact with a bat.[2] Oftentimes, the bite wound from a bat is so small that the person may not know they were bitten and therefore does not seek medical attention and PEP.[85] Other times, they may know of the bite or other contact with a bat but do not realize the

---

BOX 2.3
Fundamental Facts: Rabies in Humans*

Traditional stages of rabies include an incubation period, prodromal period, acute neurologic period, coma, and death (see Stages and Associated Clinical Signs and Symptoms in Humans section; Table 2.2).

The incubation period is one of the most variable of all diseases. A commonly cited incubation period is 3 weeks to 3 months; it could be days or years (see Length of incubation period in humans section).

The clinical signs and symptoms during the prodromal stage are nonspecific, such as anorexia, fatigue, fever, headache, malaise, nausea, sore throat, and vomiting. Dysphagia may develop. Paresthesia is frequently reported (see Clinical signs and symptoms of the prodromal period in humans section; Table 2.2).

The acute neurologic period generally lasts 2–7 days. There can be periods of arousal (aggression, agitation, confusion, fear, and hallucinations) interrupted with periods of lucidity (see Acute neurologic period in humans section; Table 2.2).

Other examples of common clinical signs and symptoms during the acute neurologic period include aerophobia, ataxia, dysphagia, fever, hydrophobia, hyperesthesia, hypersalivation, hyperventilation, muscle fasciculation, muscle weakness, myoclonus, myoedema, paralysis, paresis, paresthesia, piloerection, priapism, dilated pupils, and sweating (see Acute neurologic period in humans section; Table 2.2).

Clinical signs and symptoms similar to those of Guillain-Barre syndrome may be the prevalent presentation (see Acute neurologic period in humans section; Table 2.2).

The case fatality rate of rabies exceeds 99.9% (see Coma and death in humans section).

Consider rabies in any case of encephalitis, myelitis, or encephalomyelitis (see Positive indicators for rabies in differential diagnoses in humans section).

There is a wide selection of potential differential diagnoses; positive indicators for rabies can help differentiate it from diseases with similar clinical signs and symptoms. Examples of positive indicators include a progressive worsening of neurologic signs; periods of arousal and altered behavior interrupted by periods of lucidity; aerophobia; severe autonomic instability/dysautonomia; dysesthesia, such as pruritus, referable to bitten area; dysphagia; hydrophobia; and paresthesia (see Positive indicators for rabies in differential diagnoses in humans and Diseases with similar clinical signs and symptoms in humans sections; Table 2.3).

*Refer to full text for detailed information, ranges of time periods, diversity of clinical signs and symptoms, and associated outliers, plus specific references.

need to apprehend the bat for testing or to seek medical attention. Therefore, they may not mention the exposure to their physician when they seek medical attention because clinical signs and symptoms have started to develop.

The clinical course of rabies in humans has many similarities to that of animals. Although terminology and categorization of stages can vary depending on the source, rabies traditionally is referred to as having five stages (see Table 2.2): incubation period (the interval between exposure and the first signs and symptoms of the prodromal period), prodromal period, acute neurologic period (which is described by some in terms of furious or paralytic forms), coma, and death.[86] As with most elements of rabies, though, there is an imprecision to these stages. The prodromal period typically is considered to have transitioned into the acute neurologic period when clinical signs and symptoms show neurologic failure or severe behavior. Additionally, it is possible to have a continuum in the acute neurologic period with furious signs and symptoms first followed by paralytic signs and symptoms or vice versa in any one case

of rabies.[2] In addition, there was a reported example in which a single rabid dog transmitted rabies to two individuals, one exposure resulting in clinical signs and symptoms associated with the furious form of rabies and the other with those of the paralytic form.[21,22]

Incubation period in humans

Even though there may be no immediate signs in the affected area, after four or six months or even longer the poison destroys the man ... I have known someone who lapsed into the condition known as hydrophobia a whole year after being bitten.

Galen (AD 131–201)[54]

Length of incubation period in humans. The paradox of the varying length of the rabies incubation period has been documented throughout history. The erratic length of time that the virus replicates in muscle tissue or skin and the time that it takes for the virus to travel from the peripheral nerves to the CNS contribute to a significantly variable length

TABLE 2.2
Traditional Stages of Rabies and Associated Clinical Signs and Symptoms in Humans[a]

Stage of Disease	Typical Duration	Examples of Clinical Signs and Symptoms
Incubation	3 weeks to 3 months; can be days or years	No clinical signs or symptoms
Prodromal[b]	2–10 days	Nonspecific: anorexia, fatigue, fever, headache, malaise, nausea, sore throat, vomiting, weakness Paresthesia and dysesthesias, including pruritus, are frequently reported Anxiety, insomnia, irritability, and nervousness may be present
Acute neurologic[c]:	2–7 days	Aerophobia, aggression, agitation, ataxia, bradycardia, confusion, dysesthesia (including pruritus), dysphagia, fever, hallucinations, hydrophobia, hyperesthesia, hypersalivation, hyperventilation, lacrimation, muscle fasciculation, muscle weakness, myoclonus, myoedema, orofacial dyskinesia and myokymia, paralysis, paresis, paresthesia, altered phonation, piloerection, priapism, dilated pupils, sphincter dysfunction, sweating, tachycardia Cardiac or respiratory arrest
Furious (classic or encephalitic) Paralytic (dumb)		Furious: Focus of clinical signs and symptoms is on hyperactivity and autonomic excess; periods of arousal interrupted by intermittent episodes of lucidity Paralytic: Clinical signs and symptoms are similar to those of Guillain-Barre syndrome but with urinary and fecal retention
Coma		Coma; respiratory and cardiac failure
Death	7–14 days from onset of clinical signs and symptoms	Typically due to shock or respiratory or cardiac arrest

[a]For more information on clinical signs and symptoms and how they manifest and ranges in duration of stages, plus specific references, refer to the text.
[b]Clinical signs and symptoms in the prodromal period can extend into the acute neurologic period.
[c]There can be a continuum of clinical signs and symptoms between furious and paralytic.

for the incubation period. In general, the incubation period has been cited as 3–8 weeks[44] or 3 weeks to 3 months,[24,87,b] but it can range from several days to several years.[30,40,87] The World Health Organization describes the incubation period as 5 days to several years, but usually 2–3 months and rarely more than a year.[7] Similar, but slightly varied, versions of these time periods, such as 1–3 months,[30,86] are referenced throughout literature. Some extremely lengthy incubation periods for rabies have been reported in humans, including 19 years and one thought to be 27 years, although the potential for another exposure having occurred closer to the onset of illness cannot be fully discounted.[30,40,86] The incubation period of rabies is one of the most unpredictable among diseases. It can vary because of the quantity of rabies virus in the saliva, type and depth of the bite wound, innervation of the bite site, distance of the bite site from the CNS, and age and immune status of the host.[86,88,89] For instance, one theory is that a bite to the face may have a shorter incubation period due to the area being more heavily innervated and/or because it is closer to the CNS.[86] However, this theory has not been supported by others (see Chapter 6).

Reports and studies on the incubation period in humans

Rabies cases in humans in the United States (1960–2010). A study of cases of rabies in the United States was conducted from 1960 through 2010. Excluding cases acquired through laboratory exposures and transplantations, the dates of definite or probable exposure of 28 cases were used to calculate a median incubation period of 41.5 days, with a range of 8–701 days.[4]

Rabies cases in humans in Bali. In a study of 104 rabies cases in humans in Bali in which 92% of the cases had a history of a dog bite, the estimated time from a dog bite to the onset of clinical signs and symptoms was 110 days (60–90 days in most cases) with a range of 12–720 days.[89] The incubation period was shorter in cases in which the bite site was on the head and neck versus those in which the bite site was located on the extremities.

Rabies cases in humans in the Philippines. In a study of 1839 rabies cases in the Philippines, where canine rabies contributes to the majority of human cases of the disease, the greatest number of cases occurred 91–365 days postexposure followed by a group of cases that occurred 31–90 days postexposure; additionally, there were some cases with an incubation period greater than 5 years and one case believed to have an incubation period of 27 years (although in this case there is a possibility of another exposure closer to the onset of illness). There were shorter incubation periods with bites to the face, head, and neck than bites to the extremities. Finger and upper extremity bites tended to have shorter incubation periods than those to the lower extremities. Multiple bites generally led to shorter incubation periods.[30]

Rabies cases in humans with lengthy incubation periods. The following are examples of cases of rabies in humans with longer than average incubation periods.

Three immigrants to the United States from Laos, the Philippines, and Mexico developed rabies with a virus variant from their country of origin with incubation periods of at least 11 months, 4 years, and 6 years, respectively, which was based on their time of immigration.[28]

A Brazilian man succumbed to rabies 8 years after immigrating to the United States; the rabies virus variant with which he was diagnosed was that of a Latin American dog. He had not traveled outside of the United States during those 8 years and family members did recollect a contact he had with an abnormally acting dog before leaving Brazil, although no bite or scratch was noted after that incident.[90]

There was a US rabies case with a longer than typical incubation period that occurred in a person who had been the recipient of a kidney transplant 17 months before developing clinical signs and symptoms of rabies. It was later determined when stored tissues from the donor were tested that the donor had died of undiagnosed rabies; testing also revealed that it was the raccoon variant of rabies virus. The incubation period in previous rabies cases involving organ transplant recipients who had died of rabies from another donor who had died of undiagnosed rabies was 6 weeks, which is a more typical length for the incubation period.[18]

Prodromal period in humans

> *Poison of a rabid dog causes no distinctive symptom on the body before the person bitten himself becomes rabid.*
>
> Galen (AD 131–201)[54]

Clinical signs and symptoms of the prodromal period in humans. The prodromal period may last for 2–10 days.[86,87] This portion of the clinical course typically includes nonspecific clinical manifestations such as **chills**,[86,91] **fatigue**,[4,86] **fever**[4,89] (which is regularly present, but episodic), **insomnia**,[39,89] **malaise**,[4,86] **myalgia**,[89] and **weakness**[4,86] (see Table 2.2).

Multiple systems can be impacted to varying extents in different cases. For example, some may have involvement of the respiratory system (**cough**,[86,91] **dyspnea**,[86] and **sore throat**[4,39]); gastrointestinal system (**anorexia**,[4,38] **dysphagia**,[86] **nausea**,[4,89] **vomiting**,[4,89] and **abdominal pain**[86,91]) (severe abdominal pain has been reported in some cases as the first disease manifestation[88]); and central nervous system (**headache**,[4,39,89] **anxiety**,[37,38] **irritability**,[86] **nervousness**,[86] and **vertigo**[86]).

Paresthesia (localized pain, burning, cold, numbness, or tingling) at the bite site frequently is reported at this stage.[22,88,89] **Dysesthesia** (e.g., pain or **pruritus** in a limb where the bite occurred) is a positive indicator for rabies.[2]

Studies of clinical signs and symptoms in humans—prodromal period

Rabies cases in humans in the United States (1960–2010).
In a study of 108 cases of rabies in humans that occurred between 1960 and 2010 in the United States (which included indigenous cases as well as imported cases in foreign nationals diagnosed and treated within the United States and its territories), the presenting signs and symptoms were nonspecific, such as fever, malaise, headache, weakness, fatigue, sore throat, and anorexia.[4]

Rabies cases in humans in Bali.
In a study of 104 rabies cases in Bali that involved rabies transmission to humans by rabid dogs, less than 50% of the patients had prodromal signs and symptoms. Of those who did, the most commonly recorded one was pain or paresthesia at the site of the bite; others that were noted were nonspecific, such as nausea, vomiting, fever, myalgia, insomnia, and headache.[89]

Acute neurologic period in humans

Clinical signs and symptoms of the acute neurologic period in humans. The acute neurologic period usually lasts 2–7 days, although it may be longer in cases of paralytic rabies.[86,91] During the acute neurologic period, signs of nervous system dysfunction follow prodromal signs and symptoms to result in hospitalization (see Table 2.2). **Objective clinical signs** include **ataxia**,[4,39] **bradycardia** and **asystole**,[2] **dysphagia** (which contributes to hydrophobia),[4,87,89] **spontaneous ejaculations**,[4,21] **fever**,[4,30,39] **hypersalivation**,[4,30,39,89] **hypertension** with **tachycardia**,[2,92,93] **hyperventilation**,[86,87] **muscle fasciculation**,[39,89] **nuchal rigidity**,[86] **paresis**,[2] **piloerection** (gooseflesh),[39,89,92] **priapism**,[4,21,39] **seizures** (rare early in disease course, movement disorders may give the appearance of seizures; if present, they are usually in the preterminal phase of the disease),[2,4,39] and **urinary** or **fecal retention** or **incontinence**.[87,89]

Traditional discipline has divided the acute neurologic period into two forms, furious and paralytic. There is contention that there is not a need to demarcate between these forms because there can be an overlap of signs and symptoms of the two forms or one can progress into the other in more of a continuum. However, the categorization does help to emphasize how differently the disease can present in patients, a phenomenon of which medical personnel need to be aware to aid in considering rabies as a differential diagnosis.

Furious rabies is also referred to as classic or encephalitic rabies. Approximations have been made that 2/3[22] to 4/5[4,28,89] of patients develop the furious form of the disease. Furious cases of rabies are categorized as those in which the focus of clinical signs and symptoms is on hyperactivity and autonomic excess[4,21,86] compared with paralytic rabies in which the focus is on paralysis.

In furious rabies, there frequently are **phases of arousal** and **hyperexcitability**, possibly with **aggression**,[4,30] **agitation/combativeness**,[4,30,89] **anxiety**,[4,86] **confusion/delirium**,[4,89] **fear/fearful facial expression**,[21,92] **panic**,[2] and **hallucinations**[4,39] interrupted by periods of lucidity.[7,30,94] There is even a tendency for the patient to engage in **roaming** and **running**.[86]

Clinical signs and symptoms that may be manifested in furious rabies are **aerophobia**,[4,30,39,87] **bradycardia**,[2,87] **dyspnea**,[89] **spontaneous ejaculations**,[21] **hydrophobia**,[4,30,39,89] **hyperesthesia** to tactile, auditory, or visual stimulation,[86,87] **hypertension**,[92,93] **lacrimation**,[87,92] **increased libido**,[87,93] **myoclonus**,[2,39,92] **ophthalmoplegia**,[87,89] **orofacial dyskinesia and myokymia** (which may be misdiagnosed as seizures),[2,93] **paresis and paralysis**,[38,86,87] **paresthesia**,[4,30,86] **altered phonation** (voice changes or barklike sounds possibly associated with vocal cord weakness),[87] **photophobia**,[89,95] **priapism**,[4,21,39] **pruritus**,[30] **dilated pupils**,[21,87] **seizures**,[86,89] **sweating**,[39,92,93] and **tachycardia**.[86,92,93]

"Hydrophobia" means "fear of water." It is rare in other diseases and, therefore, is a positive indicator for rabies.[2] Initially, patients may have dysphagia. When they attempt to swallow, they experience contraction of the muscles of inspiration (pharyngeal and diaphragmatic spasms)[7,21,93] and may be associated with epigastric pain.[87] (Aspiration can lead to secondary pneumonia.[91]) These contractions may be followed by contraction of neck muscles, causing flexion or extension of the neck, and rarely with opisthotonic posturing.[87] During the protective reflex,[86] there can be pain and an associated feeling of terror to the point that even the thought of water or being presented with a glass of water can trigger the contractions. Therefore, patients avoid drinking water even though they may have intense thirst,[86,87] which can lead to dehydration. In developing countries, rabies is sometimes diagnosed by how drastically a person reacts to being offered water.

"Aerophobia" means "fear of air." The rabies patient cannot tolerate being touched by any movement of air. Aerophobia is considered to be a positive indicator for rabies; it is so closely associated with this disease that in developing countries the fan test, in which air is either blown by a fan toward the patient or another person blows their breath toward the patient, is sometimes used to diagnose rabies; if the patient has a significant reaction to air movement, such as spasms of the pharyngeal and neck muscles, a clinical diagnosis of rabies is reached.[87] Nasal cannulae can also evoke this reaction.[4,93]

Paralytic rabies is also referred to as dumb rabies. As mentioned previously, this form is generally classified by **paralysis being the primary clinical sign throughout the illness** because furious rabies can also lead to paralysis. **Flaccid muscle weakness** develops early in the disease course.[87] Approximations have been made that 1/5[4,28,89] to 1/3[22] of patients develop this form of the disease. Clinical signs and symptoms of paralytic rabies are frequently compared with those of **Guillain-Barre syndrome** but are **accompanied by urinary and fecal retention** in contrast to Guillain-Barre.[2,93] A collection of clinical signs and symptoms that may be present in paralytic rabies includes **abdominal discomfort,**[89] **muscle weakness,**[4,21,94] **myoedema**[21,39,86] (although the importance of this sign may require additional clarification[87]), **paresis**[30,39] and **paralysis,**[4,89,96] **paresthesia,**[4,30,86] **pruritus,**[4,30,39] **sphincter dysfunction,**[87,92] **sweating,**[92] **loss of tendon reflexes,**[92,93] and **urinary incontinence**[87,89] (retention can lead to spillover incontinence).

Studies of clinical signs and symptoms in humans—acute neurologic period

Rabies cases in humans in the United States (1960–2010). In a study of 108 cases of rabies in humans that occurred between 1960 and 2010 in the United States (including indigenous cases as well as imported cases in foreign nationals diagnosed and treated within the United States and its territories), the most commonly reported clinical signs and symptoms during the course of illness in order of prevalence were fever, confusion or delirium, agitation or combativeness, paresthesia or localized pain, and dysphagia. In 144 cases of encephalitis during the same time period in which rabies was ruled out by laboratory diagnostic testing, the most commonly reported clinical signs and symptoms in order of prevalence were confusion/delirium, fever, malaise or fatigue, headache, and agitation or combativeness. When comparing the two groups, aerophobia, hydrophobia, paresthesia or localized pain, dysphagia, and localized weakness were more likely to be reported in the rabies cases than in the nonrabies cases, plus priapism or spontaneous ejaculation (which did not reach statistical significance). Clinical signs and symptoms that were more frequent in the nonrabies encephalitis cases than in the rabies cases included headache and

malaise or fatigue, seizures, and confusion or delirium, plus insomnia (which did not reach statistical significance). The following clinical signs and symptoms occurred with equal likelihood in the rabies and nonrabies cases: fever, muscle spasm, hypersalivation, anxiety, hallucinations, autonomic instability, agitation or combativeness, nausea or vomiting, and ataxia.[4]

Comparison of clinical features in dog- and bat-acquired rabies. In a study of 122 cases of rabies in humans from North America, South America, Europe, Africa, and Asia, a comparison was made of clinical signs and symptoms in cases with dog-acquired rabies versus those with bat-acquired rabies. Clinical features found to be more common in dog-acquired rabies included encephalopathy, hydrophobia, and aerophobia. Clinical features more common in bat-acquired rabies included myoclonus, tremors, cranial nerve abnormalities, abnormal motor and sensory examinations, local sensory symptoms, symptoms at the bite or scratch site, and local symptoms in the absence of a bite or scratch. The study did not find that either furious or paralytic rabies was more associated with dog- or bat-acquired rabies.[39] Recognition of the differences in the findings of dog-acquired versus bat-acquired rabies could aid in more prompt diagnosis in some cases and may be of value to keep in mind because bat-acquired rabies is more commonly associated with US indigenous cases and dog-acquired rabies is more commonly associated with cases in some developing countries. This is a reminder of the importance of determining the patient's country of origin and acquiring information on the patient's travel history.

Comparison of furious and paralytic rabies. In a study of 104 cases of rabies in humans in Bali, which involved transmission from rabid dogs, the majority of patients (close to 80%) displayed furious rabies (defined in the study as cases in which signs of hyperactivity were dominant) compared with just more than 20% with paralytic rabies (defined in the study as cases in which the patient displayed varying degrees of paralysis and lethargy). In the cases displaying furious rabies, the most common signs were agitation and confusion. Other clinical signs included hydrophobia, hypersalivation, and dyspnea, plus photophobia, piloerection, muscle fasciculation, convulsions, ophthalmoplegia, facial weakness, and dysphagia. In the cases with paralytic rabies, there were signs of flaccid paralysis, urinary incontinence, and abdominal discomfort. Some of the patients who first presented with paralytic rabies subsequently developed signs and symptoms of furious rabies. The signs ended either by progression into a coma followed by death or by abrupt death. The fatality rate of these cases was 100%.[89]

Coma and death in humans

The clinical course of rabies generally terminates with coma and respiratory and cardiac failure. Dehydration and ketosis may contribute to the demise of the patient; tachycardia followed by cardiac arrests is common.[93] Death usually ensues within 7[86] to 10 days[7] of illness (also cited up to 14 days[87,91]). This length of illness may be increased to a month or longer if intensive care is instituted[22]; without critical care, patients tend to die within 2–3 days of admission.[93] The case fatality rate of rabies exceeds 99.9%.[82,92]

In a study of 104 cases of rabies in humans in Bali in which 92% of the cases had a history of a dog bite, the mean length of medical care until death was approximately 22 h with a range of 1–220 h.[89]

In Thailand, the average survival time from clinical onset to death with partial or no intensive care support in 80 patients with furious rabies and 35 patients with paralytic rabies was 5–7 and 11 days, respectively; all had the dog rabies virus variant.[22]

In a study of cases from North America, South America, Europe, Africa, and Asia in which clinical features in cases of rabies in humans that were acquired by bats were compared with those in cases acquired by dogs, patients from either group with paralytic rabies had longer survival times than those with encephalitic rabies.[39]

Differential Diagnoses in Humans
Positive indicators for rabies in differential diagnoses in humans

It is important to consider rabies as a differential diagnosis in any case with encephalitis, myelitis, or encephalomyelitis, especially when the patient has a known history of an animal bite or comes from an area where rabies is endemic.[90] Additionally, a patient may not relate his/her present condition to a bat encounter or an animal bite that occurred previously (see Length of incubation period in humans section), so health-care personnel should ask the patient specifically about any possible exposures. Diagnosis will aid in determining the need for PEP in people potentially exposed to infectious materials of a person determined to have rabies or PEP for others who may have been exposed by the same source.[38] Confirmation of rabies also has implications for the patient and the patient's family, plus for physicians considering treatment or palliation[2]; if negative, other causes of encephalitis, some which may be treatable, can be more aggressively pursued.[38] Research for an effective treatment is ongoing, and experimental treatments are available for which a particular patient might be a viable candidate.[2] With any potential case of rabies, a prudent course of action is to seek consultation

and guidance from the state health department and the Centers for Disease Control and Prevention (CDC). Advice on treatment of rabies encephalitis is available at www.mcw.edu/rabies.

A positive indicator for rabies includes a rapidly progressive worsening of neurologic signs,[97] which is considered to be less common in other causes of encephalitis.[17] Dysphagia is also considered to be rare in other etiologies of encephalitis.[17] Other positive indicators of rabies include aerophobia,[2,4] autonomic instability,[2,97] dysesthesia referable to the bitten limb,[2] and hydrophobia.[2,4,97] See Table 2.3 for a more detailed list. There are outliers for the time frames of every stage of the disease, and patients may not recall a bite incident, especially bites from bats that can be difficult to observe. Hence, rabies can be a delinquent consideration on the differential diagnosis.

Diseases with similar clinical signs and symptoms in humans

The clinical signs and symptoms of rabies mimic those of other diseases. Complications exhibited with rabies include cardiac arrhythmias, hypotension, cardiac failure, asphyxia, pneumonia, pneumothorax, inspiratory spasm, acute respiratory distress syndrome, Cheyne-Stokes and other respiratory arrhythmias, convulsions, hypopyrexia, hyperpyrexia, diabetes insipidus, cerebral edema, gastrointestinal bleeding and stress ulceration, and Mallory-Weiss tears.[92]

Some of the other diseases and conditions with clinical signs and symptoms that reflect those of rabies include anti-N-methyl-D-asparate receptor antibody encephalitis, cerebral malaria, conversion disorder, delirium, acute psychotic disorders, postvaccinal encephalitis, herpes simplex encephalitis, scorpion and elapid (snake) envenomation, illicit drug use, organophosphate poisoning, tetanus, brachial neuritis, and *Campylobacter*-associated summer paralysis syndrome.[2] Additional diseases that might be considered in a rabies patient who has yet to be diagnosed are enterovirus-71,[21] Nipah-virus,[21] and arbovirus encephalitides (e.g., Japanese, eastern equine, and West Nile virus encephalitis).[22,93] Hypertonia is unusual in rabies, so, if present, would be more suggestive of another disease, such as West Nile.[93] Clinical signs and symptoms of paralytic rabies can be difficult to discern from those of Guillain-Barre syndrome.[2,17,86] Therefore, a person starting to exhibit clinical signs and symptoms of rabies may be sent to a variety of specialists because of differential diagnoses being considered, which stresses the need for physicians to be aware of the elusive nature of this disease. Rabies patients have been sent

---

TABLE 2.3
Positive Indicators for Rabies in Cases of Acute Progressive Encephalitis

Aerophobia[2,4] (may be masked by intubation and sedation of the patient)

Autonomic instability/dysautonomia (such as bradycardia, catecholamine surges, hypersalivation, piloerection, priapism, and sweating)[2,97]

Periods of altered behavior and cognition, arousal, and dysautonomia interrupted by periods of lucidity[2,97]

Pain, dysesthesias (including pruritus) referable to the bitten limb[2,4,97]

Dysphagia[2,4,17]

Exposure history (known animal bite, foreign travel, immigration, high-risk occupation for exposure, attic remodeling, cabin ownership, hunting or dressing game, caving, wildlife rehabilitation, organ transplantation)[2]

Negative test results for other etiologies of encephalitis[97]

Guillain-Barre-like syndrome along with urinary and fecal retention or other dysautonomia[2,93]; percussion myoedema may be associated with paralytic rabies, but not Guillain-Barre syndrome[21]

Hydrophobia[2,4,97] (may be masked by intubation and sedation of the patient)[4]

Myoclonic jerks, paresis referable to the bitten limb[2]

Rapidly progressive worsening of neurologic signs[17,97]

Orofacial dyskinesia and myokymia (often confused for seizures)[2]

Focal weakness[4]

Rabies typically would be less likely in patients who do not require hospitalization within 1 week of developing clinical signs and symptoms or in hospitalized patients surviving longer than 2 weeks[4]; absence of fever and a prolonged prodromal period of more than 2 weeks makes rabies unlikely[2]

---

to neurologists, cardiologists, rheumatologists, pulmonologists, otorhinolaryngologists, and psychiatrists.[92]

There are differentiations that may assist in determining whether to consider rabies as a differential diagnosis (see Table 2.3). For instance, the clinical signs and symptoms are similar in Guillain-Barre syndrome and paralytic rabies. However, in paralytic rabies, fecal and urinary retention are present although they are not observed in Guillain-Barre syndrome.[2,93] The same may also apply to percussion edema[21]; however, the importance of this sign has not been established.[87]

Tetanus could also result from a bite in which a puncture wound is produced, so it should readily be considered as a potential diagnosis in cases with a bite history. Tetanus resembles rabies in the form of reflex spasms; rabies patients will not have persistent rigidity or sustained contraction of axial muscles, such as those displayed in tetanus in the jaw, neck, back, and abdomen. Spasms in rabies mostly involve respiratory muscles, whereas those in tetanus involve axial muscles. Opisthotonos, which is a characteristic sign in tetanus, is rare in rabies.[21]

Examples of differential diagnoses in rabies cases in humans

In a case of rabies in a person in the United States caused by the silver-haired bat (*Lasionycteris noctivagans*) rabies virus variant in which the patient's medical history included initial signs of progressive weakness, ataxia, dysarthria, and dysphagia, diagnosis was complicated by existing conditions of dementia, an acute urinary tract infection, and a recent fall; a presumptive diagnosis of Guillain-Barre syndrome was made. Rabies was considered as a differential diagnosis after family members remembered that the patient had awakened one night to find a bat by the neck, but no bite wound was noticed at that time.[17]

Another US case associated with a bat rabies virus variant (tricolored bat, *Perimyotis subflavus*) was diagnosed with cervical muscle strain and radiculopathy based on acute onset of severe neck pain; the patient was prescribed a muscle relaxant. When signs and symptoms progressed within a day to include paresthesia, tremors, sweating, anxiety, and hallucinations, a reaction to the muscle relaxant was suspected. The course of the disease continued with fever, tachycardia, tachypnea, hypertension, and myoclonus. Laboratory tests administered for differential diagnoses before rabies was considered included a urine drug screen, tricyclic antidepressant levels, an arbovirus panel, and testing for antibodies to Rocky Mountain spotted fever, ehrlichiosis, syphilis, and herpes simplex (all were negative).[44]

In a study of 104 rabies cases in Bali that involved rabies transmission to humans by rabid dogs, some of the rabies cases were initially misidentified as cardiac maladies due to chest pain, pulmonary maladies due to breathing difficulties, dyspepsia, typhoid fever, urinary colic, paralytic ileus, or appendicitis.[89]

REVIEW

Rabies is a disease fraught with varying lengths of incubation periods and morbidity; unusual presentations of clinical signs (and symptoms in humans), with many outliers affecting clinical manifestations; and disease presentation that can mimic that of a myriad of other diseases. It is essential for medical personnel to factor the clinical signs and symptoms of rabies into their mental database of disease knowledge; this would include learning the basics of the disease and positive indicators for rabies, plus being aware of and open to all the unusual elements of case presentation. Proper diagnosis of rabies could save lives by knowing to evaluate possible exposures scenarios for the need of PEP and preventing transplantations from persons who died of rabies.

EXAMPLES OF CASES AND CASE INVESTIGATIONS

Transmission Scenarios and Postexposure Prophylaxis Considerations

1. A horse exhibiting neurologic signs, including ataxia, was tested and confirmed to be positive for rabies. During the specimen submission, it was noted that 15 horses shared a water trough with the rabid horse; only some of these horses were previously vaccinated against rabies. Although the likelihood of being considered an exposure was low to none,[g,l,m] in consideration of the possibility of infected saliva from the rabid horse contacting the mucous membranes of the other horses drinking from the trough, the rancher opted to err on the side of caution and have PEP administered to all the remaining horses.[l] Requirements can vary per state and even may be prohibited, but the PEP in Texas (where the incident occurred) for unvaccinated horses was immediate vaccination followed by boosters on the third and eighth weeks of a 90-day confinement period.[60] This was a worthwhile decision, nonetheless, as vaccination of horses is recommended.[15,31,60]

    Note: In situations such as this, the National Association of State Public Health Veterinarians recommends that restricting an entire herd if a single animal develops rabies is not necessary because multiple rabid animals in a herd and herbivore-to-herbivore transmission of rabies are rare.[31]

    Additionally, there has never been a documented case of rabies through a fomite or water[38]; the water would create a dilution effect on the virus. Rabid animals also typically lose their appetite and have difficulty drinking, making it unlikely that they would have been drinking the water. However, in a previously described case investigation, a rabid cow was found standing at a water trough and, although she was not drinking, rabies did not preclude her from possibly drooling into the water or sticking her muzzle into the water in an attempt to drink.[a] Still, the dilution effect of the water would create a notable risk reduction.

2. A rabies incident report from the mid-1990s in Texas involved a person who believed in sharing a beer with his horse (this was even before Willie Nelson and Toby Keith were singing about legendary "Beer for My Horses"[98]). When the person's horse developed rabies, which could be transmitted by infected saliva from the rabid animal contacting mucous membrane in his mouth, this person was faced with the need for PEP.[61,n]

Quandary of an Unusual Presentation of Rabies

While in Vung Tau, Vietnam, a commander of a veterinary service medical detachment was providing aid during the daily open pet clinic when the head nurse of the nearby evacuation hospital and several army nurses presented his team with a mother dog dubbed "Queenie" and eight nursing pups whose eyes were still closed, indicating a very early age. The head nurse stated that she and her colleagues had found Queenie and her pups alongside the road earlier that morning and wanted to have them examined, plus she requested that they be provided with housing while someone could be located to care for the animals. On examination, Queenie and her pups were determined to be in adequate to good condition. The one stand-out trauma was a relatively fresh, deep puncture (estimated to be 1–4 days old) of Queenie's left eye; however, she and the pups otherwise appeared within normal limits. Queenie, though, would probably need to have her eye removed. The dogs were then assigned to an isolation kennel. As news of Queenie spread, by that evening the senior ophthalmologist at the evacuation hospital expressed interest in examining Queenie's eye with his newest medical equipment in hopes of performing some diagnostic techniques on the dog's eye. Because Queenie and her litter were eating, nursing, and otherwise behaving like healthy dogs, it was decided that she would be taken to the senior ophthalmologist the next morning. On arrival at the ophthalmologist's clinic the next morning, more than 40 doctors, nurses, technicians, and administrators were waiting to meet and pet Queenie; they all disregarded warnings to not touch her. Otherwise, the appointment went well; the ophthalmologist performed his examinations and ended by stating that the penetration looked fresh but the eye could not be saved. An apparently happy Queenie was returned to her isolation kennel with her pups. She quickly checked each pup and then ate her supper and fed the pups. During evening kennel activities, the veterinary technicians and a New Zealand army corporal (who was staying there while his dog was being treated for heartworms) reported that the animals were all doing OK. Early the next morning at the 48-hour point of this event, one of the veterinary technicians found Queenie and all of her pups dead in their isolation kennel. By protocol, such unknown deaths were treated as rabies suspects due to the high rate of rabies in Vietnam at that time. Specimens were immediately sent to the medical laboratory in Saigon, and the results indicated that Queenie and her pups had died from rabies. The end result of this story is that more than 40 US military medical personnel and one New Zealand army corporal had to receive PEP.[o]

Note: This event demonstrates that although one frequently envisions the sensationalized dog foaming at the mouth and trying to attack everything in its path when considering a case of rabies, it should be remembered that there is an array of versions in which rabies can present, including a lack of typical clinical signs. One supposition was that Queenie was infected through a bite or deep scratch to her eye, and the pups were infected as she licked them clean, indicating that there does not have to be a visible wound present for an animal to become infected. (Virus-laden saliva contacting intact skin would not be an exposure, but contacting mucous membranes or any break in the skin could be.) In addition, a reminder is generated in this scenario for onlookers to follow directions when told to not touch an animal.[o]

Rabies Considerations in Unusual Encounters With Animals

High-risk animal

A young man contacted the health department enquiring about PEP. He was sitting in his underwear holding a "pet" raccoon when the animal bit him on his genitals. The man did not want to have the animal euthanatized in order to be tested, so he said at the time it had escaped. He was taken aback by learning that as much as possible (about half) of the human rabies immune globulin (HRIG) was to be injected at the bite site. On consultation, including some opposing views (such as the need to adhere to infiltration of the bite site with HRIG), it was decided that the dose of HRIG be divided with a half dose being administered in each hip.[h,p]

Note: If anatomically feasible, the full dose of HRIG should be infiltrated around and into the wound(s), but any remaining dosage should be administered intramuscular in the closest muscle mass of suitable size to accommodate the remaining volume, with the

caveat that it should not be administered in the same syringe or in the same anatomic site as the initial vaccine dose; the HRIG should be injected into muscle, not adipose tissue (for which there could be increased risk in the gluteal area). Additionally, the deltoid area is the only acceptable site of vaccination (also intramuscular) for adults and older children. For younger children, the outer aspect of the thigh may be used. Rabies vaccine should never be administered in the gluteal area.[20]

Wild animals do not make good pets, and it may even be illegal to possess certain animals as pets. Typically, a high-risk animal for transmitting rabies that has bitten a person would be euthanatized and tested for rabies,[60] so making one of these animals a pet where it has close contact with people and an increased chance for nipping or scratching someone, even if in play, increases the chances for the animal to meet an unfortunate demise.

Low-risk and no-risk animals

A doctor called the health department to inquire about the need for PEP for a man who was bitten by an armadillo (which is considered to be a low-risk animal for transmitting rabies[60]) while sticking his hand in a hole in the ground. The veterinarian at the health department who handled the call did not think this sounded like a logical assumption pertaining to the bite scenario because armadillos are edentates (have a limited number of soft teeth without enamel that are peglike molars) and would not have produced a bite wound of that nature. On further description of the wound and the significant swelling around it, it was determined that it was actually a snake bite, for which rabies is of no concern because snakes are cold-blooded animals, and rabies is a disease of warm-blooded animals.[q]

Note: This is an example of the importance of knowing the biology of the animals with which you are dealing and, if in doubt, consulting with a specialist in veterinary medicine or wildlife biology.

Animal in "other" category

Consideration was made pertaining to prescribing PEP for a person who was bitten by a feral hog during a feral hog-catching contest, in which participants were chasing feral hogs in a pen and trying to catch them. Not only did the person not know which hog was involved in the bite incident but also the hogs were sent to slaughter after the contest. Given that a person, let alone a group of people, chasing a feral animal in an enclosed area would create circumstances for a bite to be classified as provoked and that there has been a very low incidence of rabies in feral hogs, PEP was not recommended.[c,g,r]

APPENDIX

APPENDIX TABLE 2.A1
Studies and Reports on the Incubation Period in Rabid Animals

Animal	Incubation Period	Studies and Reports
Bats	3–12 weeks	Experimentally infected Mexican (now called Brazilian) free-tailed bats[a1]
	24–125 days	Bats experimentally injected with pooled salivary tissues from naturally infected bats[a1]
Cats	Range from 9 to 51 days with a median of 18 days	Study of 26 cats inoculated with street-rabies virus[a2]
	10 days to 2 months, with one case reported as 2 years; probably not beyond 6 months	Report[a3]; report[a4]
Cattle	1–2 months	Cattle naturally infected by vampire bats[a5]
	Average of 15 days	Report on experimentally induced rabies[a4]
Dogs	Range of 9–42 days with a median of 15.5 days	Study of 54 dogs inoculated with street-rabies virus[a6]
	7–125 days	Experimentally induced with range depending on dose and variant of virus[a7]
	10 days to 2 months	Report[a3]
	Several months, but probably not beyond 6 months	Report[a8]
Ferrets	Range of 17–63 days; mean of 28 days	Study of 19 domestic ferrets experimentally inoculated with a raccoon variant of rabies virus[a9]
Foxes	Longest period was death at 110 days	In experimental inoculation in foxes, the higher the infective dose administered, the shorter the incubation period[a10]
	266 days was noted	Study[a10]
	Minimum of a 15-month incubation period	Foxes in a rabies-endemic area that were trapped and held in quarantine died of rabies up to 15 months after capture, which meant a minimum of a 15-month incubation period, but the time frame for when the exposure in the wild occurred was unknown[a10]
	Range between 4 days and 15 months, with most being between 2 weeks and 3 months	Report[a4]
	Range of 11 days–15 months, although usually not exceeding 30 days	Report[a11]
Horses	Range of 6–27 days; average of 12 days	Study of 21 horses with experimentally induced rabies[a8,a12]
	Range of 2–9 weeks; can be shorter or considerably longer (such as several months)	Report[a12,a13]
Raccoons	39–79 days, but full length of the incubation period was unknown	Naturally acquired rabies in captured raccoons, so exact exposure dates were unknown[a14]
	10–107 days (10–42 days with fox rabies virus variant, 10–107 days with Florida raccoon, 18–65 days with Pennsylvania raccoon, and 10–21 days with stock virus)	Varied depending on the type of rabies virus variant with which the raccoon was experimentally inoculated[a14]
	Range of 23–92 days; mean of 50 days	Group of experimentally infected raccoons[a4]

Continued

APPENDIX TABLE 2.A1
Studies and Reports on Length of Incubation Period in Rabid Animals—cont'd

Animal	Incubation Period	Studies and Reports
Skunks	Varied between 2 weeks and 3 months; some up to 6 months	Skunks experimentally inoculated with street virus (longer period with lower doses of virus administered)[a15]
Wild animals (in general)	Rarely less than 10 days or greater than 6 months	Report[a3]

APPENDIX TABLE 2.A2
Studies and Reports on the Length of Clinical Illness in Rabid Animals

Animal	Duration of Illness (Time Between Onset of Clinical Signs and Death)	Studies and Reports
Cats	Range of 1–8 days with a median of 5	Study of 26 cats inoculated with street-rabies virus[a2]
	Died within 10 days of onset of clinical signs	Study of 58 naturally infected cats[a16]
Cattle	Average of 4 days	Report on experimentally induced rabies[a4,a8]
Dogs	Range of 1–7 days; median of 3	Study of 54 dogs inoculated with street-rabies virus[a6]
	Died within 10 days	Study of 644 naturally infected dogs[a16]
	0–14 days	Experimentally inoculated with rabies virus[a7]
	1–11 days	Report[a3]
Ferrets	Range of 1–8 days; mean of 4–5 days	Study of 19 domestic ferrets experimentally inoculated with the raccoon variant of rabies virus[a9]
Foxes	1–4 days with some reaching 9 days	Experimental inoculation[a10]
	2–4 days (usual)	Report[a3]
	0–14 days; mortality rate of 100% as there have been no reports of a fox surviving infection	Report[a11]
Horses	Range of 1–7 days; mean of 4.5 days	Study of 21 horses with naturally occurring rabies[a17]
	Range of 2–11 days; average of 5.5 days	Study of 21 horses with experimentally induced rabies (using street-rabies virus produced in foxes)[a12,a13]
	4–5 days; can be as long as 15 days (rare)	Report[a18]
Raccoons	2–8 days	Naturally infected animals[a14]
	1–13 days (1–13 days with fox rabies virus variant, 2–5 days with Pennsylvania raccoon variant, 1–7 days with stock virus, and not stated for Florida raccoon)	Study of experimentally infected animals; length varied depending on the type of rabies virus variant with which the animal was inoculated[a14]
	Range of 2–10 days; mean of 4–5 days	Experimentally infected animals[a4]
Skunks	2–3 days	Experimentally infected; varied depending on the type of rabies virus variant inoculated into the skunk[a4]
	4–9 days	Report[a3]
	1–18 days	Report[a15]

APPENDIX REFERENCES

a1. Baer GM, Smith JS. Rabies in nonhematophagus bats. In: Baer GM, ed. *The Natural History of Rabies.* 2nd ed. Boca Raton: CRC Press, Inc; 1991:341–366.

a2. Vaughn JB, Gerhardt P, Paterson JCS. Excretion of street rabies virus in the saliva of cats. *JAMA.* 1963;184(9):705–708.

a3. Pan American Health Organization. Rabies. In: *Zoonoses and Communicable Diseases Common to Man and Animals.* PAHO; 2003:246–275.

a4. Hanlon CA. Rabies in terrestrial animals. In: Jackson AC, ed. *Rabies: Scientific Basis of the Disease and Its Management.* San Diego: Academic Press, An Elsevier Science Imprint; 2013:179–213.

a5. Baer GM. Vampire bat and bovine paralytic rabies. In: Baer GM, ed. *The Natural History of Rabies.* 2nd ed. Boca Raton: CRC Press, Inc; 1991:389–403.

a6. Vaughn JB, Gerhardt P, Newell KW. Excretion of street rabies virus in the saliva of dogs. *JAMA.* 1965;193(5):363–368.

a7. Fekadu M. Canine rabies. In: Baer GM, ed. *The Natural History of Rabies.* 2nd ed. Boca Raton: CRC Press, Inc; 1991:367–387.

a8. Niezgoda M, Hanlon CA, Rupprecht CE. Animal rabies. In: Jackson AC, Wunner WH, eds. *Rabies.* San Diego: Academic Press, An Elsevier Science Imprint; 2002:163–218.

a9. Niezgoda M, Briggs DJ, Shaddock J, et al. Viral excretion in domestic ferrets (*Mustela putorious furo*) inoculated with a raccoon rabies isolate. *Am J Vet Res.* 1998;59(12):1629–1632.

a10. Blancou J, Aubert MFA, Artois M, Fox rabies. In: Baer GM, ed. *The Natural History of Rabies.* second ed. Boca Raton: CRC Press, Inc; 1991:257–290.

a11. Hellenic Center for Disease Control and Prevention. Rabies in wildlife (red fox): epidemiology, symptoms, diagnosis and prevention. HCDCP E-bulletin. http://www2.keelpno.gr/blog/?p=4067.

a12. Hudson LC, Weinstock D, Jordan T, et al. Clinical presentation of experimentally induced rabies in horses. *J Vet Med.* 1996;B(43):277–285.

a13. Wilson PJ. Rabies. In: Sprayberry KA, Robinson NE, eds. *Robinson's Current Therapy in Equine Medicine.* 7th ed. St. Louis: Elsevier-Saunders; 2015:171–172.

a14. Winkler WG, Jenkins SR. Raccoon rabies. In: Baer GM, ed. *The Natural History of Rabies.* 2nd ed. Boca Raton: CRC Press, Inc; 1991:325–340.

a15. Charlton KM, Webster WA, Casey GA. Skunk rabies. In: Baer GM, ed. *The Natural History of Rabies.* second ed. Boca Raton: CRC Press, Inc; 1991:519–549.

a16. Tepsumethanon V, Lumlertdacha B, Mitmoonpitak C, et al. Survival of naturally infected rabid dogs and cats. *Clin Infect Dis.* 2004;39:278–280.

a17. Green SL, Smith LL, Vernau W, et al. Rabies in horses: 21 cases (1970-1990). *JAVMA.* 1992;200(8):1133–1137.

a18. Green SL. Equine rabies. *Vet Clin North Am.* 1993;9(2):337–347.

REFERENCES

1. Wilkinson L. History. In: Jackson AC, Wunner WH, eds. *Rabies.* San Diego: Academic Press: An Elsevier Science Imprint; 2002:1–22.

2. Willoughby RE. Rabies: rare human infection – common questions. *Infect Dis Clin N Am.* 2015;29:637–650.

3. Wunner WH, Conzelmann KK. Rabies virus. In: Jackson AC, ed. *Rabies: Scientific Basis of the Disease and Its Management.* San Diego: Academic Press: An Elsevier Science Imprint; 2013:17–60.

4. Petersen BW, Rupprecht CE. Human rabies epidemiology and diagnosis. *Intech.* 2011. November 16. https://www.intechopen.com/books/non-flavivirus-encephalitis/human-rabies-epidemiology-and-diagnosis. Accessed 16.04.18.

5. Jackson AC. History of rabies research. In: Jackson AC, ed. *Rabies: Scientific Basis of the Disease and Its Management.* San Diego: Academic Press: An Elsevier Science Imprint; 2013:1–15.

6. Steele JH, Fernandez PJ. History of rabies and global aspects. In: Baer GM, ed. *The Natural History of Rabies.* 2nd ed. Boca Raton: CRC Press, Inc; 1991:1–24.

7. World Health Organization. WHO Expert Consultation of Rabies – Third Report. *WHO Technical Report Series.* 2018;1012:1-183.

8. Lyssa. https://www.greekmythology.com/Other_Gods/Primordial/Lyssa/lyssa.html. Accessed 26.03.18.

9. Baer GM, Neville J, Turner GS. *Rabies Etiology.* In: *Rabbis and Rabies: A Pictorial History of Rabies Through the Ages.* Mexico: Laboratorios Baer; 1996:49–61.

10. Ma X, Monroe BP, Cleaton JM, et al. Rabies surveillance in the United States during 2016. *JAVMA.* 2018;252(8):945–957.

11. Hanlon CA, Childs JE. Epidemiology. In: Jackson AC, ed. *Rabies: Scientific Basis of the Disease and its Management.* San Diego: Academic Press: An Elsevier Science Imprint; 2013:61–123.

12. Bharti OK, Chand R, Chauhan A, et al. Scratches/Abrasions without bleeding cause rabies: a 7 years rabies death review from Medical College Shimla, Himachal Pradesh, India. *Indian J Comm Med.* 2017;42(4):248–249.

13. Niezgoda M, Hanlon CA, Rupprecht CE. Animal rabies. In: Jackson AC, Wunner WH, eds. *Rabies.* San Diego: Academic Press: An Elsevier Science Imprint; 2002:163–218.

14. Kelley MF, Mahlow JC. Evaluating rabies exposure. *TX Med.* 2001;97(4):60–63.

15. Wilson PJ. Rabies. In: Sprayberry KA, Robinson NE, eds. *Robinson's Current Therapy in Equine Medicine.* 7th ed. St. Louis: Elsevier-Saunders; 2015:171–172.

16. Centers for Disease Control and Prevention. Rabies death attributed to exposure in Central America with symptom onset in a US detention facility-Texas, 2013. *MMWR.* 2014;63(20):446–449.

17. Centers for Disease Control and Prevention. Human rabies – Wyoming and Utah, 2015. *MMWR.* 2016;65(21):529–533.

18. Wallace RM, Stanek D, Griese S, et al. A large-scale, rapid public health response to rabies in an organ recipient and the previously undiagnosed organ donor. *Zoon and Pub Hlth.* 2014;61:560–570.

19. Centers for Disease Control and Prevention. Investigation of rabies infections in organ donor and transplant recipients – Alabama, Arkansas, Oklahoma, and Texas, 2004. *MMWR.* 2004;53(dispatch):1–3.

20. Centers for Disease Control and Prevention. Human rabies prevention – United States, 2008: recommendations of the Advisory Committee on Immunization Practices. *MMWR.* 2008;57(RR-3):1–28.

21. Hemachudha T, Laothamatas J, Rupprecht CE. Human rabies: a disease of complex neuropathogenetic mechanisms and diagnostic challenges. *Lancet Neurol.* 2002;1:101–109.

22. Hemachudha T, Ugolini G, Wacharapluesadee W, et al. Human rabies: neuropathogenesis, diagnosis, and management. *Lancet Neurol.* 2013;12:498–513.

23. Jackson AC, Fu ZF. Pathogenesis. In: Jackson AC, ed. *Rabies: Scientific Basis of the Disease and Its Management.* San Diego: Academic Press: An Elsevier Science Imprint; 2013:299–349.

24. Baer GM, Lentz TL. Rabies pathogenesis to the central nervous system. In: Baer GM, ed. *The Natural History of Rabies.* 2nd ed. Boca Raton: CRC Press, Inc; 1991:105–120.

25. Jackson AC. Pathogenesis. In: Jackson AC, Wunner WH, eds. *Rabies.* San Diego: Academic Press: An Elsevier Science Imprint; 2002:245–282.

26. Schneider LG. Spread of virus from the central nervous system. In: Baer GM, ed. *The Natural History of Rabies.* 2nd ed. Boca Raton: CRC Press, Inc; 1991:133–144.

27. Childs JE. Epidemiology. In: Jackson AC, Wunner WH, eds. *Rabies.* San Diego: Academic Press: An Elsevier Science Imprint; 2002:113–162.

28. Jackson AC. Human disease. In: Jackson AC, Wunner WH, eds. *Rabies.* San Diego: Academic Press, An Elsevier Science Imprint; 2002:219–244.

29. Blancou J, Aubert MFA, Artois M. Fox rabies. In: Baer GM, ed. *The Natural History of Rabies.* 2nd ed. Boca Raton: CRC Press, Inc; 1991:257–290.

30. Dimaano EM, Scholand SJ, Alera MTP, et al. Clinical and epidemiological features of human rabies cases in the Philippines: a review from 1987 to 2006. *Int J Infect Dis.* 2011;15:495–499.

31. Brown CM, Slavinski S, Ettestad P, et al. Compendium of animal rabies prevention and control, 2016. *JAVMA.* 2016;248(5):505–517.

32. Canadian Council of Chief Veterinary Officers. Recommendations of the Canadian Council of Chief Veterinary Officers Subcommittee for the Management of Potential Domestic Animal Exposures to Rabies. http://homepage .usask.ca/~vim458/virology/studpages2010/rabies/Clinic alSigns.html. Accessed 21.05.18.

33. Centers for Disease Control and Prevention. Rabies in a Dairy Cow, Oklahoma. Posted 23.12.05. http://www.cdc.gov/rabies/ resources/news/2005-12-23.html. Accessed 14.09.16.

34. Gibbons RV. Cryptogenic rabies, bats, and the question of aerosol transmission. *Ann Emerg Med.* 2002;39(5):528–536.

35. Winkler WG, Fashinell TR, Leffingwell L, et al. Airborne rabies transmission in a laboratory worker. *JAVMA.* 1973;226(10):1219–1221.

36. Constantine DG. Rabies transmission by nonbite route. *Pub Hlth Reports.* 1962;77(4):287–289.

37. Pan American Health Organization. Rabies. In: *Zoonoses and Communicable Diseases Common to Man and Animals.* PAHO; 2003:246–275.

38. Rupprecht CE, Hanlon CA, Hemachudha T. Rabies re-examined. *Lancet Infect Dis.* 2002;2:327–343.

39. Udow SJ, Marrie RA, Jackson AC. Clinical features of dog- and bat-acquired rabies in humans. *Clin Infect Dis.* 2013;57(5):689–696.

40. De Serres G, Dallaire F, Cote M, et al. Bat rabies in the United States and Canada from 1950 through 2007: human cases with and without bat contact. *Clin Infect Dis.* 2008;46:1329–1337.

41. Mayes BC, Wilson PJ, Oertli EH, et al. Epidemiology of rabies in bats in Texas (2001–2010). *JAVMA.* 2013;243(8):1129–1137.

42. Jackson AC, Fenton MB. Human rabies and bat bites. *Lancet.* 2001;357:1714.

43. Rupprecht CE. A tale of two worlds: public health management decisions in human rabies prevention. *Clin Infect Dis.* 2004;39(2):281–283.

44. Centers for Disease Control and Prevention. Human rabies-Missouri, 2014. *MMWR.* 2016;65(10):253–256.

45. Hanlon CA. Rabies in terrestrial animals. In: Jackson AC, ed. *Rabies: Scientific Basis of the Disease and its Management.* San Diego: Academic Press: An Elsevier Science Imprint; 2013:179–213.

46. Fekadu M. Canine rabies. In: Baer GM, ed. *The Natural History of Rabies.* 2nd ed. Boca Raton: CRC Press, Inc; 1991:367–387.

47. Winkler WG, Jenkins SR. Raccoon rabies. In: Baer GM, ed. *The Natural History of Rabies.* 2nd ed. Boca Raton: CRC Press, Inc; 1991:325–340.

48. Shankar V, Dietzschold B, Koprowski H. Direct entry of rabies virus into the central nervous system without prior local replication. *J Virol.* 1991;65(5):2736–2738.

49. Charlton KM, Webster WA, Casey GA. Skunk rabies. In: Baer GM, ed. *The Natural History of Rabies.* 2nd ed. Boca Raton: CRC Press, Inc; 1991:519–549.

50. Bunn TO. Cat rabies. In: Baer GM, ed. *The Natural History of Rabies.* 2nd ed. Boca Raton: CRC Press, Inc; 1991:379–387.

51. Eidson M, Matthews SD, Willsey AL, et al. Rabies virus infection in a pet guinea pig and seven pet rabbits. *JAVMA.* 2005;227(6):932–935.

52. Hudson LC, Weinstock D, Jordan T, et al. Clinical presentation of experimentally induced rabies in horses. *J Vet Med.* 1996;B(43):277–285.

53. Green SL, Smith LL, Vernau W, et al. Rabies in horses: 21 cases (1970–1990). *JAVMA.* 1992;200(8):1133–1137.

54. Baer GM, Neville J, Turner GS. *Symptoms and diagnosis. In: Rabbis and Rabies: A Pictorial History of Rabies Through the Ages.* Mexico: Laboratorios Baer; 1996:27–45.

55. Warner Brothers. *Cujo.* 1983. https://en.wikipedia.org/wiki/ Cujo_(film).

56. University of Saskatchewan. Rabies. Saskatoon, Alberta. http://homepage.usask.ca/-vim458/virology/studpages20 10/rabies/Main.html. Accessed 17.05.18.

57. Baer GM. Vampire bat and bovine paralytic rabies. In: Baer GM, ed. *The Natural History of Rabies*. 2nd ed. Boca Raton: CRC Press, Inc; 1991:389–403.

58. Baer GM, Smith JS. Rabies in nonhematophagus bats. In: Baer GM, ed. *The Natural History of Rabies*. 2nd ed. Boca Raton: CRC Press, Inc; 1991:341–366.

59. Ontario Ministry of Natural Resources. *Border Rabies Project: Sudbury to San Antonio*. Video; 1995.

60. Texas Administrative Code. *Rabies Control and Eradication*; 2013. http://texreg.sos.state.tx.us/public/readtac$ext.View TAC?tac_view=5&ti=25&pt.=1&ch=169&sch=A&rl=Y. Accessed 07.06.18.

61. Wilson PJ, Rohde RE. *The Many Faces of Rabies*. Elsevier Connect; 2016. September. https://www.elsevier.com/con nect/the-many-faces-of-rabies Accessed 15.05.18.

62. Oertli EH, Wilson PJ, Hunt PR, et al. Epidemiology of rabies in skunks in Texas. *JAVMA*. 2009;234(5):616–620.

63. Centers for Disease Control and Prevention. Information for doctors. https://www.cdc.gov/rabies/specific_groups/d octors/transmission.html. Accessed 22.01.18.

64. Briggs DJ. Public health management of humans at risk. In: Jackson AC, Wunner WH, eds. *Rabies*. San Diego: Academic Press: An Elsevier Science Imprint; 2002:401–428.

65. Vaughn JB, Gerhardt P, Paterson JCS. Excretion of street rabies virus in the saliva of cats. *JAMA*. 1963;184(9):705–708.

66. Vaughn JB, Gerhardt P, Newell KW. Excretion of street rabies virus in the saliva of dogs. *JAMA*. 1965;193(5):363–368.

67. Niezgoda M, Briggs DJ, Shaddock J, et al. Viral excretion in domestic ferrets (*Mustela putorious furo*) inoculated with a raccoon rabies isolate. *Am J Vet Res*. 1998;59(12):1629–1632.

68. Nouvellet P, Donnelly CA, De Nardi M, et al. Rabies and canine distemper virus epidemics in the red fox population of northern Italy (2006–2010). *PLoS One*. 2013;8(4):e61588.

69. Birhane MG, Cleaton JM, Monroe BP, et al. Rabies surveillance in the United States during 2015. *JAVMA*. 2017;250(10):1117–1130.

70. Wallace RM, Gilbert A, Slate D, et al. Right place, wrong species: a 20-year review of rabies virus cross species transmission among terrestrial mammals in the United States. *PLoS One*. 2014;9(10):e107539.

71. Clark KA, Neill SU, Smith JS, et al. Epizootic canine rabies transmitted by coyotes in south Texas. *JAVMA*. 1994;204(4):536–540.

72. Centers for Disease Control and Prevention. Human rabies – Puerto Rico, 2015. *MMWR*. 2017;65(52):1474–1476.

73. Centers for Disease Control and Prevention. Rabies in Puerto Rico. https://www.cdc.gov/worldrabiesday/puer to-rico.html. Accessed 22.01.18.

74. Moore DA, Sischo WM, Hunter A, et al. Animal bite epidemiology and surveillance for rabies postexposure prophylaxis. *JAVMA*. 2000;217(2):190–194.

75. Tepsumethanon V, Lumlertdacha B, Mitmoonpitak C, et al. Survival of naturally infected rabid dogs and cats. *Clin Infect Dis*. 2004;39:278–280.

76. Krebs JW, Williams SM, Smith JS, et al. Rabies among infrequently reported mammalian carnivores in the United States, 1960–2000. *J Wildl Dis*. 2003;39(2):253–261.

77. Gautret P, Blanton J, Dacheux L, et al. Rabies in nonhuman primates and potential for transmission to humans: a literature review and examination of selected French national data. *PLoS Negl Trop Dis*. 2014;8(5):e2863.

78. Stoltenow CL, Solemsass K, Niezgoda M, et al. Rabies in an American bison from North Dakota. *J Wildl Dis*. 2000;36(1):169–171.

79. Odegaard OA, Krogsrud J. Rabies in Svalbard: infection diagnosed in arctic fox, reindeer and seal. *Vet Rec*. 1981;109:141–142.

80. Blaise A, Parola P, Brouqui P, et al. Rabies postexposure prophylaxis for travelers injured by nonhuman primates, Marseille, France, 2001–2014. *Emerg Infect Dis*. 2015;21(8):1–7.

81. Johnston WF, Jesson Y, Nierenberg R, et al. Exposure to macaque monkey bite. *J Emerg Med*. 2015;49(5):634–637.

82. Rupprecht C, Kuzmin I, Meslin F. Lyssaviruses and rabies: current conundrums, concerns, contradictions and controversies. *F1000Research*. 2017;6(184):1–22 (F1000 faculty review).

83. Baby J, Subramaniam RS, Abraham SS, et al. Natural rabies infection in a domestic fowl (*Gallus domesticus*): a report from India. *PLoS Negl Trop Dis*. 2015:1–6.

84. Herriman R. *Rabies: A Comprehensive Interview with Pamela Wilson*. Outbreak News This Week; 2016. Outbreaknewstoday.com/rabies-a-comprehensive-interview-with-Pamela-Wilson-95548/. Accessed 11.06.18.

85. Centers for Disease Control and Prevention. Rabies surveillance in the U.S.: human rabies – rabies. https://www. cdc.gov/rabies/location/usa/surveillance/human_rabies.h tml. Accessed 01.06.18.

86. Fishbein DB. Rabies in humans. In: Baer GM, ed. *The Natural History of Rabies*. 2nd ed. Boca Raton: CRC Press, Inc; 1991:519–549.

87. Jackson AC. Human disease. In: Jackson AC, ed. *Rabies: Scientific Basis of the Disease and Its Management*. San Diego: Academic Press: An Elsevier Science Imprint; 2013:269–298.

88. Chacko K, Parakadavathu T, Al-Masiamani, et al. Diagnostic difficulties in human rabies: a case report and review of the literature. *Quar Med J*. 2016;(2):15. Published online 21.04.17 https://www.ncbi.nlm.nih.gov/articles/P MC5427514/. Accessed 23.08.18.

89. Susilawathi NM, Darwinata AE, Dwija IB, et al. Epidemiological and clinical features of human rabies cases in Bali 2008–2010. *BMC Infect Dis*. 2012;12(81):1–8.

90. Boland TA, McGuone D, Jindal J, et al. Phylogenetic and epidemiological evidence of multiyear incubation in human rabies. *Ann Neurol*. 2014;75(1):155–160.

91. Hattwick MAW. Human rabies. *Pub Hlth Rev*. 1974;III(3):229–274.

92. Warrell MJ, Warrell DA. Rabies: the clinical features, management, and prevention of the classic zoonosis. *Clin Med.* 2015;15(1):78–81.

93. Mani RS, Willoughby RE. Human rabies in South Asia. In: Singh SK, ed. *Neglected Tropical Diseases – South Asia.* Springer; 2017:349–371. https://doi.org/10.1007/978-3-319-68493-2_11. Accessed 24.04.18.

94. Fooks AR, Banyard AC, Horton DL, et al. Current status of rabies and prospects for elimination. *Lancet.* 2014;384:1389–1399.

95. World Health Organization. Rabies vaccines: WHO position paper–April 2018. *Wkly Epidemiol Rec.* 2018;16(93):201–220.

96. Perl DP, Good PF. The pathology of rabies in the central nervous system. In: Baer GM, ed. *The Natural History of Rabies.* 2nd ed. Boca Raton: CRC Press, Inc; 1991:163–198.

97. Centers for Disease Control and Prevention. Information for doctors. https://www.cdc.gov/rabies/specific_groups/doctors/index.html. Accessed 25.10.18.

98. Nelson WH, Keith T. Beer for My Horses. Composed by Keith and Scotty Emerick. 2003. https://en.wikipedia.org/wiki/Beer_for_My_Horses.

PERSONAL COMMUNICATIONS

a. Alexander JL. Regional Zoonosis Control Veterinarian, Department of State Health Services, Canyon, TX. Retired. Communication on 15.12.17.

b. Wallace RM. Centers for Disease Control and Prevention, OID, NCEZID. Atlanta, GA. Communication on 09.03.18.

c. Waldrup KA. Regional Zoonosis Control Veterinarian, Department of State Health Services, El Paso, TX. Communication on 21.03.18; 07.05.18.

d. Parker KP. Zoonosis Control Program Specialist, Department of State Health Services, El Paso and Austin, TX. Communication on 07.05.18.

e. Hartman F. Regional Zoonosis Control Veterinarian, Department of State Health Services, Temple, TX. Departed. Communication in January 1995.

f. Hugh-Jones ME. Professor Emeritus, Louisiana State University, Baton Rouge, LA. Author, *Flocks in Your Confiding: Some Chapters in a Life.* Communication on 14.05.18.

g. Robinson LE. Zoonosis Control Veterinarian, Department of State Health Services, Austin, TX. Communication on 21.03.18; 30.08.18.

h. Wright JH. Regional Zoonosis Control Veterinarian, Department of State Health Services, Tyler, TX. Retired. Communication on 17.05.18.

i. Garrison RD. Regional Zoonosis Control Veterinarian, Department of State Health Services, Houston, TX. Diseases in Nature Transmissible to Man. Communication on 24.05.17; 29.10.18.

j. Miller JP. Zoonosis Control Specialist, Department of State Health Services, Houston, TX. Communication on 24.05.17.

k. Johnson GD. Zoonosis Control Specialist, Department of State Health Services, Houston, TX. Communication on 29.10.18.

l. Tyler RD. Regional Zoonosis Control Veterinarian, Department of State Health Services, Harlingen, TX. Communication on 23.03.18.

m. Maass MD. Zoonosis Control Specialist, Department of State Health Services, Temple, TX. Communication on 23.03.18.

n. Hicks BN. Zoonosis Control Program Specialist, Department of State Health Services, Abilene and Austin, TX. Currently with USDA, Austin, TX. Communication on 11.04.18.

o. Johnson HCB. Director of the State Meat and Poultry Inspection Program and Manager, Meat Safety Assurance Unit, Department of State Health Services, Austin, TX. Retired. Communication on 21.09.18.

p. Davis AL. Zoonosis Control Specialist, Department of State Health Services, Tyler, TX. Retired. Communication on 16.05.18.

q. Clark KA. Director of Zoonosis Control, Texas Department of Health, Austin, TX. Retired. Communication on 19.09.17.

r. Kieffer AJ. Regional Zoonosis Control Veterinarian, Department of State Health Services, San Antonio, TX. Communication on 21.03.18.

CHAPTER 3

Rabies Epidemiology and Associated Animals

ERNEST H. OERTLI, DVM, PhD, Diplomate, ACVPM

INTRODUCTION

The description of the maintenance and spread of the disease rabies is made more complex because of the variety of host species and local ecogeography and other physical and human factors involved.[1]

- The World Health Organization (WHO) recognizes rabies as one of the most important zoonotic diseases in the world.[2-6]
- The disease is caused by a negative-strand RNA virus of the genus Lyssavirus (family Rhabdoviridae).[7]
- All warm-blooded mammal species are susceptible. Carnivora and Chiroptera contain the major reservoir host species.[8]
- The term terrestrial refers to animals that live predominantly or entirely on land and excludes bats.
- Both canine and wildlife rabies have been described for centuries.[9,10]
- It is a disease of antiquity, yet it is still underreported and considered one of the neglected diseases.[11]
- Rabies in humans reflects the extent of contact humans have with infected animal populations. Less than 5% of rabies cases in developed nations occur in dogs, but they are the main reservoir worldwide and the principal source of rabies infection in humans[6] (see Fig. 3.1). Wildlife now accounts for more than 90% of all reported rabies cases in the United States and are a worldwide concern[6,12] (see Fig. 3.2).

NOTABLE OBSERVATIONS

- It is estimated that 1 of every 2 US citizens is bitten by an animal at some time during his or her life.[13]
- When reviewing rabies cases, it makes sense to group as three geographic epidemiologic areas of rabies: (1) countries with enzootic canine rabies; (2) countries where canine rabies is under control and wildlife rabies predominates; and (3) rabies-free countries.

- The periodicity of rabies appears to be the result of density-dependent transmission in reservoir host populations.[14]
- Ecologic factors that enhance or reduce the long-term survival of rabies in reservoir species are poorly understood.[15]
- The original origin of terrestrial rabies has not been determined.[16,17]
- There is a curiosity with the disease as the rabies virus violates two of the most important rules for successful pathogens, as it kills most of the infected hosts and it has no known stage outside of its living host.
- Encroachment by humans can affect the rabies cycle characteristics as reservoir host species interact at concentrated food sources, such as pet foods, bird feeders, and garbage dumps, and domestic pets have more exposure to wildlife.[18]
- Only one confirmed natural infection of rabies in birds has ever been reported.[19]
- The Spanish explorers in South America were the first to suspect bats as vectors of rabies, but actual documentation has only been in the last 100 years.[20]
- With no definitive reporting, an estimated 10-15 million people worldwide receive rabies postexposure prophylaxis (PEP) each year after being exposed to animals with suspected rabies.[21]
- Caution is needed: (1) when wild animals do not appear shy or afraid of people; (2) nocturnal animals (such as bats, skunks, and raccoons) are out during the day; (3) animals appear paralyzed, weak, or vicious; (4) animals bite without provocation; (5) animals are making unusual vocal noises; and (6) bats are having difficulty flying and are on the ground.

OVERVIEW

The virus is classified into serotypes and genotypes. The virus has genetically evolved so that there are many

Rabies. https://doi.org/10.1016/B978-0-323-63979-8.00003-9
Copyright © 2019 Elsevier Inc. All rights reserved.

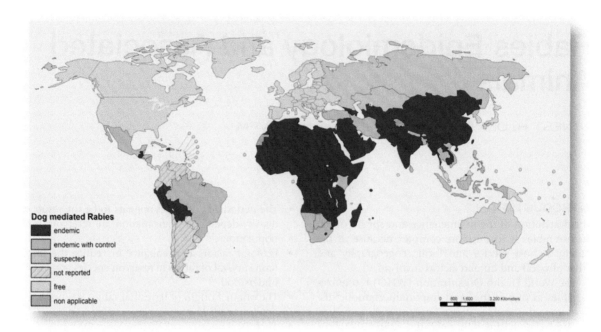

FIG. 3.1 **Dog-mediated Rabies.** Rabies Information System of the WHO (http://www.who-rabies-bulletin.org).[205]

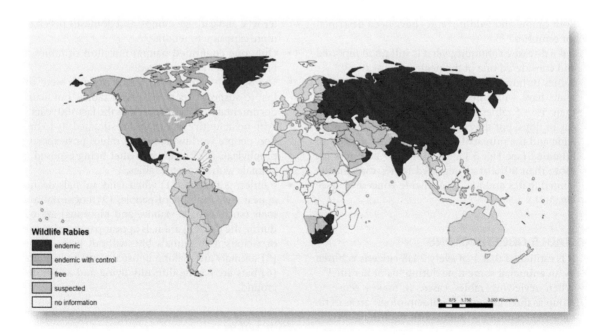

FIG. 3.2 **Wildlife-mediated Rabies.** Rabies Information System of the WHO (http://www.who-rabies-bulletin.org).[205]

variants (strains or types), each maintained in a particular reservoir host. Viral "strains or variants" are defined as virus populations maintained by a particular reservoir host in a defined geographic region that can be distinguished from other strains based on molecular and antigenic characteristics.[22] The propagation of the virus depends on the reservoir host. To explain, if a rabies variant maintained in raccoons caused rabies in a dog, it would be described as raccoon rabies in a dog, rather than canine rabies. Although it is anticipated that the dog would be a "dead end" host, because of the ability of the rabies virus to adapt to new reservoir hosts that cannot be made as an absolute statement and the dog may well infect whatever animal it bites. This propagation concern is discussed later with regard to a skunk study in Colorado.[23] Any variant can cause rabies in other species, and it has been noted that, on occasion, a virus variant adapted to one species can become established in another (big brown bat, Flagstaff, AZ).[8,24,25] A very general statement may be made that normally, each rabies variant is maintained in a particular host and usually dies out during serial passage in species to which it is not adapted. As knowledge related to this virus genus has progressed, closely-related lyssaviruses, ≥80, which are known as rabies-related lyssaviruses or non–rabies lyssaviruses, have been discovered.[26–32] Some can cause a neurologic disease identical to rabies. Clinical cases in animals and/or humans have been documented[28,29,33–49] with European bat lyssavirus (EBLV) 1, EBLV 2,[48,50] Australian bat lyssavirus,[51–54] Duvenhage virus,[55,56] Lagos bat virus,[57] Irkut virus,[58,59] and Mokola virus.[60] There are several lesser known lyssaviruses in the literature, and additional rabies-related lyssaviruses are likely to exist.[61–64] All but one or two of the identified rabies-related lyssaviruses appear to be maintained in bats, insectivorous or fruit. So far, none of these have been identified in the Western Hemisphere (see Table 3.1).

The reservoir host population, habitat, home range of host species, natural physical barriers such as rivers or mountain ranges, social behavior of host species, spillover species, rabies variant (some variants appear to be more virulent than others), other diseases of the reservoir species, and "herd immunity" status (natural or as a result of vaccination programs) are some of the factors that affect epidemiology and prevent a simple summation of disease maintenance and spread.[65,66] With the exception of Africa, Asia, and India, there has been a dramatic change in the reservoir host for rabies cases.[67,68] At one time, the highest incidence of rabies cases reported were in domestic animals, primarily canines. That would reflect the world situation in

TABLE 3.1
Rabies and Rabies-Related Lyssaviruses

Lyssavirus	Geographic Location	Neurologic Cases
Rabies	Worldwide	All warm-blooded animals
Aravan	Asia	Bats
Australian bat	Australia	Humans, bats
Bokeloh	Europe	Bats
Duvenhage	Africa	Humans, bats
European bat—1	Europe	Humans, cats, sheep, stone martens, bats
European bat—2	Europe	Humans, bats
Ikoma	Africa	Civets, bats
Irkut	Russia	Humans, bats
Khujand	Asia	Bats
Lagos bat	Africa	Cats, dogs, mongooses, bats
Lleida bat	Europe	Bats
Mokola	Africa	Humans, cats, dogs, bats
Shimoni bat	Africa	Bats
West Caucasian bat	Russia	Bats

that dogs have been regarded as the main vector of this zoonosis since ancient times and are still the source for the majority of modern day human deaths.[69-79] Vaccination programs, animal control programs, and public education have directly impacted the incidence of rabies in canines in the Americas and across Europe. Since 1960, rabies has been more frequently reported in wild than in domestic animals in the United States,[12] and that characteristic has been noted in numerous other countries.[80-86] The evolution of a disease is influenced by the population of its potential hosts. Virologists note that potential host populations vary and are subject to environmental changes, such as evolving new diseases, the ice bridge between Asia and the Americas, or global warming.[87]

The WHO considers a country to be free of rabies if there have been no indigenously acquired cases in humans or animals during the previous 2 years. The presence of a rabies-related lyssavirus does not prevent a nation from being listed as rabies free. Translocation of incubating animals, intentionally or unintentionally, is a significant factor with the mobility of the modern world.[88–91] This may include incubating humans.[92] Surveillance programs and restrictive animal movement laws are both safeguards to those countries with sound rabies control plans. In nonendemic settings, the detection of all introduced or emergent animal or human cases justifies exhaustive testing. Regulations that prohibit translocation of certain wild animal species for hunting and other purposes help reduce the likelihood of accidental introduction of rabies virus variants into rabies-free areas or introducing a new variant into an area already experiencing a rabies enzootic. The natural dispersion within the home range of an animal species can also cross borders and introduce or reintroduce the disease in a rabies-free country.[93,94] One must remember that for a rabies variant to become established, it is dependent on a corresponding species to the one being translocated/introduced or there must be a host shift.

Rabies enzootics are found in urban and sylvatic cycles. They can be totally separate or may occur concurrently. Examples: raccoon variant in raccoons in Central Park in the city of New York; domestic dog/coyote (DDC) variant in coyotes in rural South Texas[95]; and big brown bat variant in skunks and foxes in Flagstaff, Arizona, and surrounding area. Realizing the public health danger and the economic losses to livestock and pets, control efforts need to be based on good data. Surveillance of case location and laboratory identification of the specific rabies variant is essential. Disease management benefits from being able to predict, evenly roughly, the progression of epizootic cases. There are spatiotemporal epidemic models, multipatch models, and stochastic spatial models for studying the transmission dynamics of rabies.[96]

New reservoir hosts through virus adaptation is always a concern. Rabies history in Europe and the Middle East supports the conclusion that enzootic red fox rabies was a result of spillover from dog rabies epizootics. The expansion of arctic fox rabies from northern Asia into North America was one of the oldest rabies enzootics to the New World and involved both arctic and red fox. There does not appear to be any evidence that enzootic canine rabies existed in the New World until European colonization.[97] The rabies enzootics in raccoons along the US eastern seaboard and in skunks in South Central United States/North Central Mexico appear to have originated from bats. The California skunk, north central skunk, mongoose, and gray fox variants resulted from dog rabies enzootic spillovers.

PRIMARY ANIMALS ASSOCIATED WITH RABIES

Although spillover to other species occurs and human exposure may result, reservoir or maintenance species fall within the Carnivora and Chiroptera.[8]

ANIMAL RESERVOIRS IN THE UNITED STATES

In the United States, the major terrestrial reservoir host for rabies includes raccoons (*Procyon lotor*), skunks (genera *Mephitis, Spilogale,* and *Conepatus)*, foxes (genera *Vulpes, Urocyon,* and *Alopex*), and mongoose (*Herpestes auropunctatus*). The United States has numerous species of insectivorous bats that serve as extensive reservoir hosts for additional rabies variants. Bat exposures (involving bat rabies virus variants) have been responsible for most of the indigenous rabies cases in humans in the United States since the 1960s. Each year, surveillance reveals some spillover of bat variants into terrestrial species, but the numbers are normally not significant. The big brown bat variant host shift epizootic observed in skunks in Flagstaff, Arizona, was an exception.[98,99] What is normally observed is that in any region where rabies is enzootic, most cases of rabies are caused by the rabies virus variant associated with the primary terrestrial carnivore host in that region (see Table 3.2).

In the United States, the four major terrestrial reservoir host variants account for ≥ 90% of terrestrial rabies cases in any given year. Arctic fox (*Alopex lagopus*) cases are limited to Alaska, and because of the limited human population and remote environment, these cases are probably much underreported.[100] Very little spillover is noted between bat species. The norm is that a species-specific variant for that bat species is the cause. Already noted is that several enzootic terrestrial cycles are from spillover of bat rabies variants, but it has been concluded that rabies in bats exists largely independent of rabies in terrestrial animals and does not contribute to enzootic maintenance of terrestrial rabies.[10]

SPECIFIC COMMENTS ON RESERVOIR HOSTS WORLDWIDE (SEE TABLE 3.3)
Arctic Fox

Crazy foxes or polar madness cases were first recorded in 1859. This rabies variant has spread to various territorial regions within and south of the Arctic Circle including parts of Asia, Scandinavia, Russia, Alaska, Canada, and Greenland.[100–104] As climate change has occurred, there have been incursions of arctic fox into normal red fox habitat environments with resulting rabies spillover cases. These fox virus variants remain an occasional source of rabies in humans in Asia.[104] In addition, these variants were the source for independent cycling of rabies virus among raccoon dogs in Europe and Asia.[16] The arctic fox variant was involved with a major epizootic affecting red and arctic foxes in North America (northern Canada)

TABLE 3.2
Rabies Reservoir Hosts in the United States and Territories

Geographic Region	Reservoir Species Affected	Variant	Origin	Status
Alaska	Bat	Arctic fox; bat	Canine bat	Endemic
Arizona	Gray fox	Arizona gray fox	Canine	Endemic
Arizona	Skunk	South central skunk	Bat	Endemic
Arizona (Flagstaff)	Skunk	Big brown bat	Bat	Eliminated
California	Skunk	California skunk	Canine	Endemic
Continental United States	Bats	Variety of bat variants	Bat	Endemic
Eastern United States	Raccoon	Raccoon	Bat	Endemic
Eastern United States	Skunk	Raccoon	Bat	Endemic
Guam	Rabies free			
Hawaii	Rabies free			
New Mexico	Gray fox	Arizona gray fox	Canine	Epizootic
New Mexico	Skunk	South central skunk	Bat	Endemic
North Central United States	Skunk	North central skunk[a]	Canine	Endemic
Puerto Rico	Mongoose	Dog/mongoose	Canine	Endemic
South Central United States	Skunk	South central skunk	Bat	Endemic
Texas	Coyote	Domestic dog/coyote	Canine	Eliminated
Texas	Gray fox	Texas fox	Canine	Eliminated
Texas	Skunk	South central skunk	Bat	Endemic

[a]In addition to North Central United States, Tennessee and Kentucky have endemic north central skunk variant.

in the 1940s.[100] As discussed later in the red fox section, the epizootic of red fox rabies expanded from Ontario into the northeastern states of New York, New Hampshire, Vermont, and Maine. Effective control efforts initiated in Canada brought fox rabies under control in Ontario.[15]

Bats

In the continental United States, bat rabies is enzootic, and exposure to bats is the primary cause of rabies in humans.[96,105–109] In 2015 the Centers for Disease Control and Prevention (CDC) recognized that for the first time since public health surveillance for rabies began in 1944, bats were the most frequently reported rabid animal in the United States, supplanting raccoons.[110] Bats live throughout the world, except the Arctic and Antarctic,[111] and with few exceptions, rabies is endemic in their populations.[112–116] The nocturnal nature and often unseen activity of bats has contributed to the delayed recognition of their importance in disease maintenance. In addition, the limited knowledge is a result of the fact that few state laboratories identify their bat submissions nor identify the variant involved.[96,108,116–118] Rabies virus was first identified in bats in the United States in the northern yellow bat (*Lasiurus intermedius*) from Florida in 1953.[119,120] Surveillance since then has recognized rabies infection in all known species in the United States.[121] Bat rabies appears to be widespread in the 49 continental US states. Hawaii is considered to be rabies free. The incidence of rabies in bat populations may vary by species, but it is not known to be on the rise.[122,123] Bat variant rabies has been the principal cause of human deaths due to rabies in the United States for several decades and has become a significant factor in rabies in the Americas.[124,125] The spillover of bat rabies into humans is reported by Messenger[126] and Kuzmin.[127] Often the human exposures to bats occurred while the person was sleeping or otherwise unaware of a possible contact with a bat, and the bite was not reported (bat bites are small enough to go undetected) in over half of the known bat-associated cases.[125]

TABLE 3.3
Rabies Reservoir Hosts Worldwide

Geographic Region	Reservoir Species Affected	Status
Africa	Domestic dog	Endemic*
	Bats	Endemic
	Jackal	Endemic
	Kudu	Unknown
	Mongoose	Endemic
Asia	Chinese ferret-badger	Endemic
	Domestic dog	Endemic
	Raccoon dog	Endemic
	Rat	Spillover
	Wolf	Spillover
Australia	Bats	Endemic
Caribbean	Bats	Endemic
	Mongoose	Endemic
Central and South America	Bats (insectivorous and vampire)	Endemic
	Crab fox	Endemic
	Domestic dog	Endemic
Europe (Western)	Arctic fox (sub-Arctic countries)	Endemic
	Bats	Endemic
Europe (Eastern – including Russia)	Bats	Endemic
	Corsac fox	Endemic
	Domestic dog	Endemic
	Raccoon dog	Endemic
	Red fox	Endemic
	Wolf	Spillover
Middle East	Domestic dog	Endemic
	Jackal	Endemic
	Fox	Spillover
North America	Arctic fox	Endemic
	Bats	Endemic
	Coyote	Endemic
	Gray fox	Endemic
	Raccoon	Endemic
	Red fox	Endemic
	Skunk	Endemic

*Endemic cases may be widespread within a region or in very specific geographic locations. It should be noted that some species listed as spillover species periodically have significant outbreaks and may contribute to the propagation of the rabies variant.
Bacon PJ. *Population Dynamics of Rabies in Wildlife.* London and Orlando, Florida: Academic Press; 1985.

There are distinct seasonal cycles that are related to migrations and nursery (colony bats) contact. Even though there are seasonal variations in population, activity, and rabies virus circulation, the time of year should not be a consideration in treatment decisions. Hematophagous (vampire) bats are neotropical, having adapted to hot, moist, tropical climates, and are found between northern Mexico and northern Argentina.[128] *Desmodus rotundus* is the most common species of hematophagous bats and has been the cause of significant losses in the agricultural sector. It is considered a major risk to public health because of the large number of human deaths associated with it.[129-131] Texas Department of State Health Services' (TDSHS) Zoonosis Control staff has reported several cases of vampire bat rabies cases in livestock translocated from northern Mexico,[132] and there is concern that vampire bat rabies could become an important economic factor if it becomes endemic in Texas in the future.[133]

Gray Foxes

Gray foxes (*Urocyon cinereoargenteus*) have many characteristics that remind one of felines rather than canines. They can climb trees and will often be observed lying on a limb. Lifelong mating has often been attributed to the species, but that is not totally accurate. They are found in couples, and they do tend to stay together for extended periods. They are often found in close proximity to human habitations. Very adaptable, they eat a variety of food (for instance, pet food that has been left outdoors and fruit), plus prey species, including rodents, lagomorphs, and insects.

In the 1940s, an epizootic in gray foxes (the first recorded US case of rabies in foxes occurred in a gray fox in Georgia in 1940[15]) was experienced across US southern states, reaching all the way to Texas. From 1940 to 1960, gray and red foxes were the wild carnivore most commonly reported rabid in the United States. Thinning of the fox population was the primary method used to curtail the fox rabies epizootic. The basis of the thinning concept stemmed from the epidemiology of rabies. For rabies to be transmitted, animals had to be in close contact with one another (i.e., bite one another). Therefore, the lower the density of animals, the less likely the virus was to spread from one animal to another. It worked, and the gray fox population dropped from being a reservoir host and did not resume that status until 40 years later. There are currently two rabies virus variants adapted to the gray fox in the United States, and both are considered a consequence of spillover events from long-term rabies enzootics associated with dogs; they are the Texas fox variant in gray foxes[95,134] and Arizona gray fox variant.[135]

The normal lifespan of the gray fox is fairly short, averaging 4 years. The fact that at any given time two-thirds of the population are kits or young adults is a disease management consideration. The most visible sign of rabies in this species is the loss of any fear of people.[136]

The incubation period of rabies in foxes is highly variable, from days to months, with a norm of less than 30 days (see Chapter 2). The morbidity phase is normally less than 2 weeks (see Chapter 2), but a healthy looking fox could have a shedding period of virus in the saliva and be infectious before development of clinical signs.

Red Foxes

Red foxes (*Vulpes vulpes*) have demonstrated that they have no specific habitat requirements and can be found in a diverse locale, including highly urban settings.[137] Normally found as a "couple," their territory size is notably variable and population density plays an important role in determining it. At the age of 6–11 months, dispersal occurs, with males leaving earlier and traveling further.

They are responsible for the maintenance and spread of rabies in the sub-Arctic and northeastern parts of North America, sub-Arctic Asia, and in Central and Eastern Europe. The European fox rabies epizootic started in 1939 at the eastern border of Poland. This coadapted variant then spread south and west. It would appear in a pattern of clusters, decreasing the fox population but not eliminating all foxes. It reached Switzerland in 1967. Switzerland is mentioned specifically because it was there that the first field trial for the oral immunization of wildlife (foxes) was conducted. Switzerland was successful in eliminating rabies, and the lessons learned there were used in numerous other countries. Most of Western Europe has been able to eliminate the fox rabies virus variant and are classified as being rabies free by the WHO. In Alaska and several other geographic regions, rabies in red foxes represents spillover from the arctic fox host rather than a true reservoir; however, there is concern that they might become a reservoir host.

Before 1990, rabies infections in New England were attributed to red fox and bat variants. After 1993, testing showed that the red fox variant no longer existed, and instead, a raccoon rabies virus variant had moved into the region.[138] Spillover cases occur in red foxes in nearly every geographic region where the red fox species are found. The spillover variant may be, for instance, arctic fox, raccoon, DDC, Texas fox, or Arizona gray fox.

Raccoons

The raccoon rabies virus variant has caused the largest wildlife zoonotic on record.[139,140] Raccoon rabies was first observed in Florida in the 1940s, expanding northward into Georgia during the 1960s.[141] It was translocated in 1977 to West Virginia,[142] and a major outbreak in the states began.[143,144] This translocation was a result of raccoons being captured in Florida and then taken to West Virginia for hunting clubs. At least one of the captured raccoons was incubating rabies. The movement north from the Mid-Atlantic outbreak was at a rate of 30–47 km/year.[145,146] Every state on the Eastern Seaboard has been affected, and the disease reached Canada in July 1999 (Ontario), September 2000 (New Brunswick), and May 2006 (Quebec).[147] It has been documented that sylvatic rabies in raccoons is associated with low wetlands coverage, low-intensity residential land use, absence of major roads, and rivers acting as natural barriers.[82,148,149] The timing of the cases involving rabid raccoons suggest a relationship between denning and breeding and the observed outbreaks.[147] Of course, the raccoon epizootic rabies cases in Central Park, New York, Cleveland, Ohio, and Hamilton, Ontario, demonstrate the urban epizootic potential.

In the United States, the first human death associated with the raccoon variant of rabies virus was reported in Virginia in 2003. Human and companion animal exposure to rabid raccoons is enhanced by proximity to their normal foraging grounds. Raccoons exploit concentrated food sources; therefore, they are often drawn into close proximity in urban and suburban situations with Dempsey dumpsters, refuse dumps, etc.[150,151]

Skunks

Rabies in skunks is widespread throughout the Americas.[152] In the United States, the total geographic area affected by skunk rabies is approximately 3.5 million square kilometers or nearly 40% of the entire contiguous lower 48 states.[153] There are several types of skunks commonly found throughout the United States, including the striped skunk (*Mephitis mephitis*), spotted skunk (*Spilogale* spp.), hog-nosed skunk (*Conepatus leuconotus*), and hooded skunk (*Mephitis macroura*). They all not only have slightly different appearances and habits but also share many commonalities. For example, most adults grow to be about the size of a housecat or small dog. Some of the North American species have specialized diets, but most are omnivorous and eat what is readily available, including grubs, plants, small animals, and even garbage.

Striped skunks are the most common throughout North America and can be found from northern Mexico to the Northwest Territory of Canada. Their distinctive markings are used to identify them. Striped skunks have white stripes running from the tops of their heads to the tips of their tails.

Spotted skunks are most often encountered in the eastern portion of the United States where they live in woodlands and prairies. They keep a diet of field animals, insects, wild plants, and farm crops. Despite their name, spotted skunks are not actually spotted; instead, their black fur displays swirls of white stripes.

Hog-nosed skunks are typically found in the southwestern portion of the United States. They are easily identified by their stark white tails and the large, solid white stripe that runs down the length of their backs. These skunks also have relatively large noses that they use to root through the soil for food; the claws on their forefeet are adapted for digging by being larger than those on the rear feet.

Hooded skunks are desert-dwelling mammals that primarily feed on insects. They are somewhat similar in appearance to striped skunks but have longer tails and thick patches of fur around their necks. Some hooded skunks have two thin white stripes running down their backs and tails, whereas others have a single, thick stripe and solid white tail.

Spillover concerns are supported by events such as those that occurred in Colorado. After decades of apparent absence, the south central skunk (SCSK) rabies virus variant was detected in Colorado in 2007 and resulted in a large-scale epizootic in striped skunk (*M. mephitis*) populations in northern Colorado starting in 2012. Wildlife researchers attempted isolation of rabies virus from salivary gland tissues from confirmed rabid carnivores, comprising 51 striped skunks and 7 other wild and domestic carnivores collected during 2013 through 2015 in northern Colorado. They isolated rabies virus from 84.0% (158/188; 95% CI = 78.1%–88.6%) of striped skunk and 71% (17/24; 95% CI = 51%–85%) of other carnivore salivary glands. These data suggested that infected reservoir and vector species were equally likely to shed the SCSK rabies virus variant and posed a secondary transmission risk to humans and other animals.[23]

Noteworthy is the fact that skunks are the most common secondary species affected by rabies in the raccoon rabies enzootic area. Three principal areas are associated with skunk rabies virus variants: the North Central United States, the South Central United States, and California.[154-157] In 2001, Flagstaff, Arizona, reported a new skunk rabies virus variant, which arose from a bat variant.[98]

In temperate climates, cases are typically observed throughout the year, with the spiking fall and spring distribution of positive skunks apparently reflecting the spring breeding season and the fall dispersal of juveniles.[154,157,158] The different skunk species behave differently. There are distinct behavioral differences in the regional skunk populations that reflect food sources, hibernation of those in northern climates, home range variations between urban skunks and those in open rural environments, and species (striped, hog-nosed, hooded, and spotted). In some geographic areas, the distribution of rabies in cattle has been demonstrated to be similar to that of skunks, and it can be concluded that skunks are directly associated with rabies in farm animals.[159]

Coyotes

The coyote (*Canis latrans*) is widespread and can be found from Panama throughout North America. They are medium-sized carnivores in the dog family (Canidae). One of the most adaptable animals in the world, the coyote can change its breeding habits, diet, and social dynamics to survive in a wide variety of habitats.[160] The coyote is one of eight species of the genus *Canis*. Four of these are the jackals of Europe, Africa, and Asia. Other members of the genus include the gray wolf (*Canis lupus*), the red wolf (*Canis rufus*), and all breeds of the domestic dog (*Canis familiaris*). Although some coyotes are diagnosed as rabies positive each year, normally they are spillover variant cases. However, that has not always been the case. Coyotes served as a reservoir host for the DDC rabies variant in a major epizootic in South Texas. From 1988 through 1994, 531 cases of canine rabies caused by the DDC rabies virus variant were reported in Texas. Of those cases, 270 were in coyotes (*C. latrans*), and 216 were in domestic dogs (*C. familiaris*); the remainder involved other wild and domestic animals. The epizootic began in South Texas along the US-Mexico border and expanded to include 18 contiguous counties. Unlike previous rabies epizootics that were controlled with focused rabies vaccination clinics directed at domestic pets, this epizootic involved a wild canine species.[161,162] A massive oral rabies vaccination program was implemented, and it proved so successful that on September 7, 2007, the CDC declared the United States free of canine rabies.[163] There is still a concern that the DDC variant may still be circulating in northern Mexico.

Mongooses

The sugarcane plantations introduced the small Indian mongoose (*H. auropunctatus*) into the Caribbean in an effort to control rodent populations in the cane fields. The mongoose proved to be ineffective at rodent control, but because of its high reproductive rate and adaptability, the species flourished. A canine rabies virus variant adapted to the species, and the mongoose has emerged as a rabies reservoir in some, but not all, of the introduced areas. Cuba, Grenada, Hispaniola, and Puerto Rico currently report mongoose rabies cases.[164,165] It is unclear whether the variant had already adapted to the mongoose in India or if it occurred on the islands. There was also a case of rabies in a human via a bite from a rabid mongoose.[166] The other enzootic involving mongoose occurs in southern Africa and is found in the yellow mongoose (*Cynictis penicillata*).[81] Very little is known about the pathogenicity and true distribution of this rabies virus mongoose biotype. Molecular clock analysis estimates the age of the mongoose biotype to be approximately 200 years old, which is in concurrence with literature describing rabies in mongooses since the early 1800s.[17]

Raccoon Dogs

The raccoon dog (*Nyctereutes procyonoides*), also known as the mangut, is a canid indigenous to East Asia. It is the only extant species in the genus *Nyctereutes*. It is considered a basal canid species, resembling ancestral forms of the family. Among the Canidae, the raccoon dog shares the habit of regularly climbing trees only with the North American gray fox, another basal species. The raccoon dog is named for its superficial resemblance to the raccoon, to which it is not closely related. In the early 1920s, this member of the Canidae was introduced by the fur industry from Eastern Asia into the European part of Russia.[104] Because of their reproductive capability and tremendous adaptability, they have spread quickly. The animal is now found in the Baltic States, Eastern Europe, Scandinavia, and parts of Central and Western Europe. In some regions, the population density exceeds that of the red fox.

Hibernation of raccoon dogs in the cold season may influence the epidemiology of the disease within the species. The raccoon dog is a major factor in the epidemiology of rabies in Eastern and Northern Europe and is now the second most important wildlife reservoir of rabies after the red fox.

Jackals

Several species of jackals (*Canis aureus, Canis mesomelas*, and *Canis adustus*) have served as reservoir hosts of rabies variants. The golden jackal (*C. aureus*) represented a major reservoir host in Israel and surrounding Middle East region and some areas in Asia. There are three species of jackals reported as reservoir hosts in Africa and Asia. Side-striped (*C. adustus*) and black-backed (*C. mesomelas*) jackals have been principal reservoirs in Africa, and the golden jackal is a reservoir host in Asia. Initiated by rabid dogs, once initiated the

epidemics are maintained by the jackals independent of other species.[167] It has been noted that the epidemics begin as single foci and spread centrifugally. The outbreaks appear to be limited by geographic features and jackal interface boundaries.[167]

Wolves

Being one of the top predators in the food chain is reflected in the fear that humans have for wolves. The many books, legends, and tall tales have captured fear of them everywhere they are found. The fear of wolves can be attributed partially to the fact that rabid wolves, like rabid dogs, lose all fear of human beings. In locales where wolves are part of the fauna and rabies is enzootic, rabid wolves have been known to attack numerous people in one incident. It is also not uncommon to find offspring of wildlife and domestic species. These hybrids create a conundrum when involved with a bite to a human. There is no approved rabies vaccine for these animals because they are considered wildlife.

Rabies is a significant concern with some of the endangered species of wolves. Major rabies epizootics involving canine rabies virus variant in the Ethiopian wolf (*Canis simensis*) packs were extremely detrimental to restoration efforts. A sparse population was reduced even more with the epizootic rabies deaths.[168] The same concern to a much lesser degree has been observed with the Mexican gray wolf (*Canis lupus baileyi*) in Arizona and New Mexico.[169] Rabies in wolves still survives in some Asian and Middle East countries, usually as a spillover of canine rabies.

Kudus

In southern Africa, an epizootic involving kudu (*Tragelaphus strepsiceros*) occurred in 1977. About 50,000 died from rabies over an 8-year period. The epizootic appears to have been transmitted orally and resulted from exposure through grazing on thorn trees.[170,171] A number of clinical signs have been observed in kudu infected with rabies, the most common of which is loss of fear.[170,171] An infected kudu often appears completely oblivious to its surroundings; it loses its fear of both domestic animals and man and has often been observed walking into houses and garages and even approaching vehicles.

Ferret-Badgers

Common throughout Asia, this species is not known to be a reservoir host for any rabies virus variant, and most health officials believe canine rabies spillover causes epizootics. Southeast China experiences rabies cases in this species every year. In 2012, Taiwan, which had been rabies free for 52 years, reported a rabies epizootic in ferret-badgers (*Melogale moschata*). It is still to be determined if this is a spillover from a canine variant or if there has been a mutation and the ferret-badger is now a reservoir host for the new variant.[172] The rabies outbreak also spilled over into other animals. Of tested animals, health authorities found 158 of 512 ferret-badgers, 1 of 138 shrews, and 1 of 908 dogs with positive rabies test results.[173]

Nonhuman Primates

Nonhuman primates (NHPs) cause an overwhelming number of injuries reported by travelers returning to the United States. They rank second only to dogs in injuries caused and are actually number one for travelers to Southeast Asia.[174] Tourists in Brazil also appear to be at risk of visiting locations where NHPs are encountered.[175] These animals are often imported for both zoo exhibits and personal pets. There are several examples of NHPs incubating rabies when imported.[88]

HIGH-RISK VERSUS LOW-RISK ANIMALS FOR RABIES

To preface the information regarding low-risk animals for rabies, one must pay heed to the fact that the CDC warns that "all" bites from wild or domestic animals that cannot be tested or observed should be evaluated and determined as to potential for being an exposure to rabies. Small mammals such as squirrels, rats, mice, shrews, hamsters, guinea pigs, gerbils, chipmunks, opossums, armadillos, rabbits, and hares are hardly ever found to be infected with rabies and have not been known to cause rabies among humans in the United States.[176-179] Bites by these animals are usually not considered a risk of rabies unless the animal was sick or behaving in an unusual manner and rabies is widespread in the area. Although domestic livestock are not considered to be low risk, they are considered to be less of a risk than Carnivora and Chiroptera species.

CASES ASSOCIATED WITH LOW-RISK ANIMALS

Examples of exceptions include the fact that Chinese and Thailand health officials include rats as a reservoir for rabies in their region and recommend PEP for rat bites.[180,181] New York state health officials have reported an unusual set of low-risk animal species (guinea pig and rabbits) succumbing to rabies and exposing several humans.[182] The New York City health department said that the state has not found a squirrel with rabies since it began its surveillance program

in 1992 and that there have been no known transmissions from squirrels to humans in the United States. Although some rodents, such as rats, squirrels, beavers, and woodchucks, can and do become infected with rabies, there is very little naturally occurring rabies in rodents, and the risk of rabies from rodent bites remains very low.[178]

Reports of rabies in rodents in the United States usually are woodchucks (*Marmota monax*)[176] or beavers (*Castor canadensis*).

LIVESTOCK

Of domestic livestock in the United States, cattle are the most reported species with rabies. Second most reported are horses, then goats, sheep, and rarely swine.[183] Outbreaks of rabies have been documented in a wide variety of species: sheep[184]; equine[185-188]; domestic buffalo[189]; camels and cattle[190]; and multiple other livestock species.[191,192]

Cases of rabies in herbivores occur every year, but the exposure risk to humans is also considered to be very low. Individuals with cuts or abrasions who are exposed to herbivore saliva have been documented to succumb to the disease, but it is rare and there are not many examples of this occurring.[193,194] Generally, the exposure that caused these spillover cases goes unnoticed, as it is occurring in areas such as pastures, barns, and stalls when the animals are either turned out to graze or are put up for the night. The point is being unobserved.

The CDC summary reports indicate that an average of 150 rabid cattle have been reported to CDC in the United States each year since 1990.[193] In 2015, there were 85 cattle and 14 horses reported rabid.[110] Rabid dairy cattle always raise many questions about rabies exposure potential. The amount of virus present in milk is a concern,[195,196] so viability and infectivity of rabies virus in milk is also unknown; transmission of rabies virus in unpasteurized milk is theoretically possible but not likely. Regardless of the amount of viable rabies virus that may be shed in cow's milk, the theoretical risk for transmission of rabies from this route can be eliminated if all dairy products are pasteurized before consumption.

Mass human exposures often result from exposures to rabid livestock through such settings as petting zoos or raw milk consumption. Public health officials must balance knowledge of rabies epidemiology, risk for transmission, and pathogenesis with the perceived risk for death when evaluating exposed persons in these mass human exposures to rabid animals. Often, the combination of public concern, including the nearly

100% case-fatality ratio of rabies, counterbalanced with the virtually complete effectiveness of PEP, prompts administration of human rabies immune globulin and vaccine, even if the circumstances do not meet the criteria for exposure.

SPECIES WITH SPILLOVER RABIES

With the exception of mongoose (which is a reservoir host but has a limited number of positive cases each year), Table 3.4 represents some of the spillover species that have been recorded with rabies in the United States.

Almost without exception, every species of wildlife known, both free-ranging and captive, have been documented[197] with rabies; similarly, there is documentation of rabies in domestic livestock, both range and confinement (feedlot, show) animals. The same is true in other geographic areas of the world.[198–202]

DOGS, CATS, AND DOMESTIC FERRETS

Since 1981, cases of rabies in cats have exceeded cases in dogs in the United States. This is a reflection of both the fact that many states have mandatory vaccination laws for dogs, but do not require cats to be vaccinated against rabies and there are a large number of feral cat colonies.[203,204] After the first epizootic of raccoon rabies occurred in the eastern portion of the United States, the odds of diagnosing a rabid cat was 12 times greater than for the period before the epizootic.[204] The last ferret reported to CDC as positive for rabies was in 1992. No ferret has ever been reported to have been the source for a rabies case in a human. Even though it is well documented that control of rabies in dogs through programs of animal vaccination and elimination of stray dogs can reduce the incidence of rabies in humans, exposure to rabid dogs is still the cause of more than 90% of human exposures to rabies and of more than 99% of human deaths due to rabies worldwide.[6]

CONCLUSION

History has shown that the rabies cycle can be broken and the disease eliminated, but that to do so requires a significant fiscal and time commitment. Long-term cooperation between countries and agencies is a must as the disease does not recognize borders, has proven to be resilient, and will reemerge if control efforts are relaxed. The fact that the rabies virus will mutate and find new reservoir hosts contributes to the difficulty in

TABLE 3.4 Documented US Rabies Cases as a Result of Spillover
Species
Mongoose (*Herpestes javanicus*)
Cat (*Felis catus*)
Coyote (*Canis latrans*)
Bobcat (*Lynx rufus*)
Dog (*Canis lupus familiaris*)
Otter (*Lontra canadensis*)
Badger (*Taxidea taxus*)
Wolf (*Canis lupus*)
Ringtail (*Bassariscus astutus*)
Domestic ferret (*Mustela putorius furo*)
Coati (*Nasua narica*)
Mink (*Mustela vison*)
Weasel (*Mustela* spp.)
Fisher (*Martes pennant*)
Wolf-dog hybrid (*Canis lupus–Canis lupus familiaris*)
Puma (*Puma concolor*)
Bear (*Ursus* spp.)
Lesser panda (*Ailurus fulgens*)
Ocelot (*Leopardus pardalis*)
Javelina (*Pecari tajacu*)
Captive/free-ranging deer (*Odocoileus virginianus*)
Woodchuck (*Marmota monax*)
Beaver (*Castor canadensis*)
Rabbit (*Lagomorpha* spp.)
Bushbuck (*Tragelaphus sylvaticus*)
Goat (*Caprinae* spp.)
Sheep (*Ovis aries*)
Cow (*Bos taurus*)
Horse (*Equus ferus caballus*)
Pig (*Sus* spp.)
Eurasian wild boar (*Sus scrofa*)
Guinea pig (*Cavia porcellus*)

eradication. Domestic animal rabies vaccination, animal control programs, and public health education of the general public regarding rabies all help prevent human cases. Oral rabies vaccination programs are very successful in addressing wildlife rabies.

REFERENCES

1. Steele J, Fernandez P. History of rabies and global aspects. In: Baer GM, ed. *The Natural History of Rabies.* 2nd ed. Boca Raton (FL): CRC Press; 1991:1–26.
2. World Health Organization. *WHO Expert Consulatation on Rabies.* World Health Organization; 2004.
3. World Health Organization. *World Health Organization Expert Committee on Rabies, First Report* World Health Organization. Technical Report Series, 931. Geneva: WHO; 2005:1–87.
4. World Health Organization. *Expert Consultation on Rabies. Second Report* World Health Organization Tech. Rep. Ser., 982. ; 2013:1–139.
5. World Health Organization. *Rabies Bulletin Europe;* 2016. Available from: http://www.who-rabies-bulletin.org.
6. World Health Organization. *Expert consultation on Rabies. Third Report.* World Health Organization Tech Rep Ser No 1012. World Health Organization; 2018. World Health Organization Rabies fact sheets. http://www.who.int/en/newsroom/fact-sheets/detail/rabies.
7. Virology.net. http://www.virology.net/big_virology/bvrnarhabdo.html.
8. Badrane H, Tordo N. Host switching in lyssavirus history from the Chiroptera to the Carnivora orders. *J Virol.* 2001;75:8096–8104.
9. Theodorides J. *Histoire De La Rage.* Paris: Masson; 1986:289.
10. Baer GM, ed. *The Natural History of Rabies.* Boca Raton (FL): CRC Press; 1991.
11. Blancou J. *History of Surveillance and Control of Transmissible Animal Diseases.* Paris: Office International des Epizootics; 2003:193–219.
12. Wyatt J. Rabies-update on a global disease. *Pediatr Infect Dis J.* 2007;26:351–352.
13. Goldstein E. Bite wounds and infection. *Clin Infect Dis.* 1991;14:633–640.
14. Morters M, Restif O, Hampson K, et al. Evidence-based control of canine rabies: a critical review of population density reduction. *J Anim Ecol.* 2013;82(1):6–14.
15. MacInnes CD, Smith SM, Tinline RR, et al. Elimination of rabies from red foxes in eastern Ontario. *J Wildl Dis.* 2001;37(1):119–132.
16. Bourhy H, Kissi B, Audry L, et al. Ecology and evolution of rabies virus in Europe. *J Gen Virol.* 1999;80(10):2545–2557.
17. Bourhy H, Reynes JM, Dunham EJ, et al. The origin and phylogeography of dog rabies virus. *J Gen Virol.* 2008;89:2673–2681.
18. Parkhurst KA. Other animals: vertebrates as pests. In: Latimer JG, Close D, eds. *Compilers. Pest Management Guide: Home Grounds and Animals.* Blacksburg, VA: VA Coop Ext Pub 456-018 (ENTO-36P); 2015:8-1-8.10.
19. Baby J, Mani RS, Abraham SS, et al. Natural rabies infection in a domestic fowl (*Gallus domesticus*): a report from India. *PLoS Neglected Trop Dis.* 2015;9(7).
20. Banyard A, Hayman D, Johnson N, et al. *Bats and Lyssaviruses.* [Chapter 12]. https://rabiessurveillanceblueprint.org/IMG/pdf/banyard_et_al_2011.pdf.
21. Tsekoa T. *Rabies Antibodies for Passive Post-exposure Prophylaxis. Global Vaccine and Immunization Research Forum;* 2016. http:www.who.int/immunization/research/forums and initiatives/4_TTsekoa_Rabies_antibodies_gvirf16.pdf.
22. Nadin-Davis S. Molecular epidemiology. 2nd ed. *Rabies.* Academic Press; 2007:69–122.
23. Jimenez I, Spraker T, Anderson J, et al. Isolation of rabies virus from the salivary glands of wild and domestic carnivores during a skunk rabies epizootic. *J Wildl Dis.* 2018. https://doi.org/10.7589/2018-05-127. [Epub ahead of print].
24. Kuzmin I, Shi M, Orciari L, et al. Molecular inferences suggest multiple host shifts of r rabies viruses from bats to mesocarnivores in Arizona during 2001–2009. *PLoS Pathog.* 2012;8(6):e1002786.
25. Streicker D, Altizer S, Velasco-Villa A, et al. Variable evolutionary routes to host establishment across repeated rabies virus host shifts among bats. *Proc Natl Acad Sci USA.* 2012;109(48):19715–19720.
26. Arai YT. Epidemiology of rabies virus and other lyssaviruses. *Nippon Rinsho Jpn J Clin Med.* 2005;63:2167–2172.
27. Greene CE, Rupprecht CE. Rabies and other lyssavirus infections. In: Greene CE, ed. *Infectious Diseases of the Dog and Cat.* St Louis: Elsevier Saunders; 2006:167–183.
28. Harris S, et al. European bat lyssaviruses: distribution, prevalence and implications for conservation. *Biol Conserv.* 2006;131:193–210.
29. Fooks A, Brookes S, Healy D, et al. Detection of antibodies to European bat Lyssavirus type-2 in Daubenton's bats in the UK. *Vet Rec.* 2004;154:245–246.
30. Nel L, Rupprecht C. Emergence of lyssaviruses in the old world: the case of Africa. *Curr Top Microbiol Immunol.* 2007;315:161–193.
31. Dietzgen R, Calisher CH, Kurath G, et al. Rhabdoviridae. In: King A, Adams MJ, Carstens EB, et al., eds. *Virus Taxonomy: Classification and Nomenclature of Viruses: Ninth Report of the International Committee on Taxonomy of Viruses.* San Diego (CA): Elsevier; 2011:654–681.
32. Calisher CH, Ellison JA. The other rabies viruses: the emergence and importance of lyssaviruses from bats and other vertebrates. *Trav Med Infect Dis.* 2012;10:69–79.
33. Freuling C, Beer M, Conraths F, et al. Novel lyssavirus in Natterer's bat, Germany. *Emerg Infect Dis.* 2011;17(8):1519–1522.
34. Picard-Meyer E, Bruyere V, Barrat J, et al. Development of a hemi-nested RT-PCR method for the specific determination of European bat lyssavirus 1 comparison with other rabies diagnostic methods. *Vaccine.* 2004;22:1921–1929.
35. Picard-Meyer E, Robardet E, Arthur L, et al. Bat rabies in France: a 24-year retrospective epidemiological study. *PLoS One.* 2014;9(6):e98622. https://doi.org/10.1371/journal.pone.0098622.
36. Marston D, Horton D, Ngeleja C, et al. *Ikoma* lyssavirus, highly divergent novel lyssavirus in an African civet. *Emerg Infect Dis.* 2012;18(4):664–667.
37. Arechiga N, Moron S, Berciano J, et al. Novel lyssavirus in bat, Spain. *Emerg Infect Dis.* 2013;19(5):793–795.

38. Miia J, Tiina N, Tarja S, et al. Evolutionary trends of European bat lyssavirus type 2 including genetic characterization of Finnish strains of human and bat origin 24 years apart. *Arch Virol.* 2015;160(6):1489–1498.

39. Van der Poel W, Lina P, Kramps J. Public health awareness of emerging zoonotic viruses of bats: a European perspective. *Vector Borne Zoonotic Dis.* 2006;6:315–324.

40. Horton D, Banyard A, Marston D. Antigenic and genetic characterization of a divergent African virus, Ikoma lyssavirus. *J Gen Virol.* 2014;95(5):1025–1032.

41. Freuling C, Grossmann E, Conraths F, et al. First isolation of EBLV-2 in Germany. *Vet Microbiol.* 2008;131:26–34.

42. Jakava-Viljanen M, Lilley T, Kyheroinen E, et al. First encounter of European bat lyssavirus type 2 (EBLV2) in a bat in Finland. *Epidemiol Infect.* 2010;138(11):1581–1585.

43. Muller T, Cox J, Peter W, et al. Spill-over of European bat lyssavirus type 1 into a stone marten (*Martes foina*) in Germany. *Zoonoses and Public Health.* 2004;51(2):49–54.

44. Warrilow D, Smith I, Harrower B, et al. Sequence analysis of an isolate from a fatal human infection of Australian bat lyssavirus. *Virology.* 2002;297:109–119.

45. Gould A, Kattenbelt J, Gumley S, et al. Characterisation of an Australian bat lyssavirus variant isolated from an insectivorous bat. *Virus Res.* 2002;89:1–28.

46. Amengual B, Whitby J, King A, et al. Evolution of European bat lyssaviruses. *J Gen Virol.* 1997;78:2319–2328.

47. Lumio J, Hillbom M, Roine R, et al. Human rabies of bat origin in Europe. *Lancet.* 1986;1(8477):378.

48. Nathwani D, McIntyre P, White K, et al. Fatal human rabies caused by European bat Lyssavirus type 2 infection in Scotland. *Clin Infect Dis.* 2003;37:598–601.

49. Brookes S, Aegerte J, Smith G, et al. European bat lyssavirus in scottish bats. *Emerg Infect Dis.* 2005;11(4):572–578.

50. Fooks A, McElhinney L, Pounder D, et al. Case report: isolation of a European bat lyssavirus type 2a from a fatal human case of rabies encephalitis. *J Med Virol.* 2003;71(2):281–289.

51. Gould A, Hyatt A, Lunt R, et al. Characterization of novel lyssa virus from Pteropid bats in Australia. *Virus Res.* 1998;54:165–187.

52. Hanna J, Carney I, Smith G, et al. Australian bat lyssavirus infection: a second human case, with a long incubation period. *Med J Aust.* 2000;172(12):597–599.

53. McColl K, Tordo N, Aguilar-Setien A. Bat lyssavirus infections. *Rev Sci Technol.* 2000;19(1):177–196.

54. Francis JR, Nourse C, Vaska VL, et al. Australian bat lyssavirus in a child: the first reported case. *Pediatrics.* 2014;133(4):e1063–e1067.

55. Paweska J, Blumberg L, Liebenberg C, et al. Fatal human infection with rabies-related Duvenhage virus, South Africa. *Emerg Infect Dis.* 2006;12(12):1965–1967.

56. van Thiel P, de Bie R, Eftimov F, et al. Fatal human rabies due to Duvenhage virus from a bat in Kenya: failure of treatment with coma-induction, ketamine, and antiviral drugs. *PLoS Neglected Trop Dis.* 2009;3:e428.

57. Kuzmin I, Niezgoda M, Franka R, et al. Possible emergence of West caucasian bat virus in Africa. *Emerg Infect Dis.* 2008;14:1887–1889.

58. Kuzmin I, Hughes G, Botvinkin A, et al. Phylogenetic relationships of Irkut and West Caucasian bat viruses within the Lyssavirus genus and suggested quantitative criteria based on the N gene sequence for lyssavirus genotype definition. *Virus Res.* 2005;111:28–43.

59. Liu Y, Zhang S, Zhao J, et al. Isolation of Irkut virus from a Murina leucogaster bat in China. *PLoS Neglected Trop Dis.* 2013;7(3):e2097.

60. Kgaladi J, Wright N, Coertse J, et al. Diversity and epidemiology of Mokola virus. *PLoS Neglected Trop Dis.* 2013. https://doi.org/10.1371/journal.pntd.0002511.

61. Arai YT, Kuzmin IV, Kameoka Y, et al. New lyssavirus genotype from the lesser mouse-eared bat (*Myotis blythi*), Kyrghyzstan. *Emerg Infect Dis.* 2003;9(3):333–337.

62. Kuzmin I, Orciari L, Arai Y, et al. Bat lyssaviruses (*Aravan* and *Khujand*) from Central Asia: phylogenetic relationships according to N, P and G gene sequences. *Virus Res.* 2003;97(2):65–79.

63. Kuzmin I, Mayer A, Niezgoda M, et al. Bat virus, a new representative of the Lyssavirus genus. *Virus Res.* 2010;149:197–210.

64. Nadin-Davis S, Fehlner-Gardiner C. Lyssaviruses-current trends. *Adv Virus Res.* 2008;71:207–250.

65. Carey A, McLean R. The ecology of rabies: evidence of co-adaptation. *J Appl Ecol.* 1983;20:777–800.

66. Wandeler A. Oral immunization of wildlife. In: Baer GM, ed. *The Natural History of Rabies.* 2nd ed. Boca Raton, Florida: CRC Press Inc.; 1991:485–503.

67. Rupprecht C, Hanlon C, Hemachudha T. Rabies reexamined. *Lancet Infect Dis.* 2002;2:327–343.

68. Rupprecht C, Hanlon C, Slate D. Control and prevention of rabies in animals: paradigm shifts. *Dev Biol.* 2006;125:103–111.

69. Sehgal S, Bhatia R. *Rabies: Current Status and Proposed Control Programme in India.* New Delhi: National Institute of Communicable Diseases; 1985.

70. Kim J, Hwang E, Sohn H, et al. Epidemiological characteristics of rabies in South Korea from 1993 to 2001. *Vet Rec.* 2005;157:3–56.

71. Knobel D, Cleaveland S, Coleman P, et al. Reevaluating the burden of rabies in Africa and Asia. *Bull World Health Organ.* 2005;83:360–368.

72. Tang X, Luo M, Zhang S, et al. Pivotal role of dogs in rabies transmission, China. *Emerg Infect Dis.* 2005;11(12):1970–1972.

73. Cleaveland S, Hampson K, Kaare M. Living with rabies in Africa. *Vet Rec.* 2007;161:293–294.

74. Sugiyama M, Ito N. Control of rabies: epidemiology of rabies in Asia and development of new-generation vaccines for rabies. *Comp Immunol Microbiol Infect Dis.* 2007;30:273–286.

75. Gruzdev K. The rabies situation in Central Asia. *Dev Biol.* 2008;131:37–42.

76. Seimenis A. The rabies situation in the Middle East. *Dev Biol.* 2008;131:43–53.

77. Tenzin, Ward MP. Review of rabies epidemiology and control in South, South East and East Asia: past, present and prospects for elimination. *Zoonoses Public Health.* 2012;59(7):451–467.

78. Vigilato M, Clavijo A, Knobl T, et al. Progress towards eliminating canine rabies: policies and perspectives from Latin America and the Caribbean. *Philos Trans R Soc Lond B Biol Sci.* 2013;368(1623):20120143.

79. Singh R, Singh K, Cherian S, et al. Rabies-epidemiology, pathogenesis, public health concerns and advances in diagnosis and control: a comprehensive review. *Vet Q.* 2017;37(1):212–251.

80. Wallace R, Gilbert A, Slate D, et al. Right place, wrong species: a 20-year review of rabies virus cross species transmission among terrestrial mammals in the United States. *PLoS One.* 2014;9:e107539.

81. Chaparro F, Esterhuysen J. The role of the yellow mongoose (*Cynictis penicillata*) in the epidimology of rabies in South Africa-preliminary results. *Onderstepoort J Vet Res.* 1993;60:373–377.

82. Smith G. The role of the badger *(Meles meles)* in rabies epizootiology and the implications for Great Britain. *Mamm Rev.* 2002;32:13–26.

83. Vanaga S, van der Heide R, Joffe R, et al. Rabies in wildlife in Latvia. *Vector Borne Zoonotic Dis.* 2003;3:117–124.

84. Holmala K, Kauhala K. Ecology of wildlife rabies in Europe. *Mamm Rev.* 2006;36:17–36.

85. Maciulskis P, Lukauskas K, Sederevicius A, et al. Epidemiology of enzootic rabies in Lithuania. *Med Weter.* 2006;62:769–772.

86. Niin E, Laine M, Guiot A, et al. Rabies in Estonia: situation before and after the first campaigns of oral vaccination of wildlife with SAG2 vaccine bait. *Vaccine.* 2008;26:3556–3565.

87. Acevedo-Whitehouse K, Gulland F, Greig D, et al. Disease susceptibility in California sea lions. *Nature.* 2003;422:35.

88. Richardson J, Humphrey G. Imported rabies in nonhuman primates. *Lab Anim Sci.* 1971;26:1081–1082.

89. Centers for Disease Control and Prevention. Translocation of coyote rabies—Florida, 1994. *MMWR (Morb Mortal Wkly Rep).* 1995;44:580–583.

90. Rosatte R. Emergency response to raccoon rabies introduction into Ontario. *J Wildl Dis.* 2001;37(2):265–279.

91. Castrodale L, Walker V, Baldwin J, et al. Rabies in a puppy imported from India to the USA, March 2007. *Zoonoses P H.* 2008;55(8–10):427–430.

92. Carrara P, Parola P, Brouqui P, et al. Imported human rabies cases worldwide, 1990– 2012. *PLoS Neglected Trop Dis.* 2013;7(5):e2209.

93. Freuling C, Hampson K, Selhorst T, et al. The elimination of fox rabies from Europe: determinants of success and lessons for the future. *Philos Trans R Soc Lond Biol Sci.* 2013;368(1623):20120142.

94. Stevenson B, Goltz J, Massé A. Preparing for and responding to recent incursions of raccoon rabies variant into Canada. *Can Commun Dis.* 2016:125–129. Rep 42.

95. Rohde RE, Neill SU, Clark KA, et al. Molecular epidemiology of rabies epizootics in Texas. *J Clin Virol.* 1997;8:209–217.

96. Rohde R, Mayes B. Molecular diagnosis and epidemiology of rabies. In: Hu P, Hedge M, Lennon PA, eds. *Modern Clinical Molecular Techniques.* New Edition. NY: Springer Press; 2012.

97. Leonard J, Wayne R, Wheeler J, et al. Ancient DNA evidence for old world origin of new world dogs. *Science.* 2002;298:1613–1616.

98. Leslie M, Messenger S, Rohde R, et al. Bat-associated rabies virus in skunks. *Emerg Infect Dis.* 2006;12(8). www.cdc.gov/eid.

99. Blanton J, Palmer D, Rupprecht C. Rabies surveillance in the United States during 2009. *JAVMA.* 2010;237(6):646–657.

100. Tabel H, Corner A, Webster W, et al. History and epizootiology of rabies in Canada. *Can Vet J.* 1974;15(10):271–281.

101. Mork T, Prestrud P. Arctic rabies—a review. *Acta Vet Scand.* 2004;45:1–9.

102. Johnston D, Fong D. Epidemiology of Artic fox rabies. Wildlife rabies control. In: *Proceedings of the International WHO Symposium on Wildlife Rabies Control, Geneva, 1990 and Report of the WHO Seminar on Wildlife Rabies Control, Geneva 1990.* Wells Wells Medical Cop; 1992:45–49.

103. Odegaard O, Krogsrud J. Rabies in Svalbard: infection diagnosed in arctic fox, reindeer and seal. *Vet Rec.* 1981;109:141–142.

104. Shao X, et al. Genetic evidence for domestic raccoon dog rabies caused by Arctic-like rabies virus in Inner Mongolia, China. *Epidemiol Infect.* 2011;139:629–635.

105. Blanton J, Palmer D, Dyer J, et al. Rabies surveillance in the United States during 2010. *JAVMA.* 2011;239(6):773–783.

106. Blanton J, Krebs J, Hanlon C, et al. Rabies surveillance in the United States during 2005. *JAVMA.* 2006;229:1897–1911.

107. Patyk K, Turmelle A, Blanton J, et al. Trends in national surveillance data for bat rabies in the United States: 2001–2009. *Vector Borne Zoonotic Dis.* 2012;12:666–673.

108. Rohde R, Mayes B, Smith J, et al. Bat rabies, Texas, 1996–2000. *Emerg Infect Dis.* 2004;10(5).

109. Theimer T, Dyer A, Keeley B, et al. Ecological potential for rabies virus transmission via scavenging of dead bats by mesocarnivores. *J Wildl Dis.* 2017;53(2):382–385.

110. Rabies Watch. *Update: Rabies Surveillance in the U.S. Fall;* 2017. Issue #6.

111. Reis N, Peracchi A, Pedro W, et al., eds. *Morcegos Do Brasil. Ne´ lio R. dos Reis.* Londrina, Brasil; 2007:1–253.

112. Uieda W, Harmani NM, Silva MM. Rabies in insectivorous bats (mollisidae) of southeastern Brazil. *Rev Saude Publica.* 1995;29:393–397.

113. Pounder D. Bat rabies. *BMJ.* 2003;326(7392):726.

114. Stantic-Paylinic M. Public health concerns in bat rabies across Europe. *Euro Surveill.* 2005;10(11):217–220.

115. Lina P, Hutson A. Bat rabies in Europe: a review. *Dev Biol.* 2006;125:245–254.

116. Mayes BS, Wilson PJ, Oertli EH, et al. Epidemiology of rabies in bats in Texas (2001–2010). *JAVMA.* 2013;243:1129–1137.

117. Smith J, Orciari L, Yager P. Molecular epidemiology of rabies in the United States. *Semin Virol.* 1995;6:387–400.

118. Liesener A, Smith K, Davis R, et al. Circumstances of bat encounters and knowledge of rabies among Minnesota residents submitting bats for rabies testing. *Vector Borne Zoonotic Dis.* 2006;2:208–215.

119. Venters H, Hoffert W, Schatterday J, et al. Rabies in bats in Florida. *Am J Public Health Nation's Health.* 1954;44(2):182–185.

120. Schatterday J, Galton M. Bat rabies in Florida. *Vet Med.* 1954;49:133–155.

121. Streicker DG, Turmelle AS, Vonhof MJ, et al. Host phylogeny constrains cross-species emergence and establishment of rabies virus in bats. *Science.* 2010;329:676–679.

122. Bleck TP, Rupprecht CE. Rabies. In: Richman DD, Whitley RJ, Hayden FG, eds. *Clinical Virology.* New York: Churchill Livingstone; 1997:879–897.

123. Brass DA. *Rabies in Bats—Natural History and Public Health Implications.* Ridgefield, CT: Livia Press; 1994.

124. Dantas-Torres F. Bats and their role in human rabies epidemiology in the Americas. *J Venom Anim Toxins Incl Trop Dis.* 2008;14(2):193–202.

125. DeSerres G, Dallaire F, Cote M, et al. Bat rabies in the United States and Canada from 1950 through 2007: human cases with and without bat contact. *Clin Infect Dis.* 2008;46:1329–1337.

126. Messenger S, Smith J, Orciari L, et al. Emerging patterns of rabies deaths and increased viral infectivity. *Emerg Infect Dis.* 2003;9:151–154.

127. Kuzmin I, Bozick B, Guagliardo S, et al. Bats, emerging infectious diseases, and the rabies paradigm revisited. *Emerg Health Threats J.* 2011;4:10.3402.

128. Greenhall A. Ecology and bionomics of vampire bats in Latin America. In: Greenhall A, Artois, Fekadu M, eds. *Bats and Rabies.* Lyon, France: Fondation MarcelMe´rieux; 1993:3–57.

129. Mayen F. Haematophagous bats in Brazil, their role in rabies transmission, impact on public health, livestock industry and alternatives to an indiscriminate reduction of bat population. *J Vet Med.* 2003;50:469–472. Series B.

130. Schneider M, Romijn P, Uieda W, et al. Rabies transmitted by vampire bats to humans: an emerging zoonotic disease in Latin America? *Pan Am J Public Health.* 2009;25:260–269.

131. Condori-Condori RE, Streicker DG, Cabezas-Sanchez C, et al. Enzootic and epizootic rabies associated with Vampire bats, Peru. *Emerg Infect Dis.* 2013;19(9):1463–1469.

132. Texas Department of State Health Services. Zoonosis Control Branch. Rabies Surveillance in Texas. 2008 Summary of Cases by County and Year. https://dshs.texas.gov/IDCU/disease/rabies/Cases.doc.

133. Anderson A, Shwiff S, Shwiff S. Economic impact of the potential spread of vampire bats into south Texas. In: Timm RM, O'Brien JM, eds. *Proc. 26th Vertebr. Pest Conf.* Davis: U. of Calif. 2014:305–309.

134. Texas Department of State Health Services. *Rabies in Texas: A Historical Perspective.* Available at: www.dshs.state.tx.us/idcu/disease/rabies/history/historyInTexas.pdf.

135. Velasco-Villa A, Reeder S, Orciari L, et al. Enzootic rabies elimination from dogs and reemergence in wild terrestrial carnivores, United States. *Emerg Infect Dis.* 2008;14(12):1849–1854.

136. *Northeast Wildlife Disease Cooperative.* https://www.northeastwildlife.org/disease/rabies.

137. Steck F, Wandeler A, Bichsel P, et al. Oral immunization of foxes against rabies. Laboratory and field studies. *Comp Immunol Microbiol Infect Dis.* 1982;5:165–171.

138. Chang H, Eidson M, Noonan-Toly C, et al. Public health impact of reemergence of rabies, New York. *Emerg Infect Dis.* 2002;8(9).

139. Childs JE, Curns AT, Dey ME, et al. Predicting the local dynamics of epizootic rabies among raccoons in the United States. *Proceedings of the National Academy of Science USA.* 2000;97:13666–13671.

140. Kirby R. Rabies: an old disease of new importance. *Clin Microbiol Newsl.* 1995;17:1–4.

141. Kappus K, Bigler W, McLean R, et al. The raccoon an emerging rabies host. *J Wildl Dis.* 1970;6(4):507–509.

142. Nettles V, Shaddock J, Sikes R, et al. Rabies in translocated raccoons. *American J Pub Health.* 1979;69:601–602.

143. Wilson M, Bretsky P, Cooper G, et al. Emergence of raccoon rabies in Connecticut, 1991-1994: spatial and temporal characteristics of animal infection and human contact. *Am J Trop Med Hyg.* 1997;57:457–463.

144. Rupprecht C. *Epidemiology of Raccoon Rabies. Wildl Rabies Control.* Kent, UK: Wells Medical; 1992:42–44.

145. Jenkins S, Winkler W. Descriptive epidemiology from an epizootic of raccoon rabies in the middle Atlantic states, 1982-1983. *Am J Epidemiol.* 1987;126(3):429–437.

146. Moore DA. Spatial diffusion of raccoon rabies in Pennsylvania, USA. *Prev Vet Med.* 1999;40:19–32.

147. Rosatte R, Sobey K, Donovan D, et al. Behavior, movements, and demographics of rabid raccoons in Ontario, Canada: management implications. *J Wildl Dis.* 2006;42(3):589–605.

148. Recuenco S, Eidson M, Cherry B, et al. Factors associated with endemic raccoon (*Procyon lotor*) rabies in terrestrial mammals in New York State, USA. *Prev Vet Med.* 2008;86:30–42.

149. Jones M, Curns A, Krebs J, et al. Environmental and human demographic features associated with epizootic raccoon rabies in Maryland, Pennsylvania, and Virginia. *J Wildl Dis.* 2003;39(4):869–874.

150. Dalgish J, Anderson S. A field experiment on learning by raccoons. *J Mammal.* 1979;60:620–622.

151. Prange S, Gehrt S, Wiggers E. Demographic factors contributing to high raccoon densities in urban landscapes. *J Wildl Manag.* 2003;67:324–333.

152. Charlton KM, Webster WA, Casey GA. Skunk rabies. In: Baer GM, ed. *The Natural History of Rabies.* 2nd ed. Boca Raton, FL: CRC Press; 1991:307–324.

153. Krebs J, Mondul A, Rupprecht C, et al. Rabies surveillance in the United States during 2000. *JAVMA.* 2001; 219:1687–1689.

154. Gremillon-Smith C, Woolf A. Epizootiology of skunk rabies in North America. *J Wildl Dis.* 1988;4:620–626.

155. Greenwood R, Newton W, Pearson G, et al. Population and movement characteristics of radio-collared striped skunks in North Dakota during an epizootic of rabies. *J Wildl Dis.* 1997;33:226–241.

156. Kuzmina N, Lemey P, Kuzmin I, et al. The phylogeography and spatiotemporal spread of South-central skunk rabies virus. *PLoS One.* 2013;8(12):e82348.

157. Oertli EH, Wilson PJ, Hunt PR, et al. Epidemiology of rabies in skunks in Texas. *JAVMA.* 2009;234(5):616–620.

158. Rosatte R. Seasonal occurrence and habitat preference of rabid skunks in southern Alberta. *Can Vet J.* 1984;25:142–144.

159. Blanton J, Palmer D, Christian K, et al. Rabies surveillance in the United States during 2007. *JAVMA.* 2008;233(6):884–897.

160. National Geographics. *Coyotes.* https://www.nationalgeographic.com/animals/mammals/c/coyote.

161. Fearneyhough M, Wilson P, Clark K, et al. Results of an oral rabies vaccination program for coyotes. *JAVMA.* 1998;212(4):498–502.

162. Sidwa T, Wilson P, Moore G, et al. Evaluation of oral rabies vaccination programs for control of rabies epizootics in coyotes and gray foxes: 1995–2003. *JAVMA.* 2005;227(5):785–792.

163. Centers for Disease Control and Prevention. *U.S. Declared Canine-Rabies Free;* 2007. https://www.cdc.gov/media/pressrel/2007/r070907.htm.

164. Everard C, Everard J. Mongoose rabies in the caribbean. *Ann N Y Acad Sci.* 1992;653:356–366.

165. Krebs J, Smith J, Rupprecht C, et al. Rabies surveillance in the United States during 1996. *JAVMA.* 1997; 15(211(12)):1525–1539.

166. Styczynski A, Tran C, Dirlikov E, et al. Human rabies – Puerto Rico, 2015. *MMWR (Morb Mortal Wkly Rep).* 2017;65:1474–1476. https://doi.org/10.15585/mmwr.mm6552a4.

167. Bingham J, Foggin CM, Wandeler AI. The epidemiology of rabies in Zimbabwe. 2.Rabies in jackals (*Canis adustus* and *Canis mesomeles*). *Onderstepoort J Vet Res.* 1999;66:11–23.

168. Randall D, Williams S, Kuzmin I, et al. Rabies in endangered ethiopian wolves. *Emerg Infect Dis.* 2004;10(12):2214–2217.

169. U.S. Fish and Wildlife Services. *Mexican Wolf Recovery Program.* https://www.fws.gov/southwest/es/mexicanwolf/pdf/wolfdzinfofinal.pdf.

170. Barnard BJH, Hassel RH, Geyer HJ, et al. Nonbite transmission of rabies in kudu (*Tragelaphus strepsiceros*) Onderstepoort. *J Vet Res.* 1982;49:191–192.

171. Schneider L, Barnard B, Schneider H. Application of monoclonal antibodies for epidemiological investigations and oral vaccination studies. I. African viruses. In: Kuwert E, Merieux C, Koprowski H, Bagel K, eds. *Rabies in the Tropics.* Berlin: Springer-Verlag; 1985:47–59.

172. Chang J, Tsai K, Hsu W, et al. Rabies virus infection in ferret badgers (*Melogale moschata subaurantiaca*) in Taiwan: a retrospective study. *J Wildl Dis.* 2015;51(4):923–928.

173. *MMWR Morb Mortal Wkly Rep.* 2014;63(8):178.

174. Gautret P, Blanton J, Dacheux L, et al. Rabies in non-human primates and potential for transmission to humans: a literature review and examination of selected French national data. *Negl PLoS Trop Dis.* 2014;8: e2863.

175. Machado G, Antunes J, Uieda W, et al. Exposure to rabies virus in a population of free- ranging capuchin monkeys (*Cebus apella nigritus*) in a fragmented, environmentally protected area in southeastern Brazil. *Primates.* 2012;53: 227–231.

176. Fishbein D, Belotto A, Pacer R, et al. Rabies in rodents and lagomorphs in the United States, 1971–1984: increased cases in the woodchuck (*Marmota monax*) in mid-Atlantic states. *J Wildl Dis.* 1986;22:151–155.

177. Moro M, Horman J, Fischman HR, et al. The epidemiology of rodent and lagomorphs rabies in Maryland, 1981 to 1986. *J Wildl Dis.* 1991;3:452–456.

178. Winkler W, Jenkins S. Raccoon rabies. In: Baer GM, ed. *The Natural History of Rabies.* second ed. Boca Raton, FL: CRC Press. Inc.; 1991. 325-240.

179. Childs JE, Colby L, Krebs JW, et al. Surveillance and spatiotemporal associations of rabies in rodents and lagomorphs in the United States, 1985–1994. *J Wildl Dis.* 1997;33:20–27.

180. Smith P, Lawhaswasdi K, Vick W, et al. Enzootic rabies in rodents in Thailand. *Nature.* 1968;217:954–955.

181. Kamoltham T, Tepsumethenon V, Wilde H. Rat rabies in phetchabun province, Thailand. *J Trav Med.* 2002;9(2):106–107.

182. Eidson M, Matthews S, Willsey A, et al. Rabies virus infection in a pet Guinea pig and seven pet rabbits. *JAVMA.* 2005;(227):6.

183. Dyer JL, Yager P, Orciari L, et al. Rabies surveillance in the United States during 2013. *JAVMA.* 2014;245: 1111–1123.

184. Zhu Y, Zhang G, Shao M, et al. An outbreak of sheep rabies in Shanxi province, China. *Epidemiol Infect.* 2011;139: 1453–1456.

185. Green SL. Equine rabies. *Vet Clin N Am Equine Pract.* 1993;9:337–347.

186. Green SL. Rabies. *Vet Clin N Am Equine Pract.* 1997;13: 1–11.

187. Weese J. A review of equine zoonotic diseases: risks in veterinary medicine. *Proc Annual Convention AAEP*. 2002;48:362–369.

188. Wilkins P, Piero F. Rabies. In: Sellon DC, Long MT, eds. *Equine Infectious Diseases*. Philadelphia (PA): Saunders, Elsevier Inc.; 2007:185–191. [Chapter 19].

189. Jindal N, Narang G. An outbreak of rabies in buffaloes in Haryana. *Indian Vet J*. 1998;75:839–840.

190. Liu Y, Zhang H, Zhang SF, et al. Rabies outbreaks and vaccination in domestic camels and cattle in Northwest China. *PLoS Neglected Trop Dis*. 2016;10(9):e0004890.

191. Meltzer M, Rupprecht C. Review of the economics of the prevention and control of rabies. Part 2: rabies in dogs, livestock and wildlife. *Pharmacoeconomics*. 1998;14:481–498.

192. Ye F, Yanyan S, Mingyang Y, et al. Livestock rabies outbreaks in Shanxi province, China. *Arch Virol*. 2016;161:2851–2854.

193. Krebs J, Smith J, Rupprecht C, et al. Rabies surveillance in the United States during 1997. *JAVMA*. 1998;213(12):1713–1728.

194. Bender J, Schulman S. Reports of zoonotic disease outbreaks associated with animal exhibits and availability of recommendations for preventing zoonotic disease transmission from animals to people in such settings. *JAVMA*. 2004;224:1105–1109.

195. Debbie JG, Trimarchi CV. Pantropism of rabies virus in free-ranging rabid red fox Vulpes fulva. *J Wildl Dis*. 1970;6:500–506.

196. Afshar A. A review of non-bite transmission of rabies virus infection. *Br Vet J*. 1979;135:142–148.

197. Krebs J, Wheeling J, Childs J. Rabies surveillance in the United States during 2002. *JAVMA*. 2003;223(12):1736–1748.

198. Bögel K, Schaal E, Moegle H. The significance of martens as transmitters of wildlife rabies in Europe. *Zbl Bakteriol*. 1977;238:184.

199. De Mattos CC, De Mattos CA, Loza-Rubio E, et al. Molecular characterization of rabies virus isolates from Mexico: implications for transmission dynamics and human risk. *Am J Trop Med Hyg*. 1999;61:587–597.

200. David D, Yakobson B, Smith JS, et al. Transmission dynamics of rabies virus in Thailand: implications for disease control. *J Clin Microbiol*. 2000;38:755–762.

201. Blancou J. The control of rabies in Eurasia: overview, history and background. *Dev Biol*. 2008;131:3–15.

202. Botvinkin AD, et al. Rabies in the Mongolian steppes. *Dev Biologicals*. 2008;131:199–205.

203. *MMWR Morb Mortal Wkly Rep*. 1982;31(27):379–380.

204. Gordon ER, Curns AT, Krebs JW, et al. Temporal dynamics of rabies in a wildlife host and the risk of cross-species transmission. *Epidemiol Infect*. 2004;132(3):515–524.

205. *Rabies-Bulletin-Europe*. http://www.who-rabies-bulletin.org.

CHAPTER 4

Laboratory Testing

RODNEY E. ROHDE, PhD, MS, SM(ASCP)CM, SVCM, MBCM, FACSc

SCENARIO

A real-life example: a young female college student decided to "rescue a downed and sick" bat. Without understanding the risk, she retrieved the bat with bare hands and took it to the university biology department "for possible help" to save the bat. Several professors and numerous students were exposed in this scenario, and the female student disappeared before anyone even considered the risk and danger. After consultations were initiated about the situation, the bat was tested for rabies, and the result was positive. University- and city-wide campaigns were implemented to locate the young woman, with a successful outcome. This is just one example of hundreds of stories across the United States and elsewhere that highlights the critical need for rapid rabies diagnosis in the animal and sometimes human specimen.[1]

Once rabies is suspected, the proper and timely collection of samples for testing can determine whether or not further steps are needed, such as the administration of rabies postexposure prophylaxis (PEP). Moreover, the use of regional and national virus reference laboratories can aid in the diagnosis and epidemiology of the case. This is all contingent, although, on medical, public health, and animal care and control professionals knowing how, when, and why to suspect rabies and how to test for rabies and other lyssaviruses.

INTRODUCTION

The diagnosis of rabies in humans before death (antemortem) now provides hope for physicians to overcome the inertia to attempt experimental therapeutic approaches in patients. Traditional methods for antemortem and postmortem rabies diagnosis have several limitations. Advances in technology and understanding of rabies pathogenesis have led to the improvement or design of several diagnostic assays, which include methods for rabies viral antigen and antibody detection, and assays for viral nucleic acid detection and identification of specific biomarkers. These assays, augmented by traditional methods, are beginning to revolutionize rabies diagnosis across the global landscape.

Unfortunately, there are still no accurate and foolproof diagnostic tests available for the detection of lyssaviruses before onset of clinical rabies disease. Surveillance and diagnosis for rabies in animals and humans by laboratory testing are severely lacking in much of the developing world where rabies is endemic. Although the ability to diagnose rabies differs geographically, there remains the issue of physicians and other health-care professionals attempting to diagnose rabies based on clinical signs and symptoms alone. The true disease burden and public health impact due to rabies remain underestimated because of lack of simple, sensitive, specific, and cost-effective laboratory methods for rabies diagnosis. The other problem is that much of the classical testing is subjective (operator dependent) and requires high biosafety level reference laboratories that are difficult to maintain. Therefore, the impetus of this chapter is to attempt to place emphasis on helping veterinarians, physicians, and other health-care practitioners and professionals identify the best available path for laboratory techniques and research advancements in the field of rabies.

This neglected zoonosis is a preventable disease that, despite the availability of efficacious and affordable biologics, is the cause of an estimated 59,000 human deaths worldwide (mainly children) every year. Rabies is an acute and rapidly progressive encephalitis that is usually fatal once symptoms and signs begin. The disease (or syndrome) is caused by 12 lyssavirus species, including genotype 1 lyssavirus more commonly known as rabies virus. It is a worldwide disease primarily arising from an animal encounter. The only known region globally that is free of rabies and rabies-like viruses is the continent of Antarctica. Rabies is a single-stranded RNA, nonsegmented, negative-sense virus and is the only lyssavirus present in the Americas.[2] Transmission of rabies occurs when saliva containing rabies virus is introduced into an opening in the wound, usually via the bite or scratch of a rabid animal. Although rare, transmission can also occur through contamination of mucous membranes or transplantation. Rabies has the highest case fatality ratio of any

Rabies. https://doi.org/10.1016/B978-0-323-63979-8.00004-0
Copyright © 2019 Elsevier Inc. All rights reserved.

infectious disease when intervention is not initiated before development of clinical signs and symptoms. Typical treatment for viral exposure consists of wound care, passive immunization with rabies immune globulin (RIG), and a series of four doses of rabies vaccine (five doses in immunocompromised individuals in the United States).[3,4]

A differential diagnosis of rabies should be suspected for individuals with signs of encephalitis, myelitis, or encephalomyelitis. With rabies, there is a progressive worsening of the disease, so patients with these clinical signs who respond to treatment do not require rabies testing. The absence of an exposure history does not provide evidence to terminate any suspicions of a rabies diagnosis because many patients, especially in the United States, have no definitive exposure history.[5] Indeed, several recent cases of rabies in humans in the United States have been diagnosed either retrospectively or after the clinical course of the disease has progressed, despite compatible clinical observations. A heightened awareness among physicians and the medical community of possible rabies infections in cases where clinical signs are compatible with a diagnosis of rabies is critical. Cases of less severe disease or seropositivity absent any disease suggest a broader continuum of disease severity, such that laboratory testing may have to be considered earlier and in more patients with encephalitis.[6,7] In addition, medical and veterinary personnel must be aware of appropriate methods for sample collection for antemortem and postmortem diagnosis and must know how to interpret the test results.[8,9]

RABIES DIAGNOSIS

When a physician suspects a case of rabies, there are usually two decisions that come to bear. First, the decision must be made about the possibility of exposure to rabies virus so that a determination of rabies PEP in others can be made promptly (refer to Chapter 6 for guidance). The second decision is the actual laboratory diagnosis of rabies that is important for the care (limited or intensive) and isolation via infection control of the case.[10]

This chapter will focus on the methods most commonly used for the laboratory diagnosis of rabies and policies in use in North America. These include the gold standard direct fluorescent antibody (DFA) test normally applied to fresh animal brain tissue and to skin biopsy tissues (and other samples) used in human antemortem diagnosis. Diverse molecular methods, primarily based on the polymerase chain reaction

(PCR) with various sample types for human antemortem diagnosis and as a confirmatory test for other sample types, are rising in utilization. Immunohistochemical methods have traditionally been applied for rabies diagnosis of fixed tissues, but molecular methods are also being investigated regularly.

Specimen Submission for Laboratory Procedures

A patient history form detailing the clinical history of the patient should accompany the specimen, complete with the name and phone number of the physician who should be contacted with the test results.[11] All samples should be considered potentially infectious. Test tubes and other sample containers must be securely sealed (moisture-resistant tape around the cap will ensure that the containers do not open during transit). If immediate shipment is not possible, all samples, *except brain tissues*, should be stored frozen at $-20°C$ ($-4.0°F$) or below. With respect to brain tissues for testing, one should refer to their own state and local rabies-testing laboratory for specific guidelines on storage and shipment of the specimen. For example, in the Texas Administrative Code, it states to keep the specimen chilled between 32 and 45°C Fahrenheit either in a refrigerator or by packing with sufficient amounts of refrigerants (such as gel packs or similar refrigerants, but ice is not recommended) in the shipping container; the specimen should not be frozen.[12] Similarly, the recommendations in the Compendium of Animal Rabies Prevention and Control under "10. Rabies diagnosis" regarding submitting an animal specimen for rabies testing are "To facilitate prompt laboratory testing, submitted specimens should be stored and shipped under refrigeration without delay. The need to thaw frozen specimens will delay testing." Thus, brain tissues for public health testing should be refrigerated at 0–7.2°C (32–45°F), whereas surveillance specimens can be refrigerated or frozen.[13] However, in the WHO's recent report, it recommends either refrigerating or freezing the specimen.[14] The Centers for Disease Control and Prevention (CDC) provides a different perspective pertaining to shipment of a specimen by mentioning the following: "The increased growth of bacterial contaminants within the refrigerated samples may interfere with the ability to rule-out the presence of rabies virus antigen in tissues, antibodies in serum and cerebrospinal fluid (CSF), and nucleic acid in saliva or skin biopsy samples." For submissions to the CDC (must consult with and have prior approval from the CDC to submit a specimen to the CDC), fresh frozen (unfixed) tissues are preferred for rabies diagnosis. For a submission to

CDC, specimens that should be packed on dry ice and shipped frozen include fresh frozen (unfixed) tissue (e.g., brain, skin biopsy), serum, and body fluids (such as saliva and CSF). Additionally, dry ice shipments should comply with the International Air Transport Association (IATA) packing instructions 954 for UN 1845 and be shipped by a HAZMAT-certified packer. For CDC submissions, refrigeration (via gel packs) is not a preferred method for any rabies diagnostic samples and should be used as last resort when dry ice is not available.[15] Packing of clinical specimens for rabies testing should fulfill the IATA regulations for shipment of UN 3373 Biological substance Category B.

Samples should be shipped by an overnight courier in watertight primary containers and leak-proof secondary containers that meet the guidelines of the IATA. Usually, the state health department rabies laboratory receiving the specimen should be telephoned at the time of shipment (again, a consultation and prior approval is needed to submit a specimen to the CDC if deemed necessary). Information regarding the mode of shipment, expected arrival time, and courier tracking number is critical to give to the CDC.[15] In most states, it is preferable to ship by bus or other reliable carrier; the entity that will be receiving the shipment should be contacted for its recommendations.

Sample Considerations
Antemortem samples—human
If rabies is considered as a diagnosis, a variety of samples should be sent for antemortem study. These include nuchal skin biopsy, saliva, serum, and CSF. As with any disease of unknown origin, personal protective equipment and barrier protection should be used when samples are collected. This will not only protect the medical laboratory professional from exposure to rabies if the patient is infected, but it will also protect against any other potential pathogens that have yet to be identified. Rabies samples are handled as BSL-2 by the clinical laboratories. The following instructions should be used to collect samples only after consultation with the state health department, the regional reference laboratory, or the rabies laboratory at the CDC.[9,11,15]

Skin samples (5–6 mm in diameter) should be taken via biopsy from the posterior region of the neck at the hairline. A minimum of 10 hair follicles, sampled at a depth to include the cutaneous nerves at the follicle base, should be contained in the specimen. The specimen should be placed on a piece of sterile gauze moistened with sterile water and placed in a sealed container. Preservatives or additional fluids should not be added. Laboratory tests

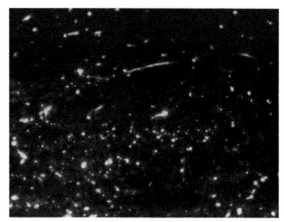

FIG. 4.1 Direct Fluorescent Antibody test. (Reprinted with permission from Rohde R. Personal photo.)

to be performed include reverse transcriptase-polymerase chain reaction (RT-PCR) of extracted nucleic acids and DFA for viral antigen (see Fig. 4.1) in frozen sections of the biopsy sample.[9,11,15]

Saliva should be collected with a sterile eyedropper pipette and placed in a small sterile container that can be sealed securely. Preservatives or additional material should not be added. Laboratory tests to be performed include detection of rabies RNA via RT-PCR and isolation of infectious virus in cell culture. Tracheal aspirates and sputum are not suitable for rabies tests.[9,11,15]

A minimum of 0.5 mL of serum or CSF should be collected; no preservatives should be added. Whole blood should not be submitted because it contains various inhibitors against nucleic acid amplification techniques. If the patient has not received vaccine or rabies immune serum, the presence of antibody to rabies virus in the serum is diagnostic and testing of CSF is unnecessary unless one is treating. Antibody to rabies virus in the CSF, regardless of the immunization history, suggests a rabies virus infection. Laboratory tests for antibody include the IFA and virus neutralization (VN).[9,11,15] Other methods to detect rabies antibody, antigen, RNA, or omics profiles are available but must be referenced against these gold standards.[16-21]

The rarity of rabies and the lack of proven treatment make brain biopsy unwarranted; however, biopsy samples negative for herpes and other types of encephalitis should be tested for evidence of rabies infection.[9,11,15,22] The biopsy sample should be placed in a sterile sealed container; preservatives or additional fluids should not be added. Laboratory tests to be performed include RT-PCR and DFA for viral antigen in touch impressions.[9,11,15]

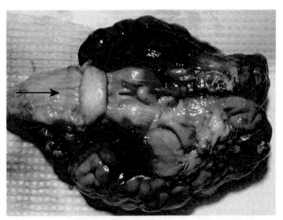

FIG. 4.2 Animal Brain Specimens for DFA Testing—Stem *(arrow)*. (Reprinted with permission from Rohde R. Personal photo.)

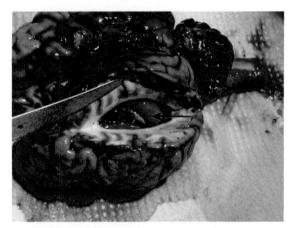

FIG. 4.4 Animal Brain Specimens for DFA Testing—Hippocampus *(arrow)*. (Reprinted with permission from Rohde R. Personal photo.)

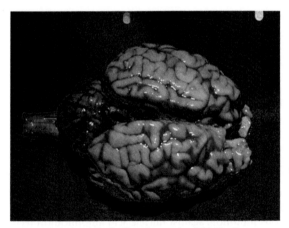

FIG. 4.3 Animal Brain Specimens for DFA Testing—Cerebellum *(arrow)*. (Reprinted with permission from Rohde R. Personal photo.)

Integrity, type, and time of collection of antemortem specimens are critical to the correct diagnosis of a rabies infection. Because of the properties of rabies pathogenesis, limited sensitivity of antemortem diagnostic tests for rabies is assumed. Different tests, repeated over time, will when combined result in a diagnosis in more than 90% of cases.[23]

Postmortem samples—animal and human
Postmortem diagnosis of rabies in animals and humans is made by the standard test: DFA staining of viral antigen in touch impressions of brain tissue. Portions of the brainstem, the cerebellum, and the hippocampus (see Figs. 4.2–4.4) should be kept refrigerated and shipped to a public health laboratory for rabies

testing.[11,15] As described above, fresh brain material should usually be refrigerated not frozen. Preservation of tissues by fixation in formalin is not recommended if rabies diagnosis is desired. However, if tissue has been placed in formalin, procedures have been described to analyze the specimen.[11,15,24] Postmortem diagnosis of rabies may also use molecular methods and immunohistochemical methods for confirmation.

Rabies virus variant typing
Reference laboratories that perform rabies virus variant characterization can offer several insights into a patient's case. The identification of the rabies virus variant may result in a clearer understanding of the type of exposure that the patient may have had with a rabid animal[8,9] or any foreign travel by the patient. In recent history, one of the most important contributions of rabies virus typing has been the discovery that most of the cases for which there is no bite exposure history have been attributed to bat rabies virus variants. Phylogeny also predicts complications and immune response kinetics during therapy with Milwaukee Protocol.

The combination of these factors led to the enhanced CDC recommendation for bat exposures in that PEP is considered in all situations in which a bat bite or direct contact with a bat may have occurred. Clarification of epizootiologic patterns including spillover will augment the creation of appropriate public health information and policy for prevention and control of rabies, including expanded resources for regional and national virus-typing laboratories.

Public health laboratories are facing critical issues, not the least of which is the problem of accurate surveillance of rabies virus variants throughout the United States and other countries. However, the successful collaboration between the CDC and the Texas Department of Health (now the Texas Department of State Health Services) rabies laboratory over the last 25 years has produced the typing data to identify and map rabies variants common to animal reservoirs in the United States and Mexico. Appropriately used, this knowledge will allow those who survey rabies to recognize when established reservoirs enlarge or expand into new areas or when different animal species become involved in cycles of rabies virus transmission. For example, it has been reported by species distribution modeling that there is support for the hypothesis that suitable habitat for vampire bats may currently exist in parts of the Mexico-US borderlands, including extreme southern portions of Texas, as well as in southern Florida. The analysis also suggests, however, that extensive expansion into the southeastern and southwestern United States over the coming ~60 years appears unlikely.[25] Regional laboratories can expand and complement the flow of national surveillance data by increasing their surveillance activities to include antigenic and molecular typing of virus samples from surrounding states.[8,9,26]

TESTING NEEDS

Laboratory assistance can aid in cases when there is no history of animal bite or exposure and hallmark clinical features, such as aerophobia or hydrophobia, are lacking. Furious and paralytic rabies are the two most common forms recognized in humans and often in animals. Typically, about 67% of cases from classical (furious) rabies and 33% from paralytic (dumb) rabies in patients and dogs are diagnosed based on its clinical signs and symptoms. Nevertheless, half of rabies cases are diagnosed at autopsy.[27] Furious rabies can overlap with NMDAR antibody encephalitis or malaria.[28,29] Paralytic forms can be clinically indistinguishable from other central nervous system cases, for example, Guillain-Barre syndrome or enterovirus D68 or neuroparalytic complications due to Semple-type antirabies vaccine from a few countries.[30-33]

Rapid diagnosis of rabies is a powerful public health tool and critical trigger to initiate prompt infection control. Although there is a multitude of important reasons for an early diagnosis, one cannot overstate the following points: a halt to unnecessary medical testing and treatment and assistance in other medical case management, such as in cases of negative rabies diagnosis; initiation of correct medical testing and treatment of

alternative more treatable diagnoses; correct and timely administration of pre- or postexposure vaccination; ultimate case closure; and light shed on the original animal exposure, which may assist in other exposure identification. Likewise, early diagnosis of rabies can assist in organ donor screening and experimental therapeutic approaches for antemortem testing, establish geographic and epidemiologic boundaries for monitoring existing and new incursions of rabies virus variants, and evaluate oral rabies vaccination for the control of wildlife rabies.[8,9,34-44] In the latter two functions, if you detected an index case of rabies in an animal in a naïve geographic area, public health measures, such as educational campaigns, could be quickly implemented and possibly help to extinguish a new epizootic before it exploded into a large-scale outbreak.

Conventional Tests

Testing for rabies dates as far back as AD 1800 when Zinke first demonstrated rabies could be transmitted to a normal animal after inoculating it with rabid animal's saliva. Negri bodies discovered by Adelchi Negri (1903) and subsequent demonstration of their diagnostic significance by his wife, Lina Negri-Luzzani, in 1913 were hallmark discoveries in the laboratory journey for rabies identification and characterization.[34]

In the following sections, basic techniques in the laboratory diagnosis of rabies are described. Where possible, limitations with testing will be covered.

Direct microscopy

"Negri bodies" (see Fig. 4.5) are infected neuronal cells of viral particles and appear as circular to oval in shape as typical eosinophilic with basophilic granules (intracytoplasmic inclusion bodies often in a rosette arrangement within the matrix and specific to rabies encephalitis). These inclusions/lesions (3–30 μm) are demonstrated by histologic tests (Seller's method) on brain smears from various areas of the brain.[45,46]

While it is a very simple, rapid test, Seller's method on unfixed tissue smears has a very low sensitivity only suitable for fresh specimens. Generally, paraffin-embedded stain sections of brain tissues are time-consuming, less sensitive, and more expensive. Histologic techniques are much less sensitive than immunologic methods, especially in the case of autolyzed specimens, and are no longer recommended for primary diagnosis, both in humans and animals.[34]

Direct fluorescent antibody test

Postmortem diagnosis of rabies in humans and animals is made by the most widely used and standard test, the DFA.

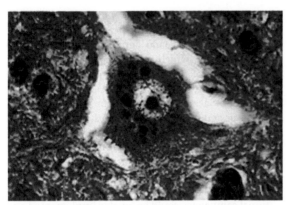

FIG. 4.5 Micrograph of Negri Bodies. Description: This micrograph depicts the histopathologic changes associated with rabies encephalitis prepared using an H&E stain. Note the Negri bodies, which are cellular inclusions found most frequently in the pyramidal cells of Ammon's horn, and the Purkinje cells of the cerebellum. They are also found in the cells of the medulla and various other ganglia. (Reprinted with permission by Source, Fair use: Centers for Disease Control and Prevention (Public Health Image Library).)

The test involves direct staining of viral antigen in touch impressions of brain tissue, including portions of the brainstem, the cerebellum, and the hippocampus. Both the World Health Organization (WHO) and World Organization for Animal Health (OIE) recommend the DFA as the gold standard for these postmortem tissues. The DFA can be used to confirm the presence of rabies antigen in cell culture or in brain tissue of mice that have been inoculated for diagnosis. The specificity and sensitivity of the test almost approach 99% in an experienced laboratory and results are available within a few hours. While it may be used on corneal smears (which, in general, are no longer recommended) and nuchal skin biopsy in suspected cases, it has been found to have limited reliability and low sensitivity for antemortem diagnosis of rabies.[9,34]

Virus isolation

The isolation of rabies virus can be very useful to characterize the molecular nature of the virus with respect to geographic placement and for determining the origin of the virus if found in an area free from rabies. Isolation of rabies virus is usually required for confirmatory diagnosis when the DFA gives a weak or uncertain result. There are two primary tests that are used to isolate rabies virus: the mouse inoculation test (MIT) and rapid tissue culture infection test (RTCIT).[47,48]

Mouse inoculation test. The MIT is performed by the intracerebral inoculation of three-to-ten mice, 3–4 weeks old (12–14 g), or a litter of 2-day-old newborn mice, with supernatant of a 10%–20% (w/v) homogenate of brain material. They are observed daily for 28 days for typical clinical signs of rabies any time after 5–7 days. Typical signs consist of initial ruffling of hair, hunchback, and dragging hind limbs followed by paralysis of limbs. A DFA of the extracted brain of the suspected mouse brain may offer confirmation of the diagnosis. Unfortunately, one disadvantage of MIT is the long interval (28 days) before a diagnosis can be confirmed. Cell culture facilities, if available, avoid the use of live animals, are less expensive, and give more rapid results with higher sensitivity. However, advantages of a positive MIT are that a large amount of virus can be isolated from a single mouse brain for strain identification purposes.[49]

Rapid tissue culture infection test. Unlike the MIT, the RTCIT is much more rapid of a test (24–48 h). Murine neuroblastoma cell line Neuro-2a is most suitable and most common for virus isolation. Chicken embryo-related (CER) and baby hamster kidney (BHK 21) are not as sensitive but may be used. Human embryonic kidney cell line (HEK 293) cells have been shown to be sensitive. Specimens are inoculated onto the cells grown in a shell vial or 96-well plates, incubated for 24 h, and stained by DFA after acetone fixation. RTCIT is a faster and cheaper alternative to MIT; however, it can be performed only in laboratories with cell culture facilities as well as a fluorescent microscope.[49]

Rapid Rabies Enzyme Immunodiagnosis

The rapid rabies enzyme immunodiagnosis is an enzyme-linked immunosorbent assay (ELISA)–based technique, which detects the rabies (N) antigen in a brain homogenate by a polyclonal or monoclonal anti-N antibody coated on the solid phase. Next, the captured antigen is detected by adding peroxidase conjugated monoclonal or polyclonal antibody raised in a different species or even better by the addition of biotinylated (N) antibody followed by streptavidin peroxidase and color development with o-phenylenediamine dihydrochloride and hydrogen peroxide. It has been shown to be as sensitive and specific as the DFA. The partial decomposition of the brain will not affect the test result; however, the requirement of brain tissue precludes its use in antemortem diagnosis.[34,50]

Antibody Confirmation

Antibody demonstration in the serum in the absence of a history of vaccination for rabies or in CSF offers indirect evidence of rabies infection. Unfortunately, interpretation of test results usually varies among individuals. In general, serologic testing for rabies is considered poor for negative predictive value early in the disease course.[10] Antibody testing is increasingly useful for antemortem diagnosis as more survivors are reported, including in retrospect in India, and is a key feature in the Milwaukee Protocol.[51,52] Serology is very useful for assessing seroconversion after vaccination and for epidemiologic studies.[6]

VN assays in cell cultures are prescribed tests for checking vaccination responses because neutralizing antibodies are considered a key component of the adaptive immune response against rabies virus. Results are expressed in international units relative to an international standard antiserum. The WHO or OIE no longer recommend the mouse neutralization test (MNT) developed in 1935 by Webster and Dawson,[53] but the rapid fluorescent focus inhibition test (RFFIT) and the fluorescent antibody virus neutralization (FAVN) test have been described for this purpose. The RFFIT is one of the most widely used substitutes to the MNT. The test requires only 20 h for completion and is slightly more sensitive than the MNT.[54] Adapted from the RFFIT, the FAVN test (1998) showed good agreement with the MNT and RFFIT.[55] Confirmation of antibody can be leveraged to monitor the immune response within the CNS, and thus a possible clearance of the rabies virus as well as immune-mediated complications in patients who are treated with the Milwaukee Protocol or other experimental therapy.[52]

At the current time, the RFFIT is considered the gold standard to estimate the titer of rabies virus neutralizing antibodies. However, limitations for the test include the need for resources such as a trained work force, cell culture, fluorescent microscopy, and adequate biosafety protocols. This test is sensitive to cytotoxicity in poor-quality sera, and nonspecific inhibitors of virus in sera may produce false-positive results.

More Recent Diagnostic Tests

Over the past decade or so, a diverse variety of molecular methods, mostly based on PCR, are increasingly applied to various sample types for human antemortem diagnosis and as a confirmatory test for other samples. Likewise, immunohistochemical methods traditionally applied for rabies diagnosis of fixed tissues are now being leveraged to explore for molecular tools and applications. In the following sections, representative techniques in these newer laboratory diagnostic tools of rabies are described. Where possible, limitations with testing are also included.

Direct rapid immunohistochemical test

The direct rapid immunohistochemical test (dRIT) is a rapid immunohistochemical test developed at the

CDC in Atlanta, Georgia,[56] based on detecting rabies (N) protein in suspected brain tissue using a cocktail of highly concentrated and purified biotinylated monoclonal antibody to (N) protein followed by addition of streptavidin peroxidase and substrate (H_2O_2 and amino ethyl carbazole). A positive result is demonstrated by brownish-red clusters within the neuron, along the axons, and scattered all over the brain smears. Advantages include testing time (less than an hour) with a light microscope making it applicable for field testing (fluorescent microscope is not required) with a disadvantage of refrigerated reagent storage requirement. The test has been evaluated under field conditions in Tanzania and was found to be 100% sensitive and specific compared with the DFA. The test has also undergone extensive evaluation in other countries, and 100% correlation was found with the DFA.[34] It offers an alternative to the DFA for improved decentralized laboratory-based surveillance, but commercialization of the reagents or in-house production in selected laboratories in developing countries should be considered.

Indirect rapid immunohistochemistry test

In 2013, the indirect rapid immunohistochemistry test (IRIT) method was published offering the detection and differentiation of rabies virus (RABV) variants via traditional light microscopy. Fresh-frozen brain touch impressions or cell culture monolayers fixed in buffered formalin are stained with a panel of murine antinucleoprotein monoclonal antibodies (mAb-N) and commercially available biotin-labeled goat anti-mouse antibody. The IRIT method agrees with distinct reactivity patterns associated with current and historical RABV reservoir hosts similar to the IFA test and genetic sequence analysis. Like the dRIT, this test can be performed in a field setting without expensive standard laboratory equipment rendering it as a cost-effective diagnostic test. The IRIT can be used to study the prevalence, distribution, and transmission of rabies virus variants among reservoir hosts in rabies enzootic areas.[57]

Reverse-transcription polymerase chain reaction

The RT-PCR assay is the most frequently used molecular method that seeks to detect rabies and rabies-related virus RNAs.[58] Although it is most often applied postmortem to fresh brain material from a suspect animal or human, it may also be applied to saliva, skin samples (often collected antemortem from suspect humans), salivary glands, and, virtually any other tissue or sample. If a positive amplification result occurs, sequence characterization of the product and comparison with other reference viruses can differentiate the variant type, common species transmission, and geographic locale information. Limitations include testing time (up to 2 days) and the expense, as well as the powerful sensitivity of the technique, escalating risk of cross-contamination, and subsequent erroneous findings.[34,58] Practically speaking, it is the sensitivity coupled with the gain provided by logs of amplicon, leading to the potential for cross-contamination within the testing environment from previous testing. The related issue is that amplicons can look correct by size but be nonspecific, so probe or sequence confirmation is indicated for a high consequence test.

Quantitative "real-time" PCR

The quantitative real-time PCR (qPCR)–based assays allow for the "real-time" detection and quantification of genome copies with the advantage of a closed-tube assay, which allows for a significant reduction in cross-contamination. Human saliva samples for antemortem rabies diagnosis via qPCR using SYBR Green chemistry and as a universal real-time assay for the detection of lyssaviruses have been evaluated,[59,60] but specificity must be carefully ensured.[61]

The TaqMan qPCR assays, however, ensure a high specificity because of the intrinsic hybridization reaction, detection range, and sensitivity compared with traditional nested RT-PCR.[34,60] Despite several advantages, viral genetic heterogeneity may prove to be an impediment to the development of TaqMan probe-based PCR because mismatches between the target and the probe can lead to false-negative results or decreased sensitivity.[34,62]

Increasingly broad spectrum qRT-PCR assays have been described. Two qRT-PCR assays were developed for large-spectrum detection of African rabies virus isolates. Primer and probe sets targeted highly conserved regions of the nucleoprotein (N) and polymerase (L) genes. Nonspecific amplification was absent as was cross-reaction with a range of other viruses belonging to the same taxonomic family (Rhabdoviridae), as well as negative brain tissues from various host species. Analytical sensitivity ranged between 100 and 10 standard RNA copies detected per reaction for N-gene and L-gene assays, respectively.[63] A pan-lyssavirus qPCR intended for use on postmortem brain samples is capable of detecting other lyssaviruses that cause clinical rabies. Degenerate primers and locked nucleic acid probes target the leader sequence and part of the nucleoprotein (N) gene and include an internal β-actin control. Analytical sensitivity ranged between 0 and

18 standard RNA copies. Fourteen laboratories participated in validation.[64] Effective detection and high sensitivity of these assays showed that they can be successfully applied in general research and used in diagnostic process and epizootic surveillance with proper cross-checking strategy.[63]

Automated molecular platforms

Assessing the utility of a high-throughput molecular platform, such as the Qiagen QIAsymphony SP/AS, in conjunction with quantitative reverse transcription-PCR (qRT-PCR), to augment or potentially replace the standard DFA has been evaluated. A triplex qRT-PCR assay, including assembly and evaluation for sensitivity, specificity, and ability to detect variants was performed. Additionally, a comparison was conducted between the qRT-PCR assay and gold standard DFA. More than 1000 specimens submitted for routine rabies diagnosis were tested to directly compare the two methods. All results were in agreement between the two methods, with one additional specimen detected by qRT-PCR below the limits of the DFA sensitivity. With the proper continued validation for variant detection, molecular methods have a place in routine rabies diagnostics within the United States.[65]

Rapid immunodiagnostic test and other antigen assays

The rapid immunodiagnostic test detects rabies antigen from postmortem samples and can be used for rabies diagnosis without the need for laboratory equipment. The methodology is based on a lateral flow strip test in a one-step test that facilitates low-cost, rapid identification of viral antigen. The specimen in question is added to the test device and conjugated detector antibodies attached to two different zones on a membrane indicate the presence of viral antigen. Using the same methodology and principle, dog saliva samples have been tested and evaluated for rabies viral antigen detection using a combination of purified polyclonal and monoclonal antibodies.

Another example of a rapid screening test kit for rabies has been developed using monoclonal antibodies, which recognize epitope II and III of the nucleoprotein of rabies virus, and has been improved for rabies diagnosis in animals. It is a rapid, reliable, and user-friendly test for laboratories with modest infrastructure. Although the test exhibits high sensitivity, unfortunately, the specificity is not and thus is unsuitable for diagnosis of rabies in humans.[66-69] These immunochromatographic techniques can be used as a rapid screening test in animals; however, they need to undergo considerable testing on human clinical samples to improve sensitivity and specificity before they can be recommended for diagnosis of rabies in humans.

There is an interesting rapid test for the detection of lyssaviruses belonging to all seven genotypes circulating in Europe, Africa, Asia, and Oceania based on a sandwich enzyme-linked immunosorbent assay (ELISA) platform. It would be very useful, if one was interested in a screening assay that is simple and easy to perform to detect the major genotypes.[70,71] There are additional platforms for rabies viral antigen detection, which include a dot-blot immunoassay for brain tissues[72] and an enzyme immunoassay for rapid diagnosis of rabies in humans and animals.[73] Chimeric bifunctional molecules based on alkaline phosphatase-fused antirabies virus glycoprotein scFv antibody fragment was found to be a novel in vitro tool for detecting rabies viral antigen in brain smears and demonstrated a way to avoid the heterogeneous conjugates.[74]

Diverse molecular platforms

With the ongoing advent of molecular platforms, we continue to observe a variety of unique and powerful technologies. One such platform is the utilization of three enzymes to produce many copies of RNA in isothermal conditions. This assay is nucleic acid sequence-based amplification (NASBA). The NASBA can be automated and allows for rapid and user-friendly testing of samples, and researchers report equivalent sensitivity to conventional PCR assays for rabies viral RNA detection in antemortem CSF and saliva.[75]

Another unique method of amplification of DNA with high specificity and efficiency is known as loop-mediated isothermal amplification (LAMP). The LAMP has no requirement for thermal cycling and has been used for rabies diagnosis.[19,76] In the absence of technological requirements found with RT-PCR, it can be used to create surveillance protocols in the field and in countries with less-developed laboratories.

Other alternative platforms

The ELISA-based methods, where appropriate, are being used as an alternative to RFFIT.[77] The driving force for using these methods are their simplicity, affordability, user-friendliness, timeliness, and safety features when compared with the RFFIT. Assays that do not require live virus and high-containment facilities and produce rapid results have been validated and found to correlate well with RFFIT.[78,79] The downside to these methods

is their antigen-binding nature versus functional detection of actual neutralizing antibodies.

An ELISA based on monoclonal antibodies to rabies nucleoprotein (N) and glycoprotein (G) rabies-specific immune complexes in CSF samples for rapid antemortem diagnosis of human rabies can be detected by ELISA monoclonal antibodies.[80] Another example can be seen with the Platelia Rabies II ELISA that detects rabies (G) antibodies in human serum and CSF samples and correlates well with RFFIT.[17] Despite several advantages, ELISA tests are subject to lower sensitivity and less dynamic range than neutralization tests.[81–83] The rapid neutralizing antibody detection test (RAPINA) based on immunochromatography was found to be an easy and rapid method for qualitative and semiquantitative detection of rabies-neutralizing antibodies in humans and dogs.[84] Latex agglutination tests for rabies-specific antibodies have been used.[85] Genetic engineering advancements have improved ELISA-based assays. For example, a unique double-sandwich ELISA that takes advantage of recombinant antigen preparation can detect rabies antibodies in dogs and other species.[86] Other researchers have described a first-time use of a recombinant diabody (a noncovalent dimer) for an ELISA quantification of rabies viral glycoprotein content in rabies vaccine for humans, which use the strain Pasteur vaccine variant of rabies virus and its comparison with the mouse protection test.[87]

To minimize the safety risks inherent to neutralization assays involving replicating rabies and other lyssaviruses, including field use, pseudotypes have been developed using lentiviruses expressing the predominant rabies neutralizing antigens.[88,89]

Proteomics and metabolomics are being studied as possible diagnostic tools to detect rabies. One study reported quantitative proteomic analysis in human brain tissues obtained at autopsy from confirmed cases of encephalitic and paralytic rabies to identify signature proteins that are differentially regulated using high-resolution mass spectrometry. Protein karyopherin alpha 4 (KPNA4) was overexpressed only in paralytic rabies, protein calcium calmodulin-dependent kinase 2 alpha (CAMK2A) was upregulated in paralytic rabies, and protein glutamate ammonia ligase was overexpressed both in paralytic and encephalitic rabies. Further investigation of these possible rabies "markers" in body fluids (CSF) in a larger cohort of rabies cases is warranted to determine their potential use as antemortem diagnostic biomarkers.[90]

Metabolomics of human CSF treated for rabies using proton nuclear magnetic resonance for hydrogen-1

(1H-NMR) spectroscopy identified several metabolites that differentiated rabies survivors from those who subsequently died.[21] Proteomics and metabolomics may reveal novel diagnostic and monitoring tools for rabies cases, including future therapy.

LN34 pan-lyssavirus real-time RT-PCR assay – a new gold standard?

The current reference method and gold standard for postmortem diagnosis of human and animal rabies is the DFA test. The DFA test has proven itself historically over many decades as a sensitive and reliable test. However, there are limitations and disadvantages such as the requirements of high-quality antibody conjugates, skilled medical laboratory scientists, a fluorescent microscope, and high-specimen quality. As mentioned previously, the LN34 pan-lyssavirus real-time RT-PCR assay represents a strong candidate for rabies postmortem diagnostics because of its ability to detect RNA across the diverse *Lyssavirus* genus, high sensitivity, potential for use with deteriorated tissues, and user-friendly design. Gigante et al. recently presented data from a multisite evaluation of the LN34 assay in 14 laboratories using 2978 samples (1049 DFA positive) from Africa, the Americas, Asia, Europe, and the Middle East. High diagnostic specificity (99.68%) and sensitivity (99.90%) were shown compared with the DFA test (no DFA-positive samples were negative by the LN34 assay) and the LN34 assay exhibited low variability in repeatability and reproducibility studies. Likewise, it was capable of detecting viral RNA in fresh, frozen, archived, deteriorated, and formalin-fixed brain tissue, which is a significant advantage over the DFA. The LN34 assay produced definitive findings for 80 samples that were inconclusive or untestable by DFA; 29 were positive. Five samples were inconclusive by the LN34 assay, and only one sample was inconclusive by both tests. Finally, use of the LN34 assay identified 1 false-negative and 11 false-positive DFA results. These findings demonstrate the reliability and robustness of the LN34 assay and support a role for enhancing and improving rabies diagnostics and surveillance.[64]

Challenges of diagnostic decisions

There are unique and sometimes difficult decision points on the path to a rabies diagnosis. Fig. 4.6 illustrates choosing which assay to use at a particular time in the course of a known or suspected case of rabies is an important point to consider.[91] In most cases, direct diagnosis of rabies cases using the DFA "gold" reference technique should be implemented in national reference laboratories. Only experienced teams must use direct diagnosis by molecular-based nucleic acid

amplification test assays. These research-use only assays, based on validated in-house tests, are not standardized, commercially available kits. The recent validation of the LN34 qPCR assay by 14 laboratories predicts that reference techniques may change.[64] Reference and research laboratories typically conduct any isolation of the virus (cell culture). Isolation of the virus, as well as PCR-based methods, may be used as a second-line test to confirm negative results of other tests, such as DFA in animals, or in the case of isolation to amplify live virus from original samples.

For postmortem human brain samples, the DFA and PCR-based techniques are highly effective for the detection of RABV antigen and genome, respectively. Likewise, RT-PCR and RT-qPCR are useful alternatives to the DFA for these samples. Saliva or nuchal skin biopsy samples for antemortem or postmortem diagnosis in humans may also be tested by these methods.[91] Needle biopsy methods may be merited for situations when open autopsies are disallowed.[92,93]

Choosing an assay (see Fig. 4.6) may vary depending on the nature of the sample to be tested and also its state of preservation.[94] For instance, the DFA continues to be less expensive than RT-PCR and can be used to test in-house; however, RT-PCR remains more effective when testing destroyed or decomposed samples.[95] In many rabies-endemic areas, there is no practical shipping entity to transport samples to the laboratory, which makes it difficult to maintain staff competence in conducting the DFA, and fluorescent conjugates may expire. For example, if there is no way to transport specimens to the laboratory, then the working staff may lose "laboratory practical competence" in determining true rabies positive samples from a contaminated sample because they are not reading enough tests in a given time range. User-friendliness, laboratory infrastructure, and the cost and ease of maintenance of this equipment are just some important factors to consider in choosing the proper assay.[96] Rabies is classified as a hazard group 3 pathogen[96] but a level 2 biosafety laboratory (BSL-2) is considered adequate containment for regular rabies diagnosis and other activities, as long as they are performed by duly immunized personnel and are not associated with a high potential for droplet or aerosol production and do not involve large quantities or high concentrations of infectious material.[91] BSL-2 containment is standard practice in clinical laboratories and suffices for routine laboratory diagnostics of the rare rabies patient; the laboratory should be advised to ensure optimal technique. It is important to note the advantages of RNA, proteomic and metabolomic-based assays, and pseudoviruses as avoiding the need for containment laboratories. PCR,

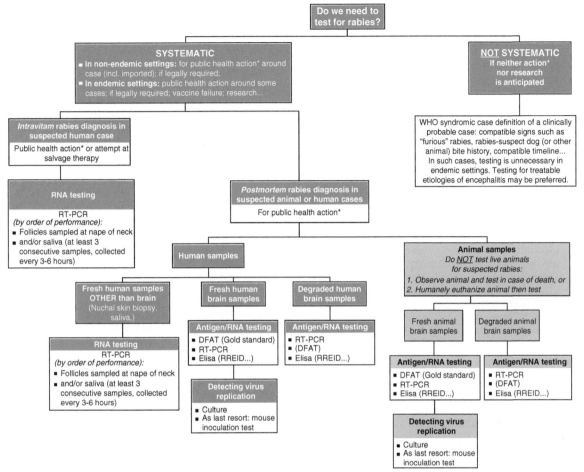

FIG. 4.6 **Proposed Rabies Testing Algorithm Based on the Objectives of Testing and the Methods to be Used in a Specialized Laboratory.** Disclaimer: Always check to ensure compliance with local testing recommendations and requirements. (Reprinted with permission from Elsevier *Int J Infect Dis*. 2016; 46:107–114.)[91]

mass spectrometry (MS), and NMR machines are far more ubiquitous than rabies reference laboratories; MS and NMR files can be disseminated electronically to reference labs.

CONCLUSIONS

Currently in the United States, vaccination of domestic animals and other public health practices have made cases of rabies in humans rare. People employed in fields associated with high risk of exposure to rabies (for example, veterinary, laboratory, and animal care and control personnel) have the added advantage of rabies preexposure vaccination. However, unknown exposures to animals (especially bats) will undoubtedly continue

to place people and animals at risk for rabies. As early clinical signs and symptoms of rabies in humans typically result in a visit to an emergency department or urgent care physicians, it is crucial that medical personnel be aware of the signs and symptoms associated with rabies infection.

Rabies testing in North America is performed yearly on more than 100,000 animal specimens by more than 100 laboratories that offer rabies diagnosis. Each positive case has ramifications for a minimum of at least one human or one domestic animal and typically involves three to ten, or even hundreds to tens of thousands of persons at public venues (for example, finding a rabid bat at a heavily frequented mall) in need of triage for potential exposure to rabies.[97]

REFERENCES

1. Rohde RE. Don't touch that bat – a rabies educational case study. In: *ASCLS – Michigan Conference, Lansing, Michigan*; 2016.

2. Bourhy H, Kissi B, Tordo N. Molecular diversity of the Lyssavirus genus. *Virology*. 1993;194:70–81.

3. Manning SE, Rupprecht CE, Fishbein D, et al. Human rabies prevention—United States, 2008: recommendations of the advisory committee on immunization practices. *MMWR Recomm Rep*. 2008;57(RR-3):1–28.

4. Rupprecht CE, Briggs D, Brown CM, et al. Use of a reduced (4-dose) vaccine schedule for postexposure prophylaxis to prevent human rabies. *MMWR Recomm Rep*. 2010;59(RR-2): 1–9.

5. Noah DL, Drenzek CL, Smith JS, et al. Epidemiology of human rabies in the United States, 1980–1996. *Ann Intern Med*. 1998;128:922–930.

6. Gilbert AT, Petersen BW, Recuenco S, et al. Evidence of rabies virus exposure among humans in the Peruvian Amazon. *Am J Trop Med Hyg*. 2012;87(2):206–215.

7. Holzmann-Pazgal G, Wanger A, Degaffe G, et al. Presumptive abortive human rabies - Texas, 2009. *MMWR (Morb Mortal Wkly Rep)*. 2010;59(7):185–190.

8. Rohde RE, Mayes BC. Molecular diagnosis and epidemiology of rabies. In: Hu P, Hedge M, Lennon PA, eds. *Modern Clinical Molecular Techniques*. New York: Springer Press; 2012:199–211.

9. Rohde RE, Wilson PJ, Mayes BC, et al. Rabies: methods and guidelines for assessing a clinical rarity. *ASCP Microbio No. MB-4 Tech Sample*. 2004:21–29.

10. Willoughby Jr RE. Rare human infection – common questions. *Infect Dis Clin*. 2015;29(4):637–650.

11. Centers for Disease Control and Prevention. *Possible Human Rabies—human Patient Form*. Available at: https://www.cdc.gov/rabies/pdf/rorform.pdf.

12. Texas Administrative Code. *Rabies Control and Eradication*; 2013. http://texreg.sos.state.tx.us/public/readtac$ext.View TAC?tac_view=5&ti=25&pt=1&ch=169&sch=A&rl=Y.

13. Brown CM, Slavinski S, Ettestad P, et al. Compendium of animal rabies prevention and control. *JAVMA*. 2016;248(5):505–517.

14. World Health Organization. *WHO Expert Consultation of Rabies – Third Report. WHO Technical Report Series*. 2018; 1012:1–183.

15. Centers for Disease Control and Prevention. *Collection of Samples for Diagnosis of Rabies in Humans*. Available at: https://www.cdc.gov/rabies/resources/specimen-submission-guidelines.html.

16. Nguyen KA, Nguyen TT, Nguyen DV, et al. Evaluation of rapid neutralizing antibody detection test against rabies virus in human sera. *Trop Med Health*. 2015;43(2):111–116.

17. Feyssaguet M, Dacheux L, Audry L, et al. Multicenter comparative study of a new ELISA, PLATELIA RABIES II, for the detection and titration of anti-rabies glycoprotein antibodies and comparison with the rapid fluorescent focus inhibition test (RFFIT) on human samples from vaccinated and non-vaccinated people. *Vaccine*. 2007;25(12):2244–2251.

18. Eggerbauer E, De BP, Hoffmann B, et al. Evaluation of six commercially available rapid immunochromatographic tests for the diagnosis of rabies in brain material. *PLoS Negl Trop Dis*. 2016;10(6):e0004776.

19. Boldbaatar B, Inoue S, Sugiura N, et al. Rapid detection of rabies virus by reverse transcription loop-mediated isothermal amplification. *J Infect Dis*. 2009;62(3):187–191.

20. Santos Katz IS, Dias MH, Lima IF, et al. Large protein as a potential target for use in rabies diagnostics. *Acta Virol*. 2017;61(3):280–288.

21. O'Sullivan A, Willoughby RE, Mishchuk D, et al. Metabolomics of cerebrospinal fluid from humans treated for rabies. *J Proteome Res*. 2013;12(1):481–490.

22. Smith JS. Rabies virus. In: Murray PR, Baron EJ, Pfaller MA, et al., eds. *Manual of Clinical Microbiology*. seventh ed. Washington, DC: American Society for Microbiology; 1999:1099–1106.

23. Willoughby Jr RE. Rabies: rare human infection - common questions. *Infect Dis Clin*. 2015;29(4):637–650.

24. Whitfield SG, Fekadu M, Shaddock JH, et al. A comparative study of the fluorescent antibody test for rabies diagnosis in fresh and formalin-fixed brain tissue specimens. *J Virol Methods*. 2001;95:145–151.

25. Hayes MA, Piaggio AJ. Assessing the potential impacts of a changing climate on the distribution of a rabies virus vector. *PLoS One*. 2018;13(2):e0192887. Available at: https://doi.org/10.1371/journal.pone.0192887.

26. Rohde RE, Neill SU, Clark KA, et al. Molecular epidemiology of rabies epizootics in Texas. *J Clin Virol*. 1997;8:209–217.

27. Hemachudha T, Ugolini G, Wacharapluesadee S, et al. Human rabies: neuropathogenesis, diagnosis, and management. *Lancet Neurol*. 2013;12:498–513.

28. Gable MS, Gavali S, Radner A, et al. Anti-NMDA receptor encephalitis: report of ten cases and comparison with viral encephalitis. *Eur J Clin Microbiol Infect Dis*. 2009;28(12):1421–1429.

29. Mallewa M, Fooks AR, Banda D, et al. Rabies encephalitis in malaria-endemic area, Malawi, Africa. *Emerg Infect Dis*. 2007;13(1):136–139.

30. Hemachudha T, Wacharapluesadee S, Mitrabhakdi E, et al. Pathophysiology of human paralytic rabies. *J Neurovirol*. 2005;11(1):93–100.

31. Gadre G, Satishchandra P, Mahadevan A, et al. Rabies viral encephalitis: clinical determinants in diagnosis with special reference to paralytic form. *J Neurol Neurosurg Psychiat*. 2010;81(7):812–820.

32. Udawat H, Chaudhary HR, Goyal RK, et al. Guillain-Barre syndrome following antirabies semple vaccine—a report of six cases. *J Assoc Phys India*. 2001;49:384–385.

33. Sheikh KA, Ramos-Alvarez M, Jackson AC, et al. Overlap of pathology in paralytic rabies and axonal Guillain-Barré syndrome. *Ann Neurol*. 2005;57(5):768–772.

34. Mani RS, Madhusudana SN. Review article – laboratory diagnosis of human rabies: recent advances. *Sci World J*. 2013:1–10.

35. Srinivasan A, Burton EC, Kuehnert MJ, et al. Transmission of rabies virus from an organ donor to four transplant recipients. *NEJM*. 2005;352(11):1103–1111.

36. Hellenbrand W, Meyer C, Rasch G, et al. Cases of rabies in Germany following organ transplantation. *Euro Surveill*. 2005;10(2):Article ID E050224.6.

37. Vora NM, Basavaraju SV, Feldman KA, et al. Transplant associated rabies virus transmission investigation team. Raccoon rabies virus variant transmission through solid organ transplantation. *JAMA*. 2013;310(4):398–407.

38. Willoughby Jr RE, Tieves KS, Hoffman GM, et al. Survival after treatment of rabies with induction of coma. *NEJM*. 2005;352(24):2508–2514.

39. Solomon T, Marston D, Mallewa M, et al. Lesson of the week: paralytic rabies after a two-week holiday in India. *Br Med J*. 2005;331(7515):501–503.

40. Sidwa TJ, Wilson PJ, Moore GM, et al. Evaluation of oral rabies vaccination programs for control of rabies epizootics in coyotes and gray foxes: 1995–2003. *JAVMA*. 2005;227(5):785–792.

41. Leslie MJ, Messenger S, Rohde RE, et al. Bat-associated rabies virus in skunks. *Emerg Infect Dis*. 2006;12(05). http://www.cdc.gov/ncidod/EID/vol12no08/05-1526.htm.

42. Mayes BC, Wilson PJ, Oertli EH, et al. Epidemiology of rabies in bats in Texas. 2001–2010. *JAVMA*. 2013;243:1129–1137.

43. Wilson PJ, Rohde RE. *8 Things You May Not Know about Rabies but Should*. Elsevier Connect; 2015. htpps://www.elsevier.com/connect/8-things-you-may-not-know-about-rabies-but-should.

44. Wilson PJ, Rohde RE. *The Many Faces of Rabies*. Elsevier Connect; 2016. htpps://www.elsevier.com/connect/the-many-faces-of-rabies.

45. Negri A. Beitrag zum Studium der Aetiologie der Tollwuth. *Zeitschrift fur Hygiene und Infections krankheiten*. 1903;43:507–527.

46. Sellers TF. Status of rabies in the United States in 1921. *Am J Public Health*. 1923;13:742–747.

47. Koprowsky H. The mouse inoculation test. In: Meslin FX, Kaplan MM, Koprowsky H, eds. *Laboratory Techniques in Rabies*. fourth ed. Geneva, Switzerland: WHO; 1996:80–87.

48. Webster WA, Casey GA. Virus isolation in neuroblastoma cell culture. In: Meslin FX, Kaplan MM, Koprowsky H, eds. *Laboratory Techniques in Rabies*. fourth ed. Geneva, Switzerland: WHO; 1996:96–104.

49. *Manual of Diagnostic Tests and Vaccines for Terrestrial Animals (OIE)*. 2013. Available from: http://www.oie.int/fileadmin/Home/eng/Health_standards/tahm/2.01.17_RABIES.pdf.

50. Perrin P, Rollin PE, Sureau P. A rapid rabies enzyme immuno-diagnosis (RREID): a useful and simple technique for the routine diagnosis of rabies. *J Biol Stand*. 1986;14(3):217–222.

51. Netravathi M, Udani V, Mani R, et al. Unique clinical and imaging findings in a first ever documented PCR positive rabies survival patient: a case report. *J Clin Virol*. 2015;70:83–88.

52. Willoughby Jr RE. *Rabies Treatment Protocol and Registry*(5); 2018. Available from: https://www.mcw.edu/departments/pediatrics/divisions/infectious-diseases/rabies-registry-website.

53. Webster LT, Dawson R. Early diagnosis of rabies by mouse inoculation: measurement of humoral immunity to rabies by mouse protection test. *PSEBM (Proc Soc Exp Biol Med)*. 1935;32:570–573.

54. Smith JS, Yager PA, Baer GM. A rapid fluorescent focus inhibition test (RFFIT) for determining rabies virus neutralizing antibody. In: Meslin FX, Kaplan MM, Koprowsky H, eds. *Laboratory Techniques in Rabies*. fourth ed. Geneva, Switzerland: WHO; 1996:181–191.

55. Cliquet F, Aubert M, Sagn´e L. Development of a fluorescent antibody virus neutralisation test (FAVN test) for the quantitation of rabies-neutralising antibody. *J Immunol Methods*. 1998;212(1):79–87.

56. Neizgoda M, Rupprecht CE. *Standard Operating Procedure for the Direct Rapid Immunohistochemistry Test for the Detection of Rabies Virus Antigen*. Atlanta: National Laboratory Training Network Course; US Department of Health and Human Services; Centers for Disease Control and Prevention; 2006.

57. Dyer JL, Niezgoda M, Orciari LA, et al. Evaluation of an indirect rapid immunohistochemistry test for the differentiation of rabies virus variants. *J Virol Methods*. 2013;190(1–2):29–33.

58. Sacramento D, Bourhy H, Tordo N. PCR technique as an alternative method for diagnosis and molecular epidemiology of rabies virus. *Mol Cell Probes*. 1991;5:229–240.

59. Nagaraj T, Vasanth JP, Desai A, et al. Antemortem diagnosis of human rabies using saliva samples: comparison of real time and conventional RT-PCR techniques. *J Clin Virol*. 2006;36(1):17–23.

60. Hayman DTS, Banyard AC, Wakeley PR, et al. A universal real-time assay for the detection of Lyssaviruses. *J Virol Methods*. 2011;177(1):87–93.

61. Nadin-Davis SA, Sheen M, Wandeler AI. Development of real-time reverse transcriptase polymerase chain reaction methods for human rabies diagnosis. *J Med Virol*. 2009;81(8):1484–1497.

62. Hughes GJ, Smith JS, Hanlon CA, et al. Evaluation of a TaqMan PCR assay to detect rabies virus RNA: influence of sequence variation and application to quantification of viral loads. *J Clin Microbiol*. 2004;42(1):299–306.

63. Faye M, Dacheux L, Weidmann M, et al. Development and validation of sensitive real-time RT-PCR assay for broad detection of rabies virus. *J Virol Methods*. 2017;243:120–130.

64. Gigante CM, Dettinger L, Powell JW, et al. Multi-site evaluation of the LN34 pan-lyssavirus real-time RT-PCR assay for post-mortem rabies diagnostics. *PLoS One*. 2018;13(5):e0197074.

65. Dupuis M, Brunt S, Appler K, et al. Comparison of automated quantitative reverse transcription-PCR and direct fluorescent-antibody detection for routine rabies diagnosis in the United States. *J Clin Microbiol*. 2015;53:2983–2989.

66. Kang B, Oh J, Lee C, et al. Evaluation of a rapid immunodiagnostic test kit for rabies virus. *J Virol Methods.* 2007;145(1):30–36.

67. Kasempimolporn S, Saengseesom W, Huadsakul S, et al. Evaluation of a rapid immunochromatographic test strip for detection of rabies virus in dog saliva samples. *J Vet Diagn Invest.* 2011;23(6):1197–1201.

68. Nishizono A, Khawplod P, Ahmed K, et al. A simple and rapid immunochromatographic test kit for rabies diagnosis. *Microbiol Immunol.* 2008;52(4):243–249.

69. Ahmed K, Wimalaratne O, Dahal N, et al. Evaluation of a monoclonal antibody-based rapid immunochromatographic test for direct detection of rabies virus in the brain of humans and animals. *Am J Trop Med Hyg.* 2012;86(4):736–740.

70. Xu G, Weber P, Hu Q, et al. A simple sandwich ELISA (WELYSSA) for the detection of lyssavirus nucleocapsid in rabies suspected specimens using mouse monoclonal antibodies. *Biologicals.* 2007;35(4):297–302.

71. Xu G, Weber P, Hu Q, et al. WELYSSA: a simple tool using mouse monoclonal antibodies for the detection of lyssavirus nucleocapsid in rabies suspected specimens. *Dev Biol.* 2008;131:555–561.

72. Madhusudana SN, Paul JPV, Abhilash KV, et al. Rapid diagnosis of rabies in humans and animals by a dot blot enzyme immunoassay. *Int J Infect Dis.* 2004;8(6):339–345.

73. Vasanth JP, Madhusudana SN, Abhilash KV, et al. Development and evaluation of an enzyme immunoassay for rapid diagnosis of rabies in humans and animals. *Indian J Pathol Microbiol.* 2004;47(4):574–578.

74. Mousli M, Turki I, Kharmachi H, et al. Genetically engineered colorimetric single-chain antibody fusion protein for rapid diagnosis of rabies virus. *Dev Biol.* 2008;131:483–491.

75. Wacharapluesadee S, Phumesin P, Supavonwong P, et al. Comparative detection of rabies RNA by NASBA, real-time PCR and conventional PCR. *J Virol Methods.* 2011;175(2):278–282.

76. Muleya W, Namangala B, Mweene A, et al. Molecular epidemiology and a loop-mediated isothermal amplification method for diagnosis of infection with rabies virus in Zambia. *Virus Res.* 2012;163(1):160–168.

77. Caicedo Y, Paez A, Kuzmin I, et al. Virology, immunology and pathology of human rabies during treatment. *Pediatr Infect Dis J.* 2015;34(5):520–528.

78. Servat A, Feyssaguet M, Blanchard I, et al. A quantitative indirect ELISA to monitor the effectiveness of rabies vaccination in domestic and wild carnivores. *J Immunol Methods.* 2007;318(1–2):1–10.

79. Muhamuda K, Madhusudana SN, Ravi V. Development and evaluation of a competitive ELISA for estimation of rabies neutralizing antibodies after post-exposure rabies vaccination in humans. *Int J Infect Dis.* 2007;11(5):441–445.

80. Muhamuda K, Madhusudana SN, Ravi V, et al. Presence of rabies specific immune complexes in cerebrospinal fluid can help in ante-mortem diagnosis of human paralytic rabies. *J Clin Virol.* 2006;37(3):162–167.

81. Cliquet F, McElhinney LM, Servat A, et al. Development of a qualitative indirect ELISA for the measurement of rabies virus specific antibodies from vaccinated dogs and cats. *J Virol Methods.* 2004;117(1):1–8.

82. Servat A, Cliquet F. Collaborative study to evaluate a new ELISA test to monitor the effectiveness of rabies vaccination in domestic carnivores. *Virus Res.* 2006;120(1–2): 17–27.

83. Welch RJ, Anderson BL, Litwin CM. An evaluation of two commercially available ELISAs and one in-house reference laboratory ELISA for the determination of human anti-rabies virus antibodies. *J Med Microbiol.* 2009;58(6):806–810.

84. Nishizono A, Yamada K, Khawplod P, et al. Evaluation of an improved rapid neutralizing antibody detection test (RAPINA) for qualitative and semiquantitative detection of rabies neutralizing antibody in humans and dogs. *Vaccine.* 2012;30(26):3891–3896.

85. Madhusudana SN, Saraswati S. Development and evaluation of a latex agglutination test for rabies antibodies. *J Clin Virol.* 2003;27(2):129–135.

86. Yang L-M, Zhao L-Z, Hu R-L, et al. A novel double-antigen sandwich enzyme-linked immunosorbent assay for measurement of antibodies against rabies virus. *Clin Vaccine Immunol.* 2006;13(8):966–968.

87. Nimmagadda SV, Aavula SM, Biradhar N, et al. Recombinant diabody-based immunocapture enzyme-linked immunosorbent assay for quantification of rabies virus glycoprotein. *Clin Vaccine Immunol.* 2010;17(8):1261–1268.

88. Nie J, Wu X, Ma J, et al. Development of in vitro and in vivo rabies virus neutralization assays based on a high-titer pseudovirus system. *Sci Rep.* 2017;7:42769.

89. Moeschler S, Locher S, Conzelmann KK, et al. Quantification of lyssavirus-neutralizing antibodies using vesicular stomatitis virus pseudotype particles. *Viruses.* 2016;8(9).

90. Venugopal AK, Ghantasala SS, Selvan LD, et al. Quantitative proteomics for identifying biomarkers for Rabies. *Clin Proteomics.* 2013;10(1):article 3.

91. Duong V, Tarantola A, Ong S, et al. Laboratory diagnostics in dog-mediated rabies: an overview of performance and a proposed strategy for various settings. *Int J Infect Dis.* 2016;46:107–114.

92. Iamamoto K, Quadros J, Queiroz LH. Use of aspiration method for collecting brain samples for rabies diagnosis in small wild animals. *Zoonoses Public Health.* 2011;58(1):28–31.

93. Tong TR, Leung KM, Lee KC, et al. Trucut needle biopsy through superior orbital fissure for the diagnosis of rabies. *Lancet.* 1999;354(9196):2137–2138.

94. Fooks AR, Johnson N, Freuling CM, et al. Emerging technologies for the detection of rabies virus: challenges and hopes in the 21st century. *PLoS Neglected Trop Dis.* 2009;3(9).

95. Beltran F, Dohmen F, Del Pietro H, et al. Diagnosis and molecular typing of rabies virus in samples stored in inadequate conditions. *J Infect Developing Countries.* 2014;8(8):1016–1021.

96. Advisory Committee on Dangerous Pathogens. *The Approved List of Biological Agents. Bootle, United Kingdom:* Health and Safety Executive; 2013. Available at: http://www .hse.gov.uk/pubns/misc208.pdf.

97. Hanlon CA, Nadin-Davis S. Chapter 11 – laboratory diagnosis of rabies. In: Jackson A, ed. *Rabies (Third Edition) Scientific Basis of the Disease and its Management.* San Diego: Academic Press, Elsevier; 2013:409– 459.

FURTHER READING

1. Wright E, McNabb S, Goddard T, et al. A robust lentiviral pseudotype neutralisation assay for in-field serosurveillance of rabies and lyssaviruses in Africa. *Vaccine.* 2009;27(51):7178–7186.

CHAPTER 5

Common Myths and Legends of Rabies

RODNEY E. ROHDE, PhD, MS, SM(ASCP)^{CM}, SV^{CM}, MB^{CM}, FACSc

INTRODUCTION

Rabies has been a part of human history for as long as it has been recorded in writing and art. From Odysseus's story to Achilles, the actual word (term) that provoked and transformed Hector to a rage and frenzy, "lyssa," is closely linked to the word "lykos" or "wolf" and is used to invoke images and feelings of an animal's anger, madness, and wolfish rage.[1] Lyssavirus is a genus of RNA viruses in the family Rhabdoviridae, order Mononegavirales. Lyssaviruses are bullet-shaped, single-stranded, negative-sense RNA viruses and the causative agents of the ancient zoonosis rabies. Africa is the likely home to the ancestors of taxa residing within the genus Lyssavirus, family Rhabdoviridae. Diverse lyssaviruses are envisioned as coevolving with bats, as the ultimate reservoirs, over seemingly millions of years (Fig. 5.1).[2]

Through eons of time, a wide range of myths and legends have developed pertaining to rabies. Many people still believe today that rabies treatment requires 20 or more shots into the stomach by some monstrously long needle. While in fact, today's treatment regimen is typically only four vaccinations (five for immunocompromised individuals) in the arm, plus a dose of humane rabies immune globulin (HRIG). This myth is but one of a long list of questions, untruths, or exaggerations about the disease known as rabies.

- Is there a way to vaccinate wildlife using a recombinant vaccine dropped from aircraft?[3–14]
- Can scientists actually determine the origin of a rabies virus variant by way of genetic testing and methodologies?[3–14]
- Are there special government laboratories that conduct specialized rabies testing?[3–14]
- Can international public health teams actually halt and remove a moving viral epizootic outbreak in a geographical area?[3–14]
- Is there a relationship between rabies and zombies?[15]

In this chapter, some of the more common misconceptions (and facts) about rabies will be described. These misconceptions are categorized under concepts of prevalence, signs and symptoms, exposure, treatment, and pop culture influence with respect to rabies.

MISUNDERSTOOD CONCEPTS OF THE PREVALENCE OF RABIES

Where exactly do most cases of rabies occur in the world? Which type of animals are often more "at risk" for contracting rabies virus, otherwise known as high-risk animals? Are there places in the world where one might travel without worrying about rabies? Do cold-blooded animals, insects, or birds have a risk for acquiring this deadly disease? There are many untruths to unpack with respect to the prevalence of rabies. Learn more in the following accounts:

- Many people believe that rabies infections only occur in poor, third-world countries. However, the truth is that rabies or rabies-like viruses are present on nearly every continent, with the exception of Antarctica. Numerous and diverse variants of lyssaviruses are found in a wide variety of animal species throughout the world, all of which may cause fatal human rabies. Rabies virus is by far the most common lyssavirus infection of humans. In the United States, only Hawaii is rabies free. Interestingly, in Hawaii and other rabies-free areas that are often islands, there are very strict laws and restrictions on the transport of animals from rabies-endemic states or countries to rabies-free geographic locations. In the United States, rabies as a disease is most prevalent along the East Coast (raccoon and bat rabies virus variants) from Florida to Maine and in Southern Arizona (Arizona gray fox) along the Mexican border. Rabies is also prevalent in Texas with south central skunk and bat rabies virus variants predominating.

Rabies. https://doi.org/10.1016/B978-0-323-63979-8.00005-2
Copyright © 2019 Elsevier Inc. All rights reserved.

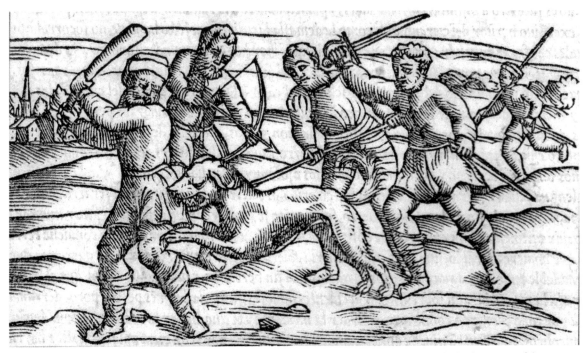

FIG. 5.1 A woodcut from the middle ages showing a rabid dog. (Reprinted with permission by source, fair use: https://en.wikipedia.org/wiki/Rabies#/media/File:Middle_Ages_rabid_dog.jpg.)

As a side note, one should always consider the risk of infectious disease when traveling to other countries by discussing travel plans with an appropriate person such as a travel physician or other health-care professional. There may be a need to plan for preexposure vaccinations (e.g., rabies, yellow fever, etc.) or medications (e.g., malaria, antibiotics) to take on their travels.[16]

- A frequent belief is that this disease kills many people in the United States. However, approximately 95% of human deaths from the disease occur in Africa and Asia, where access to health-care facilities and treatment protocols is limited. The estimated annual figure of almost 59,000 rabies fatalities in humans is probably an underestimate. Almost all cases of rabies in humans worldwide result from bites from infected dogs.[17,18] Rabies cases in humans in the United States are rare, with only one to three cases reported annually. Forty three cases of rabies in humans have been reported in the United States and its territories from January 2003 through November 2018 (Table 5.1). Almost all of the cases are attributed to bat rabies with 11 of the total cases contracted outside of the United States and its territories. Of the 43 rabies cases, there were three survivors (40 deaths). For 2018, there have been three cases, with the most recent case (death) being a 74-year-old male from Utah from bat rabies (not included in Table 1).[19]

- All warm-blooded animals can contract rabies, particularly mammals. A viral disease of the central nervous system, rabies transmits between animals, including humans, when saliva containing the virus enters an opening in the skin. Usually, the rabies virus enters through the bite of a rabid animal, but transmission can also occur when infected saliva enters through mucous membranes or a break in the skin. Viral familial relatives can be found with invertebrates and plants (distant hosts), but warm-blooded vertebrates are the hosts for the rabies virus. Among warm-blooded vertebrates, birds are susceptible to infection, but rabies predominates naturally among various mammalian populations. Only rare accounts occur in nonmammalian hosts, but in the Mammalia family, rabies cases have occurred from the armadillo to the zebra. Rabies is a significant disease of domestic and wild mammals alike, yet its zoonotic aspect is the cause of major historical infamy.[2]

TABLE 5.1

Date of onset	Date of death	Reporting state	Age (y)	Sex	Exposure*	RW†
10 Feb 03	10 Mar 03	VA	25	M	Unknown	Raccoon, eastern United States
28 May 03	5 Jun 03	PR	64	M	Bite, Puerto Rico	Dog-mongoose, Puerto Rico
23 Aug 03	14 Sep 03	CA	66	M	Bite	Bat. Ln
9 Feb 04	15 Feb 04	FL	41	M	Bite. Haiti	Dog, Haiti
27 Apr 04	3 May 04	AR	20	M	Bite (organ donor)	Bat. Tb
25 May 04	31 May 04	OK	53	M	Liver transplant	Bat. Tb
27 May 04	21 Jun 04	TX	18	M	Kidney transplant	Bat. Tb
29 May 04	9 Jun 04	TX	50	F	Kidney transplant	Bat. Tb
2 Jun 04	10 Jun 04	TX	55	F	Arterial transplant	Bat. Tb
12 Oct 04	Survived	WI	15	F	Bite	Bat, unknown
19 Oct 04	26 Oct 04	CA	22	M	Unknown. El Salvador	Dog. El Salvador
27 Sep 05	27 Sep 05	MS	10	M	Contact	Bat. unknown
4 May 06	12 May 06	TX	16	M	Contact	Bat. Tb
30 Sep 06	2 Nov 06	IN	10	F	Bite	Bat. Ln
15 Nov 06	14 Dec 06	CA	II	M	Bite, Philippines	Dog, Philippines
19 Sep 07	20 Oct 07	MN	46	M	Bite	Bat. unknown
16 Mar 08	18 Mar 08	CA	16	M	Bite. Mexico	Fox. Tb related
19 Nov 08	30 Nov 08	MO	55	M	Bite	Bat. Ln
25 Feb 09	Survived	TX	17	F	Contact	Bat. unknown
5 Oct 09	20 Oct 09	IN	43	M	Unknown	Bat. Ps
20 Oct 09	II Nov 09	Ml	55	M	Contact	Bat, Ln
23 Oct 09	20 Nov 09	VA	42	M	Contact. India	Dog. India
2 Aug 10	21 Aug 10	LA	19	M	Bite, Mexico	Bat, Dr
24 Dec 10	10 Jan 11	WI	70	M	Unknown	Bat. Ps
30 Apr II	Survived	CA	8	F	Unknown	Unknown
30 Jun II	20 Jul II	NJ	73	F	Bite. Haiti	Dog, Haiti
14 Aug II	31 Aug II	NY	25	M	Contact, Afghanistan	Dog, Afghanistan
21 Aug II	1 Sep 11	NC	20	M	Unknown (organ donor)‡	Raccoon, eastern United States
1 Sep II	14 Oct II	MA	40	M	Contact, Brazil	Dog, Brazil
3 Dec II	19 Dec II	SC	46	F	Unknown	Bat. Tb
22 Dec II	23 Jan 12	MA	63	M	Contact	Bat, My sp
6 Jul 12	31 Jul 12	CA	34	M	Bite	Bat. Tb
31 Jan 13	27 Feb 13	MD	49	M	Kidney transplant	Raccoon, eastern United States
16 May 13	11 Jun 13	TX	28	M	Unknown, Guatemala	Dog, Guatemala

Continued

TABLE 5.1—cont'd						
Date of onset	Date of death	Reporting state	Age (y)	Sex	Exposure*	RW†
12 Sep 14	26 Sep 14	MO	52	M	Unknown	Bat. Ps
30 Jul 15	24 Aug 15	MA	65	M	Bite, Philippines	Dog, Philippines
17 Sep 15	3 Oct 15	WY	77	F	Contact	Bat. Ln
25 Nov 15	1 Dec 15	PR	54	M	Bite	Dog-mongoose, Puerto Rico
5 May 17	21 May 17	VA	65	F	Bite	Dog, India
6 Oct 17	21 Oct 17	FL	56	F	Bite	Bat. Tb
28 Dec 17	14 Jan 18	FL	6	M	Bite	Bat. Tb
15 Jul 18	23 Aug 18	DE	69	F	Unknown	Raccoon, eastern United States

Dr = D rotundus. Ln = L noctivagans. My sp = Myotis species. Ps = P subflavus. Tb = T brasiliensis.
*Data for exposure history are reported when plausible information was reported directly by the patient (if lucid or credible) or when a reliable account of an incident consistent with rabies virus exposure (eg, dog bite) was reported by an independent witness (usually a family member). Exposure histories are categorized as bite, contact (eg, waking to find bat on exposed skin) but no known bite was acknowledged, or unknown (ie, no known contact with an animal was elicited during case investigation). †Variants of the rabies virus associated with terrestrial animals in the United States and Puerto Rico are identified with the names of the reservoir animal (eg, dog or raccoon), followed by the name of the most definitive geographic entity (usually the country) from which the variant has been identified. Variants of the rabies virus associated with bats are identified with the names of the species of bats in which they have been found to be circulating. Because information regarding the location of the exposure and the identity of the exposing animal is almost always retrospective and much information is frequently unavailable, the location of the exposure and the identity of the animal responsible for the infection are often limited to deduction. ‡Infection was not identified until 2013. when an organ recipient developed rabies.[19]

MISUNDERSTOOD CONCEPTS ON CLINICAL SIGNS AND SYMPTOMS OF RABIES

According to the Centers for Disease Control and Prevention (CDC), the first clinical signs and symptoms of rabies may be very similar to those of the flu including general weakness or discomfort, fever, or headache. These clinical signs and symptoms may last for days and are directly related to the difficulty of a differential diagnosis of rabies in the absence of an obvious animal bite (or other) exposure.

There may be also discomfort or a prickling or itching sensation at the site of bite, progressing within days to signs and symptoms of cerebral dysfunction, anxiety, confusion, and agitation. As the disease progresses, the person may experience delirium, abnormal behavior, hallucinations, and insomnia. The acute period of disease typically ends after 2–10 days[20] (see Chapter 2). Once clinical signs of rabies appear, the disease is nearly always fatal, and treatment is typically supportive. Disease prevention includes both passive immunity, through an injection of human rabies immune globulin, and active immunity produced via a round of injections with rabies vaccine. If a person has already begun to exhibit signs of the disease, survival is rare. To date, less than 10 documented cases of human survival from clinical rabies have been reported and only two have not had a history of pre- or postexposure prophylaxis.[20]

One of the more bizarre, but not uncommon, signs and symptoms of rabies that has been reported is male patients exhibiting hypersexual behavior. The virus sometimes acts on the limbic system of the brain causing men to show this behavior: increased sexual desire, involuntary erections, and in some reports continuous orgasms occurring at a rate of one per hour![1]

In general, most people think of dogs when the topic of animals that can carry or transmit rabies is mentioned. This may be due to the long-standing fascination with the popular media (and ancient writings) that target the canine as the primary vector for rabies. For example, if you have seen the movie *Old Yeller* or *Cujo*, then you probably understand how the popular media can influence the public to fear rabies and scrutinize the family dog for any signs of "frothing or foaming" at the mouth.[1] However, the disease affects both domestic and wild animals. Early clinical signs of the illness include fever, pain, and/or a tingling sensation around the wound.[17] However, unlike the popular notion of *Old Yeller* or *Cujo*, the most typical clinical signs of rabies are unexplained paralysis and a change in behavior (refer to Chapter 2 for details). Still, there are many reports of other strange clinical behaviors by a rabid animal.[21,22]

MISUNDERSTOOD CONCEPTS OF WHAT CLASSIFIES AS AN EXPOSURE TO RABIES

One of the difficult decisions about rabies, if not the most difficult, is "what constitutes an exposure" when trying to discern whether to treat or not to treat an individual. Likewise, there are important implications for the animal (domestic). For example, whether to quarantine the animal for observation or to euthanize an animal followed by laboratory testing for confirmation of rabies. The World Health Organization (WHO) has recommendations intended as a general guide.[23] It is recognized that, in certain situations, modifications of these procedures are warranted. Such situations include exposure of infants or mentally disabled persons and other circumstances where a reliable history cannot be obtained, particularly in areas where rabies is enzootic, even though the animal is considered to be healthy at the time of exposure.

There are other myths and legends surrounding the question of a true rabies exposure. The following are a few of the common ones:

- On a given warm summer evening in areas of Texas just as dark approaches, bats start swooping in their feeding mode of eating insects, which is an ecologic and biologic benefit. This could initiate a warning from some folks about "bats getting tangled in your hair," leading to being exposed to rabies. Of course, bats are not attracted to a person's head of hair and do not try to "nest" there, but if a bat did get tangled in someone's hair, they would receive PEP if the bat could not be tested as its too close a contact to rule out a bite occurring. However, contributing to this misconception could be media and historical writings with respect to vampire lore surrounding bats.[1] Additionally, there were even popular television series like *The Andy Griffith Show* that had an episode with Barney Fife discussing bats in caves and their potential for laying "their eggs" in a person's hair (Fig. 5.2).[24]
- Can I get rabies if I handle blood, feces, or urine? The simple answer is no in this scenario. Rabies is not transmitted through the blood, urine, or feces of an infected animal, nor is it spread airborne through the open environment. Saliva provides the primary transmission medium when the animal is in the infectious stage of rabies. For the rabies virus to get to the salivary glands, it has to travel first from the site of entry (usually a bite wound) through the animal's nervous system, then to the brain. This is what causes most rabid animals to exhibit abnormal behaviors, depending on what part of the brain is infected. Finally, the virus travels to the salivary glands during the terminal stage of rabies. It is this later stage of rabies when an animal is most infectious because the virus is in the saliva.[21,22,25]

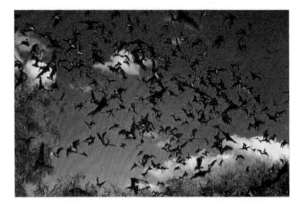

FIG. 5.2 Flying bats: this horde of flying bats could contain possible carriers of the rabies virus. (Reprinted with permission by source, fair use: Centers for Disease Control and Prevention (Public Health Image Library).)

MISUNDERSTOOD CONCEPTS ON RABIES POSTEXPOSURE PROPHYLAXIS AND TREATMENT PROTOCOLS

Treatment for rabies, one of the world's most diabolical viruses, has a long history of creative and bizarre origins. Rabies is a terrifying disease that dates as far back as the beginnings of humankind. In a sense, we humans fear rabies because it crosses the line between humanity and animal. Think about it, the disease is at the intersection of humans and animals. Somewhere deep in the psyche, one can become terrified by the thought of a bite from a rabid animal because it symbolizes the very metamorphosis of a human becoming that very rabid animal—a vampire or werewolf if you let your brain take you to that place.[1]

It should not be a surprise that humans have a long-standing and deep-seated fear of diseases with animal origins, or as science calls them, zoonotic diseases. A majority of new diseases are zoonotic. For example, swine flu, West Nile virus, anthrax, severe acute respiratory syndrome, tuberculosis, influenza, Ebola, nipah, powassan, and plague represent diseases from a wide range of eras. It is not a far reach to realize that the collective conscience of the general public has been swayed and biased by diseases with animal origins.[1] So, along with that understanding comes an almost guttural need to find ways to treat or cure those diseases. This is where some of the earliest misconceptions for treating rabies originate in our history. Let us examine some of those treatments that seem to perpetuate in time regardless of the modern advances in medicine.

- In many of the earliest recordings of the disease, the treatments centered on the wound. This makes sense when you consider that humans from early in history understood that the origin of rabies manifested in humans after a canid bite, often while the animal was drooling copious amounts of saliva (frothing at the mouth). Without listing every single early thought on treatment of these wounds, the common thread is to "bleed and cauterize (burn) the wound." For example, in early traditional Indian medicine, there is acknowledgment of the fatality of hydrophobia (fear of water in rabies patients) and a prescription of treatment for it—bleeding and cauterization of the wound. The process involved cauterizing the wound with clarified butter, which the patient is then asked to drink.[1] It is accepted even today that after an animal bite, it is wise to let it bleed, followed by rigorous washing and flushing of the wound with soap and water. However, simply closing the wound or cauterizing it will not cure one from rabies.

- Interestingly, the very pathogenesis of rabies in how it takes the central nervous system hostage to spread its deadly virions is now being studied to treat and possibly cure disease in brain cancer patients. The rabies virus, which kills tens of thousands of people a year, has a rare ability to enter nerve cells and use them as a conduit to infect brain tissue. Now, scientists are trying to mimic this strategy to ferry tumor-killing nanoparticles into brain tumors. In laymen's terms, this means using viruses to carry tiny cancer killing agents to the tumor. So far, the approach has been shown to work only in mice. If successful in people, these nanoparticles could one day help doctors send treatment directly to tumors without harming healthy cells.[26]

- Alarmingly, homeopathic and neuropathic treatments have gained some traction in the world in a variety of applications for mild to deadly diseases. Rabies is not immune to these "treatments." While there is truth that some modern day medicines and drugs come from nature (e.g., penicillin is derived from the fungus *Penicillium*), in most instances it does not replace peer-reviewed and sound clinical trial-based medical treatments or procedures. Homeopathy principles roughly state that substances that produce similar symptoms of a particular ailment can cure said ailment ("like cures like") and that diluting a substance increases its potency ("law of infinitesimals"), which brings to mind the "hair of the dog" remedy for some hangover sufferers. Recently, there was a report in which diluted saliva from a rabid dog was used to "treat" a 4-year-old boy for aggressive behavior. The first question that comes to mind is "where did the United Kingdom homeopathic pharmacy obtain rabid dog saliva?"

Regardless, the rabid dog treatment, called lyssinum (aka lyssin or hydrophobinum), is one of more than 8500 homeopathic products approved by Health Canada. There is cause for concern, including those at the US Food and Drug Administration, that such homeopathic products can be harmful and/or delay actual medical interventions and treatments. The homeopath who administered the treatment admitted that "there is no common consensus about how the remedies work" and continued to claim that it was effective and safe, plus added that the saliva was diluted to the point that it would not contain any trace of rabies virus. Most rabies experts would have concerns about this treatment.[27]

- In an earlier section of this chapter, it was mentioned that some individuals (including some in health care or other biological science majors or backgrounds) incorrectly believe that rabies treatment requires 20 or more shots into the stomach by some monstrously long needle. Actually, almost all modern treatment regimens for rabies include four key features:

  - Generous cleaning and lavage of the bite wound with soap or topical antiseptic and warm water.
  - Avoidance of wound repair. Closed bite wounds from dogs (or other animals) often become bacterially infected with early closure. The recommendation is to use very few sutures early and wait 7–14 days to more definitively close the wound.[2] Additionally, tetanus immunization boosters are indicated.
  - Human rabies immune globulin (HRIG) is essential for bridging immunity until the response to rabies vaccination occurs 10–14 days later. The HRIG is most effective when infiltrated in the wound and not intramuscularly (IM) remote from the bite wound.
  - Rabies vaccine should be a modern cell-based, inactivated vaccine. Rabies vaccine is effective when given intradermally or IM, although only the latter route is licensed in the United States. The WHO recommends several schemata for rabies immunization. In the United States, only four doses (from the original five) are now recommended (0, 3, 7, and 14 days) because an immune response is invariably present by day 14.[28] However, a fifth dose is still recommended on day 28 for individuals who are immunocompromised.[2]

Simply put, rabies usually kills its victims without early intervention. With the recent and increased attention from stories of survivors of rabies, there have been recent reports from India of natural survivors, but most often with poor functional outcomes.[29,30] The exciting new Milwaukee Protocol and its use globally has produced four survivors who have had excellent cognitive recovery and outcomes. However, two had spastic diplegia that has been described in animal survivor models of rabies.[31]

INFLUENCE OF RABIES ON POP CULTURE

It really should not be a surprise that rabies, a disease that goes back to the dawn of human civilization, continues to influence our pop culture (movies, television, art and literature, and tales told over generations). Perhaps it is because rabies has always been known to be the very transformation of a disease from animal to man that is easily observed. The CDC estimates that zoonotic diseases are very common, both in America and globally. They estimate that more than 6 out of every 10 known infectious diseases in people are derived from animals and 3 out of every 4 new or emerging infectious diseases in people are transmitted from animals.[32]

Historically, humans just did not see the connection of infectious disease to animals. Scientists and scholars blamed nearly everything but animals. Even some of the nastiest culprits of disease like smallpox (albeit this infection is not zoonotic) or Black Death (bubonic plague), which spreads to humans via respiratory droplets or by way of hitching a ride on a rat or other rodents via a flea vector, were often misunderstood regarding transmission or cause. Usually, this meant that things such as demons, bad air (literal meaning of malaria), heavenly bodies/stars, and even human behavior were the root of disease. Almost all of them were blamed on nonhuman hosts, except for rabies and anthrax. Regardless of how far one goes back in time, one did not need to look further than the consequences of what happened after a human was bitten by a "mad dog" or other animal. In addition, to add insult to injury (literally), it was often the owner's very own best friend—the dog.[1]

If one looks to the time of Greek myth, we find Lycaon, king of Arcadia, transforming into a slavering wolf with rabid and foamy jaws. In fifteenth century Spain, we read about witch-hunters called saludadores and they were known as healers of rabies. During the interim of the 15th and 18th centuries, our European counterparts were building two well-known legends— the werewolf and vampire—which had the ability to be human and animal and pass on this ability via the bite. Even as we approach the 19th century with viruses becoming more understood by science and the discovery of Pasteur's rabies vaccine, people of France were

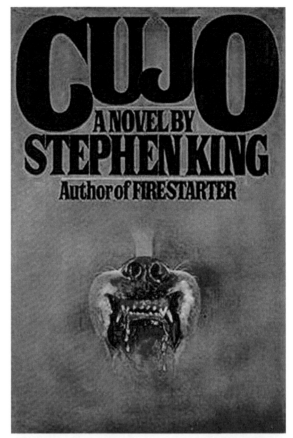

FIG. 5.3 *Cujo* book cover. (Reprinted with permission by source, fair use: https://en.wikipedia.org/wiki/Cujo#/media/File:Cujo_(book_cover).jpg.)

still transfixed and terrified by the fantasy and horror that a rabies infection converted people into maddened animals. Ironically, their horror (fantasy) had some foundation.[1]

Even after Pasteur's vaccine, which miraculously could save one from certain death by rabies if given prior to signs and symptoms, humankind's ongoing rabid fantasy about possible monster metamorphoses with rabies continues in the pop culture and is going strong to this day. One needs to look no further than even possibly American's most trusted media icon, Walt Disney, when he released *Old Yeller* or about 24 years later when the novel *Cujo* (and later film) transfixed audiences to fear rabies (Figs. 5.3 and 5.4).

Vampire movie after vampire movie arrived followed by zombie movies (*I Am Legend*, *World War Z*, etc.) and the more current television series (*The Walking Dead*, *Fear the Walking Dead*, etc.) (Fig. 5.5).

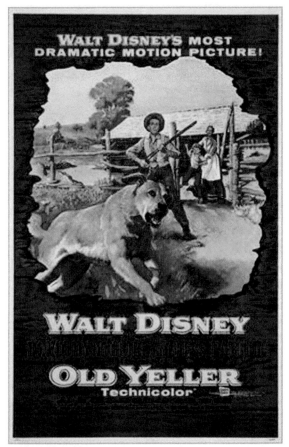

FIG. 5.4 *Old Yeller* movie poster. (Reprinted with permission by source, fair use: https://en.wikipedia.org/w/index.php?curid=41973841.)

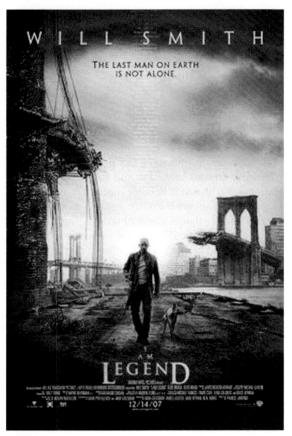

FIG. 5.5 *I Am Legend* movie teaser poster. (Reprinted with permission by source, fair use: https://en.wikipedia.org/w/index.php?curid=11659226.)

Rabies even shows up in our comedy with appearances in shows like *King of the Hill* and *Beavis and Butt-Head*, as well as in an episode of *The Office*. In the popular *Seinfeld* episode—classic TV—one of the main characters, Elaine, gets bitten by a dog, the owner evades her, she has to get PEP (the doctor tells her the shot will hurt very much), and she keeps thinking she is showing signs of rabies (spitting back water, frothing at the mouth, etc.).[1] It seems that rabies will always have a place in shaping pop culture, especially in the realm of the horror and science fiction genre. One can assume that because of this ongoing fascination with rabies in the arts and in our passing on of stories, often handing them down from one generation to the next, that we will continue to be fed misconceptions (although often based on science) about this diabolical virus known as rabies.

CONCLUSIONS

It is incumbent for all of us in the modern era to dispel these myths and legends so that we can move forward in our efforts to assist humankind and downplay the sometimes-misguided fascination with this ongoing threat. Realistically, those in the rabies medical, public health, and research community have a long way to go for increased disease survivorship and increased health literacy between health-care professionals and the public. To give just one example about our need to learn and communicate in the world of rabies, one needs to look no further than the variances in virulence and possible better outcomes from rabies virus variant phylogeny differences—the reasons for the overrepresentation of the silver-haired bat, *Lasionycteris noctivagans* (Fig. 5.6) rabies virus variant in human infections are unclear. The frequency of infection, shedding, and dissemination of rabies virus in

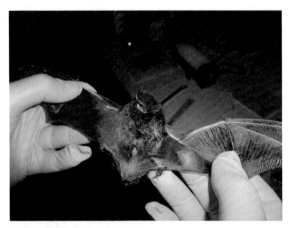

FIG. 5.6 A silver-haired bat, the type that has been responsible for numerous human rabies cases and deaths. (Reprinted with pemission by source, fair use: https://commons.wikimedia.org/wiki/File:Silver-haired_bat.JPG.)

L. noctivagans, compared with *Myotis lucifugus* and *Eptesicus fuscus*, suggests the discrepancy of human rabies cases may be due to increased infectivity in heterospecific hosts, human susceptibility, and/or behavioral factors.[33] In the interim, misconceived notions will most likely continue to be generated regarding the prevalence, signs and symptoms, diagnosis, and treatment protocols pertaining to this notorious and ancient killer known as rabies. It is incumbent upon all of us to be better stewards in the art of science communication with respect to decreasing the misunderstanding and sometimes panic surrounding this ancient disease.

REFERENCES

1. Wasik B, Rabid MM. *A Cultural History of the World's Most Diabolical Virus.* New York, NY: Penguin Books; 2012.
2. Rupprecht C, Kuzmin I, Meslin F. Lyssaviruses and rabies: current conundrums, concerns, contradictions and controversies. *F1000Res.* 2017;6:184. https://doi.org/10.12688/f1000research.10416.1.
3. Finley D. *Mad Dogs: The New Rabies Plague.* College Station, TX: Texas A&M University Press; 1998.
4. Rohde RE, Neill SU, Clark KA, et al. Molecular epidemiology of rabies epizootics in Texas. *J Clin Virol.* 1997;8:209–217.
5. Sabouraud A, Smith JS, Orciari LA, et al. Typing of rabies virus isolates by DNA enzyme immunoassay. *J Clin Virol.* 1999;12:9–19.
6. Rohde RE, Wilson PJ, Mayes BC, et al. Rabies: methods and Guidelines for Assessing a Clinical Rarity. *ASCP Microbio No. MB-4 Tech Sample;* 2004:21–29.
7. Rohde RE, Mayes BC, Smith JS, et al. Bat rabies, Texas, 1996–2000. *Emerg Infect Dis.* 2004;10(5):948–952. https://doi.org/10.3201/eid1005.030719.
8. Sidwa T, Wilson PJ, Moore G, et al. Evaluation of oral rabies vaccination programs for control of rabies epizootics in coyotes and gray foxes: 1995–2003. *JAVMA.* 2005;227(5):785–792.
9. Leslie MJ, Messenger S, Rohde RE, et al. Bat-associated rabies virus in skunks. *Emerg Infect Dis.* 2006;12(8):1274–1277. https://doi.org/10.3201/eid1208.051526.
10. Rohde RE. Rabies: an old disease for a new generation. *ASCLS Today Newsl.* 2007;21(8):14–15.
11. Rohde RE. Controlling rabies at its source: the Texas experience – oral rabies vaccination program. *ASCLS Today.* 2008;22(5):14–15.
12. Oertli EH, Wilson PJ, Hunt PR, et al. Rabies in skunks in Texas. *JAVMA.* 2009;234(5):1–5.
13. Mayes BC, Wilson PJ, Oertli EH, et al. Epidemiology of rabies in bats in Texas, 2001–2010. *JAVMA.* 2013;243(8):1129–1137.
14. Rohde RE, Mayes BC. Molecular diagnosis and epidemiology of rabies. In: Hu P, Hedge M, Lennon PA, eds. *Modern Clinical Molecular Techniques.* New York: Springer Press; 2012:199–211.
15. Rohde RE. *Invited Interview for Outbreak News Today Radio Podcast – Rabies: History, Myths and Diagnosis on Outbreak News This Week;* 2018. http://outbreaknewstoday.com/rabies-history-myths-and-diagnosis-on-outbreak-news-this-week-96853/.
16. Centers for Diseases Control and Prevention – Explore Travel Health With the CDC Yellow Book. Petersen BW, Wallace RM, Shlim DR. Chapter 3 – Infectious diseases related to travel: rabies. https://wwwnc.cdc.gov/travel/yellowbook/2018/infectious-diseases-related-to-travel/rabies.
17. Haugh L. 15 Obscure and Little Known Facts About Rabies. https://guardianlv.com/2016/06/obscure-and-little-known-facts-about-rabies/.
18. Fooks AR, Banyard AC, Horton DL, et al. Current status of rabies and prospects for elimination. *Lancet.* 2014;384:1389–1399.
19. Ma X, Monroe BP, Cleaton JM, et al. Rabies surveillance in the United States during 2017. *JAVMA.* 2018;253(12):1555–1568.
20. Centers for Disease Control and Prevention. What are the Signs and Symptoms of Rabies? https://www.cdc.gov/rabies/symptoms/index.html.
21. Wilson PJ, Rohde RE. *The Many Faces of Rabies.* Elsevier Connect; 2016. htpps://www.elsevier.com/connect/the-many-faces-of-rabies.
22. Wilson PJ, Rohde RE. *8 Things You May Not Know About Rabies – But Should.* Elsevier Connect; 2015. https://www.elsevier.com/connect/8-things-you-may-not-know-about-rabies-but-should.
23. World Health Organization. Rabies – Guide for Post-exposure Prophylaxis. http://www.who.int/rabies/human/postexp/en/.
24. Barney Fife – Bat eggs. https://www.youtube.com/watch?v=lrb3zoeKiGM.

25. 911Wildlife. Common Misconceptions About Rabies. http://www.911wildlife.com/animals/common-misconceptions-about-rabies/.

26. Blois M. How to stop brain cancer—with rabies. *Science*. 2017. http://www.sciencemag.org/news/2017/02/how-stop-brain-cancer-rabies.

27. Mole B. Homeopath "Treated" 4-yr-old Boy's Behavior Problems With Saliva From Rabid Dog. https://arstechnica.com/science/2018/04/homeopath-treated-4-yr-old-boys-behavior-problems-with-saliva-from-rabid-dog/.

28. Willoughby Jr R. Rabies: rare human infection – common questions. *Infect Dis Clin*. 2015;29:637–650.

29. de Souza A, Madhusudana SN. Survival from rabies encephalitis. *J Neurol Sci*. 2014;339:8–14.

30. Karande S, Muranjan M, Mani RS, et al. Atypical rabies encephalitis in a six-year old boy: clinical, radiological, and laboratory findings. *Int J Infect Dis*. 2015;36:1–3.

31. Feder Jr HM, Petersen BW, Robertson KL, et al. Rabies: still a uniformly fatal disease? Historical occurrence, epidemiological trends, and paradigm shifts. *Curr Infect Dis Rep*. 2012;14:408–422.

32. Centers for Disease Control and Prevention. Zoonotic Diseases. https://www.cdc.gov/onehealth/basics/zoonotic-diseases.html.

33. Davis AD, Morgan SMD, Dupuis M, et al. Overwintering of rabies virus in silver haired bats (*Lasionycteris noctivagans*). *PLoS One*. 2016;11(5):e0155542. https://journals.plos.org/plosone/article?id=10.1371/journal.pone.0155542.

CHAPTER 6

Rabies Postexposure Prophylaxis: Who, What, When, Where, Why, and How

RODNEY E. WILLOUGHBY, Jr., MD •
ERNEST H. OERTLI, DVM, PhD, Diplomate, ACVPM

INTRODUCTION

Who

This section refers to humans and domestic animals that were potentially exposed to rabies. For clarity, this section refers to both animals that were potentially exposed to rabies by other animals, and the animals that possibly exposed a human to rabies. Additionally, the term "animal" refers to a nonhuman mammal.

What

Rabies is a rapidly progressive encephalitis characterized by a prolonged and highly variable incubation period. It was the world's second vaccine-preventable disease, after smallpox, and the world's first postexposure prophylaxis by vaccine.[1] Until the advent of cell-culture-derived rabies vaccines (CCDVs) in the 1970s, vaccination required people to receive up to 21 doses for efficacy. The preceding neural tissue–derived vaccines (now only in use in Argentina, Bolivia, Algeria, and Ethiopia) were associated with very high rates of adverse events involving autoimmune encephalitis, balancing a 5%–50% risk of rabies versus 0.25%–0.5% risk of serious vaccine sequelae.[2,3] Therefore, routine preexposure vaccination (see Chapter 8) was prohibitive because of safety profile and cost, and PEP was the mediocre norm.

Rabies postexposure prophylaxis (PEP) improved considerably in the 1970s to 1990s. CCDVs and rabies immune globulin (RIG) were developed commercially. CCDVs are now given intradermally (ID) or intramuscularly (IM), requiring four to eight doses. Unfortunately, rabies remains vaccine preventable in theory rather than practice. The costs associated with low-volume production of the vaccines and polyclonal RIG remain prohibitive in most rabies-endemic regions. Only 5% of patients who require RIG in rabies-endemic countries such as China receive it.[4] Current vaccines also require a cold chain and repeated doses that are logistically challenging for populations living in remote areas.

We are experiencing a second revolution of rabies PEP. There are many promising developments that should alter the susceptibility of humans to the rabies virus. Firstly, there has been progressive modernization of antique schedules of rabies immunization, with more potent killed as well as attenuated vaccines. Secondly, routine scheduled vaccination of children against rabies in highly endemic areas has been investigated.[5-10] Thirdly, live attenuated vaccines have been engineered that promise single-dose prophylaxis of high potency.[11] Polyclonal human or horse antibodies are superseded by humanized monoclonal antibodies.[12] Passive immunization with antibodies is now targeted to the wound rather than administered systemically for exposure to dog rabies.[13] Modern antivirals promise chemoprophylaxis as alternatives or adjuncts to immunological prophylaxis.[14-16]

There have also been notable successes in reducing the exposure of rabies-susceptible populations to canine rabies, notably in the Americas through concerted public and veterinary health efforts and in selected locales elsewhere involving humane population control and vaccination of dogs.[17-19] Because of the lethality of rabies, there is little tolerance in the procedures public health officials promulgate for the handling of animals potentially exposed to rabid animals. The procedures must include a safety margin sufficient to ensure with certainty that no failures will occur. Rabies can induce necrophobia also known as

Rabies. https://doi.org/10.1016/B978-0-323-63979-8.00006-4
Copyright © 2019 Elsevier Inc. All rights reserved.

"death phobia." It is common and causes countless people unnecessary distress. These are combined emotions mixed with fear of death from rabies, which take a toll on the health and the mental peace of a person. Public health officials must be prepared and able to address concerns appropriately. Hard data from proven strategies are the basis for alleviating those concerns and fears.

The rabies virus has an unusual pattern of dissemination in the body.[20] When the virus is introduced into the body via a bite, it enters an eclipse phase during which it replicates in the muscle tissue (may also occur in skin with some bat variants). During this phase it does not stimulate an immune response, but it is susceptible to neutralization if antibodies are present. For reasons not totally understood, the incubation period can vary from days to months to years (rare). The virus enters the peripheral nerves and moves at a rate of 8–20 mm/day[21] to enter the spinal cord of the central nervous system (CNS). Replication within the CNS occurs and clinical signs appear as the neurons are cumulatively infected. Distribution to highly innervated tissues then occurs back through the peripheral nerves.[22]

Rabies virus is rapidly inactivated by desiccation under ambient conditions, so cannot be transmitted by physical contact with dead animals. Rabies is transmitted by saliva or neural tissue. Rabies virus replicates with an incubation period of days to months before salivary excretion, so cannot be transmitted by saliva from a bitten pet immediately after contact of the pet with a rabid animal (but can following exposure to moist saliva on the coat of an animal who has been in a fight with another animal that was rabid). Social grooming habits among some colony bats have been implicated in the transmission cycle for that species. There is no transmission of rabies by blood, urine, or stool. Semen has not been studied. Rabies content in breast milk and cow milk has not been sufficiently studied; pasteurization kills the rabies virus.[23] Rabies does not penetrate intact keratinized skin but can infect respiratory mucosa. If application of alcohol to the skin results in a burning sensation, then the skin is not intact. Inhalational rabies appears restricted to high-intensity laboratory exposures; two putative exposures to bat-colonized caves in the 1950s have not been replicated. However, in 2009 there was a 17-year-old Texas female diagnosed with rabies who survived and whose only known exposure was a bat cave.[24] No documented human cases have resulted from eating raw meat or drinking milk from a rabid animal, but these routes have been demonstrated

experimentally.[25,26] Processing of meat from a rabid animal will cause rabies and merits PEP.[27,28]

Not all rabid animals will transmit the virus to animals they bite.[29] Infection is affected by rabies virus variant, species of the bitten animal, species of the biting animal, presence of rabies virus in the saliva at the time of the bite, dose of the virus, location of the bite, and existing immunity against rabies. Virus shedding does not occur in all rabid animals, and the amount of virus in the saliva can vary greatly. Some animal species shed virus before clinical signs, and the duration of virus shedding can also vary greatly between species. Some other rare transmission routes have been reported.[30–33] These include scratches,[29,34] mucous membranes,[29,35] and iatrogenic disease.[29] There have been several documented human cases from organ transplants,[36–43] and aerosol transmission[29,35,44–46] has been documented. Rabies viruses have been transmitted by ingestion in experimentally infected animals,[35,47,48] and there is one documented epizootic among kudu (*Tragelaphus strepsiceros*) where rabies may have spread between animals eating leaves on thorn trees.[49] There are at least two peer-reviewed veterinary articles that suggest suspected transplacental transmission of rabies in animals.[47,50] The utilization of dogs for human sustenance is not uncommon, and translocation of animals, human exposure in capturing and transporting these animals preslaughter, handling of tissues while processing, and ingestion of undercooked meat with nervous tissue are all public health concerns with regard to rabies.[27,51–54]

When

This chapter provides information for observed or suspected exposures to humans and domestic animals. Given the cost of PEP and the time lost for medical visits, particularly in subsistence-level economies, it is critical to correctly identify exposures to infectious rabies virus.[3,55]

The WHO defines 3 grades of exposure to zoonotic rabies (see Table 6.1).[13] While category II exposures are used programmatically by some endemic countries to manage limited supplies of rabies immunoglobulin, this recommendation has been challenged by medical anecdote, animal models, and particularly for bat rabies.[34,56] All WHO category II exposures are considered category III exposures by the United States Centers for Disease Control and Prevention (CDC).[57] Bat exposures resulting in rabies regularly involve minor physical contact without perceived wounds, so should be considered category III. Based on historical epidemiology, the CDC also considers colocalization of an untested or rabid bat in the same room as sleeping

TABLE 6.1
Categories of Exposure and Recommended Postexposure Prophylaxis

WHO Category of Exposure	Type of Exposure to a Domestic or Wild Animal Suspected or Confirmed to be Rabid or Animal Unavailable for Testing	Recommended Postexposure Prophylaxis
I	Touching or feeding animals, licks on intact skin (no exposure)	**None, if reliable case history is available[a]**
II	Nibbling of uncovered skin Minor scratches or abrasions without bleeding (exposure)	**CDC: Treat as category III** Administer vaccine immediately Stop treatment if animal remains healthy throughout an observation period of 10 days[b] or is proven to be negative for rabies by a reliable laboratory using appropriate diagnostic techniques. Treat as category III if bat exposure is involved.
III	Single or multiple transdermal[c] bites or scratches Contamination of mucous membrane or broken skin with saliva from animal licks Exposures due to direct contact with bats (severe exposure)	**Administer rabies vaccine immediately and rabies immunoglobulin, preferably as soon as possible after initiation of postexposure prophylaxis. Rabies immunoglobulin can be injected up to 7 days after administration of first vaccine dose. Stop treatment if animal remains healthy throughout an observation period of 10 days[b] or is proven to be negative for rabies by a reliable laboratory using appropriate diagnostic techniques.**

[a]If an apparently healthy dog or cat in or from a low-risk area is placed under observation, treatment may be delayed.
[b]This observation period applies only to dogs, cats, and ferrets. Except for threatened or endangered species, other domestic and wild animals suspected of being rabid should be euthanized and their tissues examined for the presence of rabies antigen by appropriate laboratory techniques.
[c]Bites especially on the head, neck, face, hands, and genitals are category III exposures because of the rich innervation of these areas.
From *WHO Expert Consultation on Rabies, Third Report*. Geneva: World Health Organization; 2018. Report No.: 1012[(13)], 201–220. with permission. **US CDC recommendations are indicated in bold type**, notably that Category II exposures are treated as Category III exposures. From Use of a reduced (4-dose) vaccine schedule for postexposure prophylaxis to prevent human rabies: recommendations of the Advisory Committee on Immunization Practices (ACIP). *MMWR*. 2010;59(RR-2):6[(78)].

persons, those mentally disabled or intoxicated, and those unlikely to accurately report their exposures (young child or someone with a psychiatric disorder) to have been exposed.[57] Bats seen outside the same room, even if capable of free access to the same space as the susceptible person, are not exposures. (One must draw the line somewhere; this criterion has been effective for 19 years.) Some animal species are not reservoir hosts and almost never transmit rabies through saliva. This includes small rodents and lagomorphs, armadillos, opposums, moles, and shrews. Larger rodents such as badgers and woodchucks may transmit rabies.[26,58,59] Dogs, cats, and domestic ferrets that are healthy can be observed for 10 days. The wound should be washed immediately but PEP may be delayed during the observation period. If the animal shows clinical signs or escapes, then PEP should be started immediately. A wild animal should be euthanized immediately and its brain

tested for rabies.[57] To get a conclusive test result, see Chapter 4 for details on specimen submission guidelines. There has never been a laboratory-documented transmission of rabies between humans other than by transplantation of organs, plus a single case report of peripartum transmission.[60] Other primate bites transmit rabies.[61] Transmission between a rabid human and caregivers or at autopsy has never been confirmed.[62] Nosocomial transmission is theoretically possible when mucous membranes or open wounds are exposed to infectious saliva or nervous tissue, so PEP is recommended. Human rabies vaccines produced under good manufacturing processes are killed vaccines that cannot transmit rabies.

When an animal has been identified as possibly or confirmed rabid, then a retrospective risk assessment should be conducted to define potential exposures. Dogs, cats, and domestic ferrets should be considered infectious for 10 days before onset of clinical signs. Other animals and humans are assigned a 14-day window before signs develop. PEP should be administered, even months later.[13]

With regard to domestic animals potentially exposed to rabid animals, it is important to realize that most exposures to pets and livestock occur without owner observation. With the changing environment by encroachment on rural lands, coyotes, foxes, skunks, bats, and raccoons are commonly found in most urban and rural communities. The best prevention for rabies is vaccination. Including rabies as a core vaccine has clearly demonstrated efficacy and safety in pets, livestock, and at-risk humans.[63,64] Preexposure rabies vaccination of pets, horses, and livestock that will be in close proximity to humans should be accomplished. Other interventions, such as enforcement of existing rabies prevention laws, stray dog and cat control, sterilization of dogs and cats, and education programs on dog bite prevention, plus dangers of wildlife feeding and wildlife as pets, should be established, improved, and enforced.[65,112]

The transmission of rabies virus to animals is no different than with humans. Rabies is transmitted only when the virus is introduced through a bite wound, open cuts in skin, or onto mucous membranes such as the mouth or eyes. Nonbite exposures occur when animals chew on or eat other rabid animals, such as a cat or dog chewing on a grounded bat. As with humans, contact with blood, urine, or feces of a rabid animal does not constitute an exposure. Some bites are hard to detect, especially those by bats. It is important to determine if the altercation which potentially exposed the animal was provoked or unprovoked. Abnormal or unusual behavior should raise concerns as to the possibility of the animal in question being rabid; some examples are listed below (see Chapter 2 for detailed information on clinical signs of rabies):

- Animals active in the daytime that are normally nocturnal
- Animals with excessive salivation (drooling saliva)
- Wildlife unusually friendly to humans
- Recumbent or paralyzed animals for no apparent reason
- Animals that appear to withdraw from light or water
- Animals that are aggressive, biting at anything
- Pets that are normally affectionate who withdraw
- Livestock or pets that demonstrate unusual vocalization[66]

A classic example of rabies in a domestic animal is documented in the submitting report for a laboratory-confirmed rabid cat diagnosed in Texas in September 2018: "4-Day history of progressive neurologic disease; now cannot use hind legs, elevated third eyelids cannot defecate."[67]

Where

For people who sustain terrestrial animal bites and scratches in an area free of terrestrial rabies, PEP is not required.[13] All US states and territories contain terrestrial rabies, but some areas within states may not. Physical contact by a bat always requires PEP.[55]

The utilization of robust surveillance programs allows public health managers to use the data as part of the risk assessment. Without laboratory support, most rabies surveillance programs are ineffective. Surveillance, confirmed by laboratory results, presents a picture of disease transmission; it helps to describe both geographic and temporal trends in disease occurrence, populations affected, and changes in the rabies variant causing agents. If dependable surveillance supports it, there are situations where exposures to dogs, cats, domestic ferrets, or other domestic animals may not be considered potential rabies exposures when they occur in nonendemic terrestrial rabies regions.[57] Regardless of the rabies endemic/nonendemic geographical region, for domestic animals as with humans, PEP is generally not recommended for animals for bites, scratches, or other contacts from low-risk animals. However, these incidents should be evaluated on an individual basis, especially in unusual cases involving small rodents/lagomorphs, and definitely with large rodents such as beavers and woodchucks.

The PEP decisions can be based on the geographical area where the exposure occurred and whether it falls into a rabies endemic or rabies nonendemic status. In the United States, with the exception of Hawaii, there are no rabies-free states (bat and terrestrial). There are areas within some states where rabies is very low risk. While dog rabies has been eliminated in the United States, cross-species transmission occurs and dogs, cats, and ferrets can transmit rabies. The Flagstaff, Arizona, big brown bat epizootic in skunks[67] should cause caution to public health officials as host shifts do occur in areas where terrestrial rabies has not been observed. Even though there are seasonal variations in population, activity, and rabies virus circulation, the time of year should not be a consideration in PEP considerations.

It should be recognized that PEP consistency is not achievable in all situations. The epidemiology and risk of rabies varies across rabies-endemic countries as evidenced by the range in number and species of animal rabies cases. This variability includes the rabies virus variants, the reservoir species for rabies, and the prevalence of rabies virus in the respective reservoir species. Cost of quarantine, facilities, and availability to medical care all may come into play. These epidemiologic and practical factors are important considerations in rabies management. Unlike humans, the PEP recommendations for animals vary between countries and even between states in the United States (see Table 6.2). A sampling is provided just to show variation. Veterinarians and/or attending staff should always check with the local public health officials to ensure they are complying with legal requirements.

In many countries and states within the United States, laboratory confirmation of rabies may be limited to specific circumstances. The long quarantine periods with its cost and labor, possible destruction of the animal(s), and potential for exposure to the person caring for the animal(s) often make it prudent to confirm the rabies status even if the financial burden of laboratory testing falls on the owner of the exposed animal(s).

The incubation period for domestic animals possibly exposed to the rabies virus should not be confused with the 10-day observation period for a dog, cat, or domestic ferret that has potentially exposed a human or another animal to rabies. A dog, cat, or domestic ferret exposed to a rabid animal may develop rabies long after the exposure because the incubation period for rabies is so variable (see Chapter 2 for average incubation). A prolonged confinement is necessary to exclude the possibility of subsequent development of rabies in a dog, cat, domestic ferret, or livestock exposed to a rabid animal. In pet rodents and lagomorphs, limited knowledge of clinical signs and shedding periods is available to determine whether such observation periods would provide complete assurance of rabies status at the time of a bite. Animal and human health will be best protected by housing and maintenance of pet rodents and lagomorphs to prevent exposure to rabies virus, which means not placing their pens where they can be exposed to rabid wildlife.[68]

The variations in PEP may include what is considered an exposure, euthanasia considerations, timing of any subsequent vaccinations, and length of quarantine or confinement. The decision whether PEP is required for an animal (pet, livestock, exotic pet, zoo exhibit, etc.) should be based on an evaluation of each exposure by a competent individual. All animals bitten or possibly exposed by rabies reservoir species, such as bats, foxes, raccoons, skunks, coyotes, and mongooses in the United States and its territories or in other rabies-endemic countries as appropriate (dogs, foxes, ferret-badgers, raccoon dogs, jackals, mongooses, non-human primates, etc.)

should receive PEP if the biting animal is not available for testing. (The National Association of State Public Health Veterinarians (NASPHV) Rabies Compendium specifically mentions that any wild mammalian carnivores, skunks, and bats that are not available or suitable for testing should be regarded as rabid.) As mentioned previously, not all potential exposure events carry a significant risk of transmission and thus the implementation of PEP may not be required. Contact with a species that does not commonly transmit rabies in that geographic area and did not display any abnormal behavior may not warrant any follow-up action.

Why

Rabies is almost perfectly fatal and rarely treatable when clinically evident. Despite considerable cost, the fatal consequences and loss of disability-adjusted life years in a young population have always justified PEP economically.[69] Over time, the economics of prophylaxis have improved as vaccine doses and RIG volumes dropped and side effects were minimized.[70,71]

Rabies virus is an enveloped virus showing poor stability in the environment. Virus in wounds can be inactivated by soap and water (that strip the membrane envelope) and topical antiseptic compounds such as povidone iodine (that oxidize the virus envelope and glycoproteins).

Louis Pasteur recognized that the incubation period of human rabies (usually 2 weeks to 6 months) is longer than the time required to mount a vaccine-induced immune response to the rabies virus (7 days).[72] Natural infection by rabies viruses occurs at low levels of virus replication within the immunologically privileged peripheral nervous system and CNS, so that infection is not rapidly detected by the adaptive immune system. Most humans with rabies die without detectable immune response to the rabies virus.

Both innate (largely type 1 interferons) and adaptive immunity (largely antibodies directed at the surface G glycoprotein of the rabies virus) prevent rabies infection. The adaptive antibody response to rabies virus cross-neutralizes phylotype I lyssaviruses including European bat lyssaviruses 1 and 2, Bokeloh, Kotalahti, Aravan, Irkut, Khujand, Australian bat lyssavirus, Gannoruwa, Taiwan, and Duvenhage viruses.[13] Susceptibility to other phylotypes of lyssaviruses are not affected by PEP to rabies virus.

Administration of RIG, including human, modified equine, or monoclonal antibodies, is highly effective as sole prophylaxis in animal models and serves as an important bridge for 7 days until an endogenous antibody response to rabies vaccine appears. The maximal

TABLE 6.2
Example Comparison of Postexposure Prophylaxis Recommendations With Variations

Legal Entity	Species	Exposure	Vaccination Status	Option Euthanasia	Option Vaccinate	Quarantine
NASPHV[a] Compendium	Dogs, cats, ferrets	Yes	Current (at least 28 days)	No	Booster	45-day observation (owner)
	Dogs, cats, ferrets	Yes	Unvaccinated	Yes (but if owner says no)	Within 96 h[b]	Strict quarantine 4[c] months for dogs/cats 6 months for ferrets
	Dogs, cats	Yes	Not current document	No	Booster	45-day observation (owner)
	Dogs, cats	Yes	Not current no document	Possible case by case	Booster or serology (prior to booster)	Strict quarantine or observation based on evaluation and/or serology
	Livestock	Yes	Unvaccinated	Yes (but if owner says no)	No	6-month observation
	Livestock	Yes	Current	No	Booster	45-day observation (owner)
	Livestock, ferrets	Yes	Not current	Possible case by case	Booster	Strict quarantine or observation based on evaluation
Canada	Dogs, cats, ferrets	Yes	Current (at least 14 days)	No	Booster (within 7 days)	Booster within 7 days—none not within 7 days–3 month observation
	Dogs, cats	Yes	Unvaccinated	No	Vaccinate	Within 7 days–3 months (consider booster at 3rd week) not within 7 days–6 months (consider booster at 3rd week)
	Ferrets	Yes	Unvaccinated	No	Vaccinate	6 months (consider booster at 3rd week)
	Dogs, cats, ferrets	Yes	Not current	No	Vaccinate	Evaluation then 6 months, 3 months, or none
	Livestock	Yes	Current, not current, unvaccinated	No	Vaccinate or booster	Quarantine 60 days from exposure or 40 days from herd index case
Texas[d]	Domestic animals	Yes	Unvaccinated or not current	Yes (but if owner says no)	Vaccinate or booster	90-day confinement with additional vaccination at 3rd and 8th week
	Domestic animals	Yes	Current	Yes (but if owner says no)	Booster	45-day confinement

[a]NASPHV (National Association of State Public Health Veterinarians).
[b]Animals should still receive a vaccination even if it is longer than 96 h postexposure.
[c]Quarantine may be extended to 6 months if the vaccination is delayed past 96 h.
[d]Texas: Dr. Tom Sidwa, State Public Health Veterinarian, Zoonosis Control Branch, Texas Department of State Health Services.

dose of RIG should not be exceeded because this will interfere with vaccine take. For large wounds, RIG can be diluted with sterile saline to saturate the wound without exceeding the maximum permitted dose.

Recent case series show equivalence of RIG injected with only the limited volume required to infiltrate wounds when compared to the conventional approach of RIG dosed per kilogram of body weight, with residual RIG after wound care given IM.[73] The wound-targeted approach can result in considerable saving on RIG volume in busy clinics. It remains unclear whether this practice can be applied to vampire bat wounds. Unfortunately, contact with other bats rarely results in a defined bite, and the full amount of RIG should be administered IM. Mucosal exposures require IM administration.[13]

There are nucleoside analogs such as favipiravir that inhibit replication of a wide range of RNA viruses including rabies virus. Animal studies of favipiravir for PEP show promise.[14-16] The CNS pharmacokinetics of favipiravir in humans are unknown, but CNS penetration by passive antibodies, vaccine-induced antibodies, or drugs is not essential for PEP. Human chemoprophylaxis studies of orally available favipiravir should follow.

Modern CCDV are of superior immunogenicity and low reactogenicity relative to antecedent nerve tissue–derived vaccines that have been phased out in all but four countries. Rabies vaccines can be administered ID or IM per WHO recommendations, even if this is off-label use.[13] ID administration is off-label in the United States.

Treatment of clinical rabies remains problematic and largely dependent on a rapid development (within 7 days of hospitalization) of neutralizing antibody to the rabies virus in serum and cerebrospinal fluid (CSF).[74] This is best elicited without immunomodulation by vaccines and immune globulin products including RIG.[75] Vaccination with inactivated rabies vaccines generates primarily a Th2 response in animal models that do not produce antibodies in the CNS.[76] Dog rabies and insectivorous bat rabies viruses also do not elicit a CNS immune response in many rabid patients; vampire bat rabies does.[74] Vaccination during rabies (clinical disease) provides a small amount of killed antigen when there is an abundance of wild-type viral antigen in the brain, skin, and organs that precedes the clinical onset of rabies, so the vaccine adds little therapeutically.[57]

Prior vaccination (e.g., onset of rabies during PEP) is associated with improved survival but also severe neurological sequelae. In contrast, half of unvaccinated survivors show good outcomes.[74] Unlike human killed rabies vaccines, live-attenuated vaccines can clear rabies encephalomyelitis in animal models, associated with a Th1 immune response and CSF antibodies.[76] There are no licensed attenuated rabies vaccines for human use but the hope is that these will follow for more efficient prophylaxis as well as rabies therapy.

The efficiency of rabies virus transmission varies with both the species and the behavior of the infected animal. It is intuitive that animals with the furious form are more likely to spread rabies than animals with the paralytic form, and that carnivores are also more efficient vectors than herbivores.

Not all rabid animals will transmit the virus to animals they bite. Virus shedding is estimated to occur in 50%–90% of infected animals, and the amount of virus in the saliva varies from a trace to high titers.[77] The saliva virus load can be influenced by the species of animal and the viral variant. Shedding can begin before the onset of clinical signs. Refer to Chapter 2 for more information on rabies virus shedding in the various species.

How
Vaccine routes and schedules
In nonendemic regions, the recommendation for IM administration persists as the standard for PEP.[78] This is practical because ID administration does not provide economies of scale from sharing vaccine and RIG vials and the technique requires practice or syringe adapters for proficiency. IM sites include anterolateral thighs in children aged <2 years and deltoid muscle for other ages. The gluteal area is to be avoided.

All licensed IM vaccine products are considered suitable by the WHO for ID use.[13] In bite centers and clinics with high weekly volumes of PEP administration, use of ID vaccination is effective and efficient. Recommended ID sites include deltoids, lateral thighs, and suprascapular areas for optimal delivery to regional lymph nodes.

Recent WHO recommendations that RIG volumes can be limited to injection of the wound sites are programmatically efficient but not yet the US recommendation.[13,79] Insectivorous bat contact rarely results in a defined bite, and the full amount of RIG should be administered IM. Vampire bat bite wounds often involve the face, head, neck, hands, and feet. Fingertips, noses, ears, and other small, sensitive sites can be infiltrated effectively and should be, given that the alternative is a highly fatal disease. Infiltration should be done carefully to avoid compartment syndrome in the injected areas. There is no experience using less than the maximal per kilogram dosing of RIG for bat rabies.

During mass exposures to a rabid animal, temporary limitations of rabies vaccine and RIG may occur. The ID route and RIG administration restricted to the wound only are ideal under this circumstance if the shortage cannot be remedied within days.

Timing of prophylaxis for humans

1. PEP including (a) proper wound washing, (b) RIG, and (c) CCDV is almost 100% effective in preventing rabies, even with severe wounds.
2. Rabies virus is rapidly inactivated by topical disinfectants and soap and water, which should be used emergently, given the high densities of rabies virus (10^4 pfu/mL) in saliva and of receptors for rabies virus in motor end plates (8.0×10^9 receptors/mm^2).[80,81]
3. Bites to the highly innervated face, head, neck, hands, and genitals are considered particularly high risk due to their innervation, but this is contradicted by the absence of propagation of rabies virus via sensory nerves in humans and by data supporting the severity scoring of dog bites to hands in Haiti (Table 6.3).[3,13,56] An alternative explanation for increased susceptibility is that the face, head, and neck contain many small muscle groups that provide ready access by rabies virus to receptors in the motor end plates that cluster in the belly of human muscles.[82] The more small the muscles, the more rabies receptors. Longer muscles in the extremities are less susceptible to infection unless the bite coincides with the belly of the muscle.
4. Many vaccinated patients progress to rabies because RIG was not administered.[4] RIG is a crucial bridge providing neutralization of rabies virus until vaccine-induced immunity develops in 7 days.
5. After initiating vaccination series, there is no benefit to RIG after 7 days.
6. RIG should be injected into the wound several hours before suturing to allow diffusion of immunoglobulin within the tissues and preclude inoculating infectious rabies viruses deeper into the wound.[13] When RIG is not immediately available, wound margins are best left unsutured or loosely approximated by a limited number of sutures until RIG is administered. Severe bite wounds are best treated by daily dressing changes followed by secondary closure to avoid bacterial infection, tetanus, or rabies. Later wound repair under controlled conditions also results in a more cosmetic outcome.
7. Rabies vaccine and RIG can be used during pregnancy and lactation.
8. There are numerous WHO-approved rabies vaccine schedules (Table 6.4).[13] There is only one option in the United States. Note that some modern schedules obviate the day 3 dose and others are complete by 7 days with only three visits. At least 1 prime and 1 booster dose are required to guarantee prolonged immunological memory. (Rabies virus incubation periods have been documented to extend up to 8 years.) Rabies vaccine reliably generates neutralizing rabies antibodies by 14 days after start of the vaccine schedule.[78] No further doses are needed after 14 days with the US regimen.[78] For immunocompromised individuals, an additional dose at day 28[78] may be needed (Table 6.4).[72]

   Due to the highly variable and prolonged incubation period for human rabies, it is never too late to receive RIG and rabies vaccine after a confirmed rabies exposure.[13] Among rabies cases, 2%–3% had an incubation period >1 year. WHO recommends a cutoff of 12 months for suspected or probable exposures.[13] Prophylaxis schedules can be resumed at any time without the need to restart the vaccine series. Vaccinations started with one rabies vaccine product or route can be completed by another product or route that should then be used to complete the series.[13]
9. PEP is always indicated after a rabies exposure, even when the patient has been previously vaccinated.[13,57] For persons at high and recurrent risk, preexposure prophylaxis is recommended and will lead to simplified PEP with later exposures to rabies. The anamnestic response from prior vaccination requires no bridging RIG and provides superior titers with more even tissue delivery.
10. For persons traveling to rabies-endemic areas where exposure to rabid or wild animals is probable (bite incidence > 5% per annum) and access to RIG and CCDV is haphazard, preexposure prophylaxis is recommended.[13] Ironically, persons residing in rabies-endemic areas meeting these parameters should receive preexposure prophylaxis (and simplified PEP to follow exposures), but rabies vaccine is not included in routine vaccine schedules except for high-risk areas in Peru and the Philippines.[83] An expansive recommendation for preexposure prophylaxis exists for India.[84]
11. Duration of vaccine-induced and immunological memory is likely lifelong. Given the fatality of rabies, booster doses are recommended for repeat rabies exposures and every 2 years for those whose occupation puts them at frequent risk of exposure.

TABLE 6.3
Severity Scoring of Dog Bites and Risk of Death From Rabies

Exposure Consideration	Probability of Rabies Based on Clinical Categorization of Bite (Babes)	OBJECTIVE RISK MATRIX							Advanced Surveillance Program Capacity	
		Limited Surveillance Program Capacity						Dog Healthy and Available for Quarantine	Dog Healthy 10 Days Post-Bite	Tested Negative
		Dog Symptomatic	Dog Dead At Follow-up	Dog Bite Was Not Provoked	Stray Dog	Dog Bit Multiple People	Dog Not Vaccinated			
Bite to head/neck	45.00%	27.99%	17.87%	6.75%	6.26%	4.77%	2.12%	0.04%	0.00%	0.00%
Multiple severe bite wounds	27.50%	17.11%	10.92%	4.13%	3.82%	2.92%	1.29%	0.02%	0.00%	0.00%
Bites to young children	27.50%	17.11%	10.92%	4.13%	3.82%	2.92%	1.29%	0.02%	0.00%	0.00%
Bites to extremities	5.00%	3.11%	1.99%	0.75%	0.70%	0.53%	0.24%	0.00%	0.00%	0.00%
Minor bites (no break in skin)	1.00%	0.62%	0.40%	0.15%	0.14%	0.11%	0.05%	0.00%	0.00%	0.00%
Category II	1.00%	0.62%	0.40%	0.15%	0.14%	0.11%	0.05%	0.00%	0.00%	0.00%
Medley et al. probability of rabies[2]		62.20%	39.70%	15.00%	13.90%	10.60%	4.70%	0.08%	0.00%	0.00%

[1]Risk levels illustrated by Green (Low), Yellow/Orange (Moderate), and Red (High).
[2]Probability of rabies as calculated from the data sets used in this study. "Dog Bite Was Not Provoked" was a best guess estimate at 15%.
From Medley A, Millien M, Blanton J, et al. Retrospective cohort study to assess the risk of rabies in biting dogs, 2011–2015, Republic of Haiti. *Trop Med Infect Dis.* 2017;2(2):14(3), with permission (open access).[3]

TABLE 6.4
WHO-Recommended Postexposure Regimens

PEP Regimen	Duration of Course (days)	No. of Injection Sites Per Clinic Visit (days 0,3,7,14,21–28)
WHO-RECOMMENDED INTRAMUSCULAR REGIMEN[a]		
2 weeks	**14**	**1-1-1-1-0**
3 weeks	21	2-0-1-0-1
WHO-RECOMMENDED INTRADERMAL REGIMEN[b]		
1 week, 2 sites	7	2-2-2-0-0
Alternative Intradermal Regimens		
1 week, 4 sites	7	4-4-4-0-0
4 weeks, 2 sites	21–28	2-2-2-0-2
4 weeks, 2 sites	21–28	4-0-2-0-1

[a]US CDC recommended regimen; vaccines licensed for this indication and route.
[b]As of print time for this book, unpublished: Tarantola et al.
From *WHO Expert Consultation on Rabies, Third Report*. Geneva: World Health Organization; 2018. Report No.: 1012[(13)], with permission. **US CDC recommendations are indicated in bold type.**
From Use of a reduced (4-dose) vaccine schedule for postexposure prophylaxis to prevent human rabies: recommendations of the Advisory Committee on Immunization Practices (ACIP). *MMWR.* 2010;59(RR-2):6[(78)].

12. Administration of PEP to a clinically rabid patient has demonstrated consistent ineffectiveness and may worsen outcome in rabies survivors.[57]

Serological and virological testing

There is no laboratory test that detects rabies virus replication during the incubation period (see Chapter 4). Given the near 100% efficacy of PEP in normal hosts, there is no need for confirmatory serology. There is no known titer proven to be protective in humans; such a trial would be unethical. In patients with antibody- or cell-mediated immunocompromise, the immune response should be confirmed 2–4 weeks after final vaccination to assess need for one additional dose of vaccine. Individuals working with high concentrations of rabies or other phylotype I lyssaviruses should be tested every 1–2 years to ensure adequate immune response and to detect unnoticed exposures that require risk mitigation.

Given the near lifelong immunity to rabies following preexposure prophylaxis or PEP, booster doses are not required for people living in or traveling to high-risk areas without a defined exposure. For those previously immunized (2 or more doses), no RIG is indicated upon later rabies exposure. ID or IM booster doses should be given on days 0 and 3. Alternatively, a 4-site ID vaccine can be given on day 0 only.[13] The US regimen is restricted to IM doses given on days 0 and 3.

Challenges and contraindications to postexposure prophylaxis

There are no contraindications to PEP, including newborns, pregnancy, lactation, or immunocompromise.[13] A previous severe reaction to a rabies vaccine requires use of an alternative vaccine product.

The main challenge is that rabies is a zoonosis. Globally, rabies control depends on veterinary/agricultural expenditures for population control and rabies vaccination of dogs. A rabies eradication blueprint is available online, building on notable successes.[17–19,85] Vaccination of cats is epidemiologically important in many countries.[86]

The second challenge is economic, including poor funding and logistics and kleptocracy. This is unfortunate because expenditures on animal and rabies vaccines provide considerable economic benefit.[69] Gavi, the Vaccine Alliance that advises the WHO on preferred drugs provided at discount to eligible countries, recommended inclusion of the rabies vaccine on the prioritized short list for endemic disease prevention.[87] Safety issues center on poorly manufactured and counterfeit rabies vaccines.[88] Nerve-tissue derived vaccines with poor safety profiles remain in use in four countries.[13]

Prioritization of limited rabies immune globulin or vaccine

When supplies of RIG or rabies vaccine are limited by temporary shortages, local unavailability, or stretched by a mass exposure, then supplies must be prioritized. Wound cleaning and disinfection are never in short supply and are key practices with proven effectiveness. RIG can be stretched for canine rabies by limiting injections to the wound site, without use of the standardized dose per kilogram.[89] RIG should also be prioritized to patients with bites from an animal with confirmed or probable rabies; bites to the head, neck, and hands; severe immunodeficiency (no response to vaccines); multiple bites; deep wounds; or a bite, scratch, or exposure of mucous membranes from a bat.[13] Patients benefit from PEP even with delays, so temporary shortages should be corrected so that PEP is applied urgently and appropriately.

Special considerations pertaining to exposure to rabid bats

Bat exposures require special consideration based on differences in rabies biology and recommended PEP. The following points are reiterated:

When:

1. Insectivorous bat exposures resulting in rabies regularly involve minor physical contact without perceived wounds, so should be considered category III.

2. Based on national epidemiology, the United States CDC also considers colocalization of an untested or rabid bat in the same room as sleeping persons, those mentally disabled or intoxicated, and those unlikely to accurately report their exposures (young child or someone with a psychiatric disorder) to have been exposed.[57] Bats seen outside the same room, even if capable of free access to the same space as the susceptible person, are not exposures. (One must draw the line somewhere; this criterion has been effective for 19 years.)

3. For persons traveling to rabies-endemic areas where exposure to rabid or wild animals is probable (bite incidence > 5% per annum) and access to RIG and CCDV is haphazard, preexposure prophylaxis is recommended.[13] Persons resident in rabies-endemic areas meeting these parameters should receive preexposure prophylaxis, as is done in Peru and the Philippines.[83]

Why:

4. The adaptive immune response to rabies virus cross-neutralizes bat-associated phylotype I lyssaviruses including European bat lyssaviruses 1 and 2, Bokeloh, Kotalahti, Aravan, Irkut, Khujand, Australian bat lyssavirus, Gannoruwa, Taiwan, and Duvenhage viruses.[13]

5. The wound-targeted approach can result in considerable saving on RIG volume. It remains unclear whether this practice can be applied to vampire bat wounds. Unfortunately, insectivorous bat contact rarely results in a defined bite to infiltrate with RIG.

How:

6. Insectivorous bat contact rarely results in a defined bite and the full amount of RIG should be administered IM.

7. Vampire bat bite wounds often involve the face, head, neck, hands, and feet. Fingertips, noses, ears, and other small, sensitive sites can be infiltrated effectively and should be, given that the alternative is a highly fatal disease. Infiltration should be done carefully to avoid compartment syndrome in the injected areas. There is no experience using less than the maximal per kilogram dosing for bat rabies.

Rabies postexposure prophylaxis management in animals

In animal interactions, activities that could pose a risk for exposure include bites, licking, or other direct contact between saliva and mucous membranes or broken skin, and sharing eating or drinking utensils. While the risk is low, ingestion and scratches involving moist saliva containing rabies virus have been documented as causing transmission.[29,35,47] By a vast majority, bites are the mode of transmission of rabies virus. However, there are rare reports of transmission by other routes. Aerosol transmission has been documented under special circumstances with an unusually high density of aerosolized, viable virus particles. Rabies viruses have been transmitted by ingestion in experimentally infected animals. Some authors have speculated that ingestion might play a role in rabies transmission among animals. In one epizootic among kudu (*Tragelaphus strepsiceros*), the virus may have spread between animals when they fed on thorn trees.[49] Skunks, raccoons, and foxes are often found at cave entrances feeding on downed bats. It would not be unreasonable to assume that some exposures to rabies occur as a result. As with humans, when domestic animals are found in situations in which a bat is physically present (dead or alive) and one cannot reasonably exclude the possibility of a bite exposure, PEP should be given unless prompt capture and testing of the bat has excluded rabies virus infection.[90]

As with humans, the incubation period for animals varies with the amount of virus transmitted, virus variant, site of inoculation (bites closer to the head in general have a shorter incubation period), preexisting conditions which affect host immunity, and nature of the wound. See Chapter 2 regarding variations in incubation periods. It is very important to note that variations do occur between species and within species. The recommended confinement periods for exposed animals are directed at the normal incubation periods.

The ultimate goal of animal PEP is to protect public health. When a domestic animal has possibly been exposed to rabies, it is critical that the owners be educated about the potential health risks to themselves, their family, the public, and other domestic animals. In a perfect public health world, these risks would be eliminated by promptly euthanizing the exposed animal(s). However, due to emotional attachment, financial concerns, and other considerations, this is seldom the option chosen by owners. Additionally, utilizing just that option contributes to needless euthanasia of animals, especially in situations in which an exposure cannot be definitively confirmed. If the owners are educated regarding the risks and they acknowledge that they would like to keep the exposed animal alive, then they need to also be educated on the PEP requirements and possible clinical signs of the disease. Postexposure management of animals is variable by jurisdiction, bite circumstance, availability of the biting animal, and vaccination status of the bitten animal; there may be a mandate for an animal control officer, veterinarian, or animal owner to have oversight of the animal during this time. In all cases, PEP requirements should be diligently enforced to ensure compliance.

If possible and without exposing oneself (wear gloves in case moist saliva from the biting animal is present), PEP consists of immediate wound cleansing and disinfection. Wound cleansing cannot be overemphasized. Immediate and thorough washing of all bite wounds and scratches with soap and water (and an iodine-based antiseptic, if available) is a critical measure for preventing rabies. In experimental animals, simple local wound cleansing has been shown to markedly reduce the likelihood of rabies.[91] Tetanus vaccination in horses and measures to control bacterial infection in all animals should be provided as indicated.

The PEP is highly effective if it is begun soon after exposure. One issue in the United States is that there is not a USDA-licensed vaccine for every species. Refer to the latest edition of the publication titled *The Compendium of Animal Rabies Prevention and Control* by the NASPHV for a list of approved rabies vaccines for a specific species. There are no licensed rabies vaccines currently available for wild animals or hybrids of wild and domestic animals or even for some domestic animals, such as goats and pigs. Administration of products which are not labeled for use in a species is called off-label/extra-label usage (while the term off-label is frequently used, extra-label is the correct definition.) The administration of a rabies vaccine in a species for which no licensed vaccine is available is at the extra-label discretion of the veterinarian; however, it should be remembered that an animal receiving a rabies vaccine under these conditions is not considered to be vaccinated against rabies virus in potential rabies exposure situations.

Vaccines are most effective if they are administered starting as soon as possible after the exposure. There is no effective veterinary treatment once the clinical signs develop. Once it has been determined that an exposure occurred, the vaccination status of the exposed animal must be accomplished. Vaccination status falls into three categories: (1) unvaccinated, (2) currently vaccinated, or (3) out-of-date vaccination. The category of current vaccination status must be based on the legal authority where the exposure occurred. An animal's vaccination status may vary by the ordinance/law of the municipality, county, or state. In the United States, the legislative authority granted to local governments varies by state. Forty of the fifty states apply the principle known as Dillon's Rule in some form to determine the bounds of a municipal government's legal authority.[92] There are state constitutions that allow counties or municipalities to enact ordinances without the legislature's permission and are said to provide home-rule authority. There are some states that have limitations on what kind of local government or population size must exist to be able to exercise home rule; a Dillon's Rule state that allows for home rule in specified circumstances applies Dillon's Rule to matters or governmental units where home rule is not specifically authorized. The National League of Cities identifies Dillon's Rule states and states that follow Dillon's Rule but also permit home rule for some jurisdictions.[93] Each state defines for itself what powers it will grant to local governments. In these states, the state grants cities, municipalities, and/or counties the ability to pass laws to govern themselves as they deem appropriate for their area (so long as they obey the state and federal constitutions). This allows the city or county to pass more restrictive laws; however, state or federal minimum requirements must still be met. Just an example (not a fact) can be found in that the fictional city of Xavier, Texas, ordinance may require annual rabies vaccination regardless of the vaccine used, while Golf County (the fictional county in which Xavier is located) and the state of Texas may require that the owner comply with the vaccine label (for example, 1 year or 3 years) to maintain current vaccination status.

In a mobile society that often travels with their pets, this can create problematic situations. In the United States, current vaccination means the administration of a rabies vaccine suitable to the species, and the vaccine has to be administered according to the manufacturer's instructions not later than the expiration date on the package.[94]

There are variations in recognition as to the length of time between vaccination and an anticipated protective response. This variation is noted between rabies ordinances which may state that current vaccination begins 14,[95] 28,[94] or 30 days[96] following primary vaccination and continue for the period stated in the manufacturer's instructions. The immune response to the rabies vaccination can be detected by day 7[97] and peaks at day 28.[94] The variation on recognition of what constitutes a current rabies vaccination is based on the somewhat

Infection

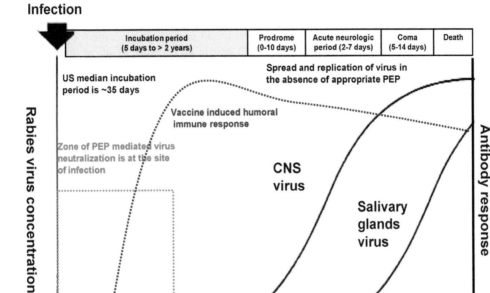

FIG. 6.1 Humoral immune response and rabies virus concentration timelines (refer to Chapter 2). *CNS*, central nervous system; *HRIG*, human rabies immune globulin; *PEP*, postexposure prophylaxis. (Used with permission by Moore S. *Humoral Immune Response Ad Rabies Virus Concentration Timelines*. Kansas State Veterinary Diagnostic Laboratory.[98])

subjective decision of where in the immune response the animal has protection against the rabies virus. Most rabies public health managers choose the conservative peak end of the immune response—28 days. (The animal must have been vaccinated at least 28 days prior to exposure to be considered currently vaccinated.) While Fig. 6.1 depicts the human humoral immune response and rabies virus concentration timelines in response to PEP, it is also reflective of the nonhuman animal immune response to preexposure vaccination.[99,100] Of course, there is no administration of human rabies immune globulin to animals, plus the timelines of disease stages in Fig. 6.1 are reflective of those found in the course of rabies in humans versus those in animals.

Some previously vaccinated animals may be overdue on a rabies vaccination by days, months, or years (or considered not currently vaccinated because the vaccine was administered too recently). Several studies have been accomplished to assist in the management of animals potentially exposed to rabies. Results indicated that dogs with out-of-date vaccination status were not inferior in their antibody response following booster rabies vaccination compared with dogs with

current vaccination status. Findings supported immediate booster vaccination followed by observation for 45 days of dogs, cats, and domestic ferrets with an out-of-date vaccination status that are exposed to rabies, as is the current practice for dogs, cats, and domestic ferrets with current vaccination status.[101] Booster vaccinations for the bitten animals are recommended after exposure to bats and other wildlife unless the animal is available for testing.

Recommendations for the postexposure handling of domestic animals that have been exposed or potentially exposed to rabies may vary slightly. Examples of the existing protocols that are most often referenced are provided as follows (also see Table 6.2):

1. The **National Association of State Public Health Veterinarians; Compendium of Animal Rabies Prevention and Control** recommendations[102] as of 2018 are as follows:

   Dogs, cats, ferrets, and **livestock** that are currently vaccinated (if it has been administered a licensed rabies vaccine in accordance with the label directions and at least 28 days have elapsed since the animal's initial vaccination) should immediately receive veterinary medical care for assessment, wound cleansing, and booster vaccination. The animal should be kept under the owner's control and observed for 45 days.

Dogs, cats, and **ferrets** that have never been vaccinated should be euthanized immediately. There are currently no USDA-licensed biologics for PEP of previously unvaccinated domestic animals, and there is evidence that the use of vaccine alone will not reliably prevent the disease in these animals. If the owner is unwilling to have the animal euthanized, the animal should be placed in strict quarantine for 4 (dogs and cats) or 6 (ferrets) months. Strict quarantine in this context refers to confinement in an enclosure that precludes direct contact with people and other animals. A rabies vaccine should be administered at the time of entry into quarantine to bring the animal up to current rabies vaccination status. Administration of vaccine should be done as soon as possible. It is recommended that the period from exposure to vaccination not exceed 96 h. If vaccination is delayed, public health officials may consider increasing the quarantine period for dogs and cats from 4 to 6 months, taking into consideration factors such as the severity of exposure, the length of delay in vaccination, current health status, and local rabies epidemiology.

Dogs and **cats** that are overdue for a booster vaccination and that have appropriate documentation of having received a USDA-licensed rabies vaccine at least once previously should immediately receive veterinary medical care for assessment, wound cleansing, and booster vaccination. The animal should be kept under the owner's control and observed for 45 days. If booster vaccination is delayed, public health officials may consider increasing the observation period for the animal, taking into consideration factors such as the severity of exposure, the length of delay in booster vaccination, current health status, and local rabies epidemiology.

Dogs and **cats** that are overdue for a booster vaccination and without appropriate documentation of having received a USDA-licensed rabies vaccine at least once previously should immediately receive veterinary medical care for assessment, wound cleansing, and consultation with local public health authorities. The animal can be treated as unvaccinated, immediately given a booster vaccination, and placed in strict quarantine.

Or alternatively, prior to booster vaccination, the attending veterinarian may request guidance from the local public health authorities in the possible use of prospective serologic monitoring. Such monitoring would entail collecting paired blood samples to document prior vaccination by providing evidence of an anamnestic response to booster vaccination. If an adequate anamnestic response is documented, the animal can be considered to be overdue for booster vaccination and observed for 45 days. If there is inadequate evidence of an anamnestic response, the animal is considered to have never been vaccinated and should be placed in strict quarantine.

Ferrets that are overdue for a booster vaccination should be evaluated on a case-by-case basis, taking into consideration factors, such as the severity of exposure, time elapsed since last vaccination, number of previous vaccinations, current health status, and local rabies epidemiology, to determine need for euthanasia or immediate booster vaccination followed by observation or strict quarantine.

Livestock that have never been vaccinated should be euthanized immediately. Animals that are not euthanized should be confined and observed on a case-by-case basis for 6 months.

Livestock overdue for a booster vaccination should be evaluated on a case-by-case basis, taking into consideration factors such as severity of exposure, time elapsed since last vaccination, number of previous vaccinations, current health status, and local rabies epidemiology, to determine need for euthanasia or immediate booster vaccination followed by observation or strict quarantine.

Livestock herd management in general: Multiple rabid animals in a herd and herbivore-to-herbivore transmission of rabies are uncommon. Therefore, restricting the rest of the herd if a single animal has been exposed to or infected with rabies is usually not necessary. Rabies virus is widely distributed in the tissues of rabid animals. Tissues and products from a rabid animal should not be used for human or animal consumption or transplantation. However, pasteurization and cooking will inactivate rabies virus. Therefore, inadvertently drinking pasteurized milk or eating thoroughly cooked animal products does not constitute a rabies exposure. Handling and consumption of uncooked tissues from exposed animals might carry a risk for rabies transmission. Persons handling exposed animals, carcasses, and tissues should use appropriate barrier precautions. State and local public health authorities, state meat inspectors, and the USDA Food Safety and Inspection Service should be notified if exposures occur in animals intended for commercial use. Animals should not be presented for slaughter in a USDA-regulated establishment if such animals originate from a quarantine area and have not been approved for release by the proper authority. If an exposed animal is to be custom slaughtered or home slaughtered for consumption, it should be slaughtered immediately after exposure and all tissues should be cooked thoroughly.

Other mammals exposed to a rabid animal should be euthanized immediately. Animals maintained in USDA-licensed research facilities or accredited zoological parks should be evaluated on a case-by-case basis in consultation with public health authorities. Management options may include quarantine, observation, or administration of rabies biologics.

2. The **Canadian Council of Chief Veterinary Officers Subcommittee for the Management of Potential Domestic Animal Exposures to Rabies**[95] recommendations as of 2018 are as follows:

Dogs, cats, and **ferrets** are considered currently vaccinated if they have been administered a licensed rabies vaccine in accordance with the label directions and at least 14 days have elapsed since the animal's vaccination. The time between the animal's vaccination and the labeled duration of immunity of the vaccine must not have elapsed. Both primary (animal has not received the label recommended second vaccination) and fully vaccinated animals are considered currently vaccinated. Currently vaccinated dogs, cats, and ferrets that have been exposed, or potentially exposed, to rabies should receive a postexposure vaccination immediately. Currently vaccinated animals that receive a postexposure vaccination within 7 days of exposure do not require quarantine. Owner education and follow-up should still occur. Currently vaccinated animals that do not receive a postexposure vaccination within 7 days of exposure should be quarantined for a period of 3 months (with the possible exception of animals that received a vaccination shortly before exposure—these animals would not be quarantined).

Dogs, cats, and **ferrets** exposed to rabies that have no known history of previous rabies vaccination should be vaccinated immediately and quarantined for a period of 3 months. Consideration should be given to the administration of a second rabies vaccination in the third week following exposure. If not vaccinated within 7 days of the exposure event, these animals should be quarantined

for 6 months. Note: The committee recognizes that the World Organization for Animal Health (OIE) considers the incubation period for rabies to be 6 months.[103] Under normal circumstances, when an animal is under a public health observation period following a bite to a human, it should not be vaccinated. Uncommonly, an animal both is potentially exposed to rabies and bites a human. In these infrequent circumstances, rabies vaccination should be administered to the animal immediately.

Dogs, cats, and **ferrets** that are out of date on their vaccination should be given a booster vaccination (preferably within 7 days) and assessed on a case-by-case basis. All other things being equal, a shorter duration since the animal's vaccination status lapsed, a higher number of previous rabies vaccinations, minimal delay between exposure and revaccination, and better overall health status of the animal would each generally be expected to result in better immunity. The expected level of protection against rabies should be assessed and the animal placed under a 6-month, 3-month, or no quarantine as deemed appropriate.

All **livestock** species, regardless of vaccination status, that are exposed or potentially exposed to rabies should be quarantined for 60 days from the time of exposure, if known, or 40 days from the time of the first diagnosis if the index case is within the herd/group. While specific evidence is lacking to support the use of postexposure rabies vaccination in livestock species, evidence does support this practice in dogs and cats. Postexposure vaccination of livestock species immediately following an exposure event may similarly reduce the risk of these animals developing rabies. For the purposes of this recommendation, horses, donkeys, and their hybrid offspring are considered to be "livestock species."

Livestock herd management in general: Livestock animals that are not exhibiting any clinical abnormalities consistent with rabies can be slaughtered for human consumption under standard procedures within 7 days of exposure to rabies. After this time, animals should not be slaughtered for human consumption until after completion of the appropriate quarantine period. Milk from quarantined animals can continue to enter standard processing channels but should not be used in raw milk products. The conditions of livestock quarantines should be set on a case-by-case basis with consideration given to the type of livestock and intended use, with the primary goals of minimizing direct contact with people and other animals outside of the quarantined group and ensuring handler safety should the animal(s) develop neurological disease.

3. In the United States, several **states have variations** in the handling of exposed domestic animals. One of those states (Texas)[65] is highlighted because of its significant database and documentation substantiating the effectiveness of its policies.[104-106] For domestic animals that have never been vaccinated against rabies that have been exposed to rabies, the Texas PEP Protocol has been particularly helpful. In this situation, the domestic animal should be vaccinated against rabies as soon as possible after the exposure with booster vaccines given 3 weeks postexposure and 8 weeks postexposure. The domestic animal should be strictly isolated for 90 days. This protocol has been extremely successful in preventing rabies signs and contagion when rabies vaccination had not been previously administered. The **Texas PEP Protocol** recommendations (**Texas Administrative Code 169.30**[107]) as of 2018 are as follows:

Currently vaccinated animals (domestic animals for which a USDA-licensed rabies vaccine is available, at least 30 days have elapsed since initial vaccination, and the time elapsed since the most recent vaccination has not exceeded the recommended interval for the booster vaccination as established by the manufacturer) that have been bitten by, directly exposed by physical contact with, or directly exposed to the fresh tissues of a rabid animal shall be: (1) euthanatized;

or (2) immediately given a booster rabies vaccination and placed in confinement for 45 days.

Never or not currently vaccinated animals (domestic animals for which a USDA-licensed rabies vaccine is available) that have been bitten by, directly exposed by physical contact with, or directly exposed to the fresh tissues of a rabid animal shall be: (1) euthanatized;

or (2) immediately vaccinated against rabies, placed in confinement for 90 days, and given booster vaccinations during the third and eighth weeks of confinement. For young animals, additional vaccinations may be necessary to ensure that the animal receives at least two vaccinations at or after the age prescribed by the USDA for the vaccine administered.

Other animals: In situations where none of the requirements of this section are applicable, the recommendations contained in the latest edition of the publication titled *Compendium of Animal Rabies Prevention and Control*, published by the National Association of State Public Health Veterinarians, should be followed. The administration of a rabies vaccine in a species for which no licensed vaccine is available is at the discretion of the veterinarian; however, an animal receiving a rabies vaccine under these conditions will not be considered to be vaccinated against rabies virus in potential rabies exposure situations.

Algorithms for the management of potential exposure to rabies

Algorithms are routinely used to attempt to guide the management of scenarios involving potential exposure to rabies in a standardized methodology (see Figs. 6.2 and 6.3 [animal]; 6.4–6.6 [human]).

The potential of wildlife exposure, the vaccination status of the animal, the day-to-day care, and the health status of the animal must be considered in PEP. Regardless of whether it is a domestic or wild animal that caused the potential exposure, the availability of the animal for quarantine or testing is paramount to any postexposure evaluation.

Several US states require that any dog, cat, or domestic ferret that bites another animal be confined for a minimum of 10 days following the bite or that the animal be euthanized and the head submitted to a laboratory for examination for rabies (For example: North Dakota Enforcement Authority 23-36-03 [paragraph 5]).[111] In any area not rabies free, unprovoked bites by pet animals, especially in areas classified as endemic for terrestrial rabies, should be addressed by enforcement of 10-day observation (dog, cat, domestic ferret) or euthanasia and testing of the biting animal, plus PEP for the victim, depending on the availability of the biting animal. Even provoked bites occurring in terrestrial rabies-endemic areas should also be addressed with a degree of care. A biting dog, cat, or domestic ferret that shows neurologic signs of illness during the observation period should be humanely euthanized and submitted for testing. If this occurs, the PEP taken for the exposed animal should be reevaluated to ensure PEP procedures are correct and compliant. Indoor/outdoor cats tend to be more often in close physical contact with wildlife, including those species (particularly raccoons) responsible for transmitting rabies throughout the Eastern Seaboard.[64] Many states and countries will not provide laboratory testing if a human is not involved in the biting incident. The most conservative public health practice if possible is to have any animal suspected of being rabid be destroyed immediately without injury to the head and be submitted to a laboratory approved for rabies testing. This surveillance practice can enhance rabies-management decisions immensely.

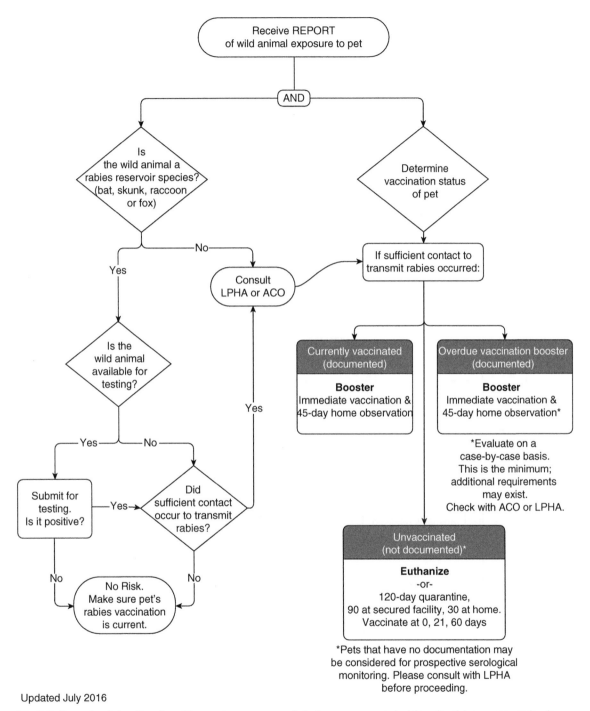

FIG. 6.2 Example of algorithm for rabies postexposure prophylaxis management decisions involving exposures by domestic animals (used with permission Colorado Disease Control and Environmental Epidemiology Division).[108] Note: PEP protocols for animals potentially exposed to rabies can vary per state. *ACO* = animal control officer; *LPHA* = Local Public Health Agency.

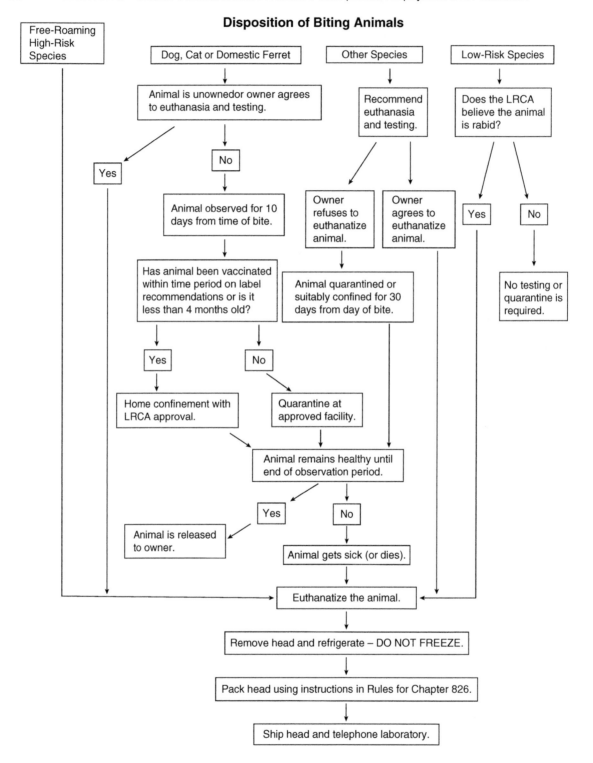

FIG. 6.3 Example of algorithm for rabies postexposure prophylaxis management decisions involving exposures by animals (Texas Department of State Health Services)[65]: https://dshs.texas.gov/idcu/health/zoonosis/education/training/aco/manual).

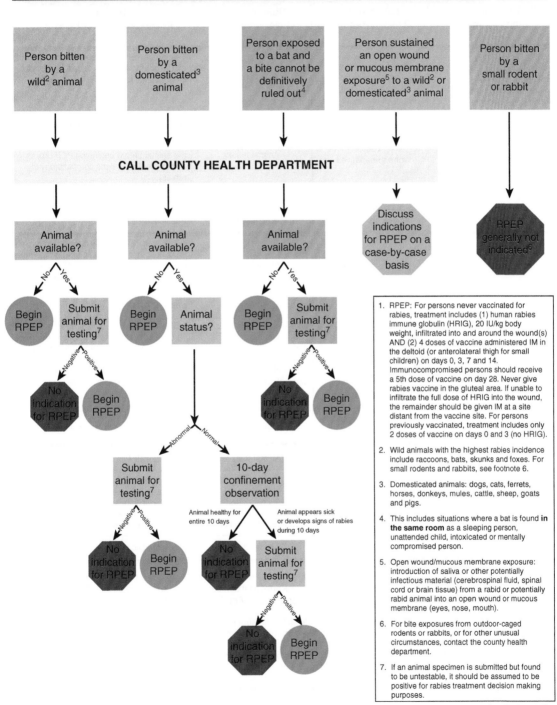

FIG. 6.4 Example of algorithm for rabies postexposure prophylaxis management decisions involving exposures to humans (New York Department of Health: https://www.health.ny.gov/publications/3028.pdf).[109]

These guidelines can help determine if PEP is needed after a potential rabies exposure. An exposure is defined as 1) an animal bite (or scratch) that breaks the skin or 2) exposure of broken skin (bled or had serous drainage within the past 24 hours) or mucous membranes to saliva or cerebrospinal fluid. Stool, blood, urine, and skunk spray do not contain rabies virus.

Risk Category of Biting Animal	Laboratory Testing Result	Quarantine/ Observation or Testing	Human Postexposure Prophylaxis
Low (rabbits, opossums, and armadillos, plus mice, rats, squirrels, nutria, shrews, prairie dogs, beavers, gophers, and other rodents)	Testing is not required unless the Local Rabies Control Authority (LRCA) or physician has cause to believe the animal is rabid.	Not applicable	Testing or PEP is not required unless the LRCA or physician has cause to believe the biting animal is rabid.
High[1] (Bats[2], coyotes, foxes, raccoons, skunks) or type of biting animal is unknown	Positive or non-negative[3]	Animal tested	Administer PEP (usually acceptable to wait up to 72 hours for test results or efforts to locate the animal before beginning PEP unless animal displayed signs compatible with rabies).
	Negative	Animal tested	PEP not administered.
	Animal not available	Not possible	Administer PEP.
Dog, Cat, Domestic Ferret[4]	Positive	Animal tested	Administer PEP (usually acceptable to wait up to 72 hours for test results or efforts to locate the animal before beginning PEP unless animal displayed signs compatible with rabies).
	Negative	Animal tested	PEP not administered.
	Not tested pending outcome of quarantine (animal placed in quarantine or home confinement until end of a 10-day observation period).	Animal placed in quarantine or home confinement until end of a 10-day observation period. If animal shows clinical signs of rabies, it should be immediately euthanized and tested.	PEP not administered if animal is available for 10-day observation. If animal shows clinical signs of rabies, it should be immediately euthanized and tested; PEP could be started immediately without waiting for test results and discontinued if test is negative.
	Animal not available or non-negative[3]	Not possible	Consult public health professional.
All Other Warm-Blooded Animals	Positive	Animal tested	Administer PEP.
	Negative	Animal tested	PEP not administered.
	Non-negative[3]	Animal tested	Consult public health professional.
	Not tested	30-day observation[5]	Consult public health professional.
	Animal not available	Not possible	Consult public health professional.

1. Refer to Texas Administrative Code, Sections 169.27(e) and (h) or consult with the Local Rabies Control Authority for your area pertaining to exemptions to mandatory euthanasia for certain high-risk animals that meet captivity parameters as specified in state law: http://texreg.sos.state.tx.us/public/readtac$ext.ViewTAC?tac_view=5&ti=25&pt=1&ch=169&sch=A&rl=Y
2. In incidents involving bats, PEP may be appropriate even in the absence of demonstrable bite, scratch, or mucous membrane exposure in situations in which there is reasonable probability that such exposure may have occurred (e.g., sleeping individual awakes to find a bat in the room, a person witnesses a bat in the room with a previously unattended child, mentally challenged person, intoxicated individual, etc.).
3. "Non-negative" includes all specimens not suitable for testing (destroyed, decomposed, etc.).
4. The decision whether a dog, cat, or domestic ferret should be euthanized and tested or quarantined rests with the Local Rabies Control Authority.
5. The Local Rabies Control Authority may authorize a 30-day observation period in lieu of testing.

FIG. 6.5 Example of algorithm for rabies postexposure prophylaxis management decisions involving exposures to humans (Texas Department of State Health Services)[96]: http://www.dshs.texas.gov/idcu/disease/rabies/information/prevention/pamphlet/). Note: Cerebrospinal fluid as an exposure source is currently under review.

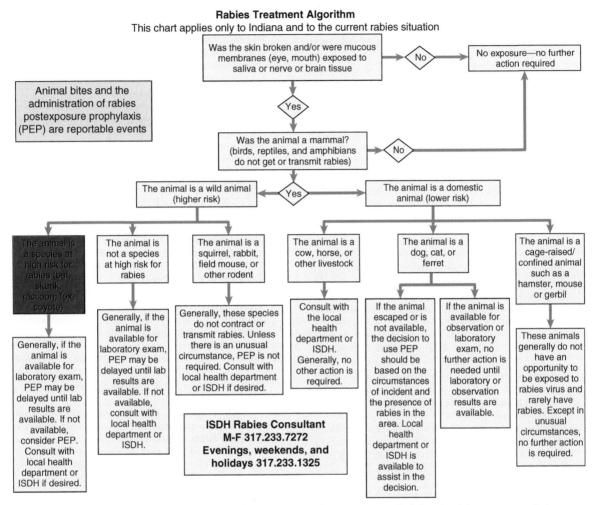

FIG. 6.6 Example of algorithm for rabies postexposure prophylaxis management decisions involving exposures to humans (Indiana Department of Health)[110]: https://www.in.gov/isdh/files/rabies_treatment_algorithm.pdf).

CONCLUSION

In those areas where human rabies deaths are still attributed to dogs, programs addressing required vaccination of dogs and cats, impoundment of stray dogs and cats, population control measures, and quarantine of potentially rabid animals, will be beneficial in reducing the number of cases. RIG is a crucial bridge providing neutralization of rabies virus until vaccine-induced immunity develops in 7 days. The costs associated with low-volume production of the vaccines and polyclonal RIG remain prohibitive in most rabies-endemic regions. Current vaccines also require a cold chain and repeated doses that are logistically challenging for populations living in remote areas. There is no RIG for domestic animals and vaccine plus quarantine must be utilized. Whether human or domestic animal, the sooner PEP is started, the more effective it is. The decisions pertaining to PEP are made much simpler when the biting animal has been captured. Likewise, PEP decisions for an exposed animal are simpler if it has been previously vaccinated. Literature searches on rabies PEP/quarantine failures reveal that there are very few failures in either humans or domestic animals when postexposure protocols are followed in a compliant and timely fashion. The published PEP algorithms help public health officials, physicians, and veterinarians make standardized responses.

REFERENCES

1. Rappuoli R. Inner workings: 1885, the first rabies vaccination in humans. *Proc Natl Acad Sci USA.* 2014;111(34):12273.
2. Hemachudha T, Phanuphak P, Johnson R, et al. Neurological complications of Semple type rabies vaccine: clinical and immunological studies. *Neurology.* 1987;37:550–556.
3. Medley A, Millien M, Blanton J, et al. Retrospective cohort study to assess the risk of rabies in biting dogs, 2011-2015, Republic of Haiti. *Trop Med Infect Dis.* 2017;2(2):14.
4. Zhang Y, Zhang S, Li L, et al. Ineffectiveness of rabies vaccination alone for post-exposure protection against rabies infection in animal models. *Antivir Res.* 2016;135:56–61.
5. Hemachudha T, Mitrabhakdi E, Wilde H, et al. Additional reports of failure to respond to treatment after rabies exposure in Thailand. *Clin Infect Dis.* 1999;28(1):143–144.
6. Ravish H, Srikanth J, Ashwath D, et al. Pre-exposure prophylaxis against rabies in children: safety of purified chick embryo cell rabies vaccine (Vaxirab N) when administered by intradermal route. *Hum Vaccines Immunother.* 2013;9(9):1910–1913.
7. Pengsaa K, Limkittikul K, Sabcharoen A, et al. A three-year clinical study on immunogenicity, safety, and booster response of purified chick embryo cell rabies vaccine administered intramuscularly or intradermally to 12- to 18-month-old Thai children, concomitantly with Japanese encephalitis vaccine. *Pediatr Infect Dis J.* 2009;28(4):335–337.
8. Shanbag P, Shah N, Kulkarni M, et al. Protecting Indian Schoolchildren against rabies: pre-exposure vaccination with purified chick embryo cell vaccine (PCECV) or purified verocell rabies vaccine (PVRV). *Hum Vaccine.* 2008;31(5):4.
9. Sabcharoen A, Lang J, Chanthavanich P, et al. Safety and immunogenicity of a three dose regimen of two tetravalent live-attenuated dengue vaccines in five- to twelve-year-old Thai children. *Pediatr Infect Dis J.* 2004;23(2):99–109.
10. Lang J, Duong G, Nguyen V, et al. Randomised feasibility trial of pre-exposure rabies vaccination with DTP-IPV in infants. *Lancet.* 1997;349(9066):1663–1665.
11. Schutsky K, Curtis D, Bongiorno E, et al. Intramuscular inoculation of mice with the live-attenuated recombinant rabies virus TriGAS results in a transient infection of the draining lymph nodes and a robust, long-lasting protective immune response against rabies. *J Virol.* 2013;87(3):1834–1841.
12. Gogtay N, Munshi R, Ashwath D, et al. Comparison of a novel human rabies monoclonal antibody to human rabies immunoglobulin for postexposure prophylaxis: a phase 2/3, randomized, single-blind, noninferiority, controlled study. *Clin Infect Dis.* 2018;66(3):387–395.
13. *WHO Expert Consultation on Rabies, Third Report.* Geneva: World Health Organization; 2018. Report No.: 1012.
14. Banyard A, Mansfield K, Wu G, et al. Re-evaluating the effect of Favipiravir treatment on rabies virus infection. *Vaccine.* November 10, 2017. https://doi.org/10.1016/j.vaccine.2017.10.109.
15. Virojanapirom P, Lumlertdacha B, Wipattanakitcharoen A, et al. T-705 as a potential therapeutic agent for rabies. *J Infect Dis.* 2016;214(3):502–503.
16. Yamada K, Noguchi K, Komeno T, et al. Efficacy of favipiravir (T-705) in rabies postexposure prophylaxis. *J Infect Dis.* 2016;213(8):1253–1261.
17. Vigilato MA, Cosivi O, Knobl T, et al. Rabies update for Latin America and the Caribbean. *Emerg Infect Dis.* 2013;19(4):678–679.
18. Lapiz SM, Miranda ME, Garcia RG, et al. Implementation of an intersectoral program to eliminate human and canine rabies: the Bohol Rabies Prevention and Elimination Project. *PLoS Neglected Trop Dis.* 2012;6(12):e1891.
19. Reece J, Chawla S, Hiby A. Decline in human dog-bite cases during a street dog sterilisation programme in Jaipur, India. *Vet Rec.* 2013;172(18):473.
20. Dietzschold B, Li J, Faber M, et al. Concepts in the pathogenesis of rabies. *Future Virol.* 2008;3(5):481–490.
21. Hemachudha T, Laothamatas J, Rupprecht C. Human rabies: a disease of complex neuropathogenetic mechanisms and diagnostic challenges. *Lancet Neurol.* 2002;1:101–109.
22. Singh R, Singh K, Cherian S, et al. Rabies – epidemiology, pathogenesis, public health concerns and advances in diagnosis and control: a comprehensive review. *Vet Q.* 2017;37:212–251.
23. Mitchell C, Guerin L, Pasieka A. Antibody production in milk serum after virus instillation of goat mammary gland VI. "Sham infection" with special reference to rabies. *Can J Comp Med.* 1974;38(1):14–17.
24. Centers for Disease Control and Prevention, Presumptive abortive human rabies—Texas, 2009. *Morb Mortal Wkly Rep.* 2010;59(07):185–190.
25. Reagan R, Yancy F, Chang S, et al. Transmission of street rabies virus strain (V308) to suckling hamsters during lactation. *Proc Soc Exp Biol Med.* 1955;90(1):301–302.
26. Nicholson K, Bauer S. Enteric inoculation with ERA rabies virus: evaluation of a candidate wildlife vaccine in laboratory rodents. *Arch Virol.* 1981;67(1):51–56.
27. Ekanem E, Eyong K, Philip-Ephraim E, et al. Stray dog trade fuelled by dog meat consumption as a risk factor for rabies infection in Calabar, southern Nigeria. *Afr Health Sci.* 2013;13(4):1170–1173.
28. Nguyen A, Nguyen D, Ngo G, et al. Molecular epidemiology of rabies virus in Vietnam (2006-2009). *Jpn J Infect Dis.* 2011;64(5):391–396.
29. Rupprecht C, Stohr K, Meredith C. Rabies. In: Williams ES, Barker IK, eds. *Infectious Diseases of Wild Mammals.* third ed. Ames, IA: Iowa State U. Press.; 2001:3–36.
30. Constantine D. Rabies transmission by nonbite route. *Publ Health Rep.* 1962;77:287–289.
31. Helmick C, Tauxe R, Vernon A. Is there a risk to contacts of patients with rabies? *Rev Infect Dis.* 1987;9(3):511–518.

32. Fekadu M, Endeshaw T, Alemu W, et al. Possible human-to-human transmission of rabies in Ethiopia. *Ethiop Med J.* 1996;34:123–127.

33. Dutta J. Rabies transmission by oral and other non-bite routes. *J Indian Med Assoc.* 1998;96(12):359.

34. Bharti O, Chand R, Chauhan A, et al. Scratches/abrasions without bleeding" cause rabies: a 7 years rabies death review from Medical College Shimla, Himachal Pradesh, India. *Indian J Community Med.* 2017;42(4):248–249.

35. Charlton K. In: Campbell JB, Charlton KM, eds. *The Pathogenesis of Rabies.* Boston, MA: Kluwer Academic Publishers; 1988:101–150.

36. Javadi M, Fayaz A, et al. Transmission of rabies by corneal graft. *Cornea.* 1996;15(4):431–433.

37. Centers for Disease Control and Prevention, Investigation of rabies infections in organ donor and transplant recipients — Alabama, Arkansas, Oklahoma, and Texas. 2004. *Morb Mortal Wkly Rep.* 2004;53(26):586–589.

38. Dietzschold B, Koprowski H. Rabies transmission from organ transplants in the USA. *Lancet.* 2004;364(9435):648–649.

39. Dietzschold B, Koprowski H. Screening of organ and tissue donors for rabies. *Lancet.* 2005;365(9467):1305.

40. Hellenbrand W, Meyer C, Rasch G, et al. Cases of rabies in Germany following organ transplantation. *Euro Surveill.* 2005;10(2):52–53.

41. Srinivasan A, Burton E, Kuehnert M, et al. Transmission of rabies virus from an organ donor to four transplant recipients. *N Engl J Med.* 2003;352(11):1103–1111.

42. Bronnert J, Wilde H, Tepsumethanon V, et al. Organ transplantations and rabies transmission. *J Trav Med.* 2007;14(3):177–180.

43. Vora N, Basavarju S, Feldman K, et al. Raccoon rabies virus variant transmission through solid organ transplantation. *JAMA.* 2013;310(4):398–407.

44. Winkler W, Fashinell T, Leffingwell L, et al. Airborne rabies transmission in a laboratory worker. *JAMA.* 1973;226(10):1219–1221.

45. Gibbons R. Cryptogenic rabies, bats, and the question of aerosol transmission. *Ann Emerg Med.* 2002;39:528–536.

46. Sikes R. Rabies. In: Davis JW, Karstad LH, DO Trainer, eds. *Infectious Diseases of Wild Mammals.* second ed. Ames, IA: Iowa State U. Press; 1981:3–17.

47. Afshar A. A review of non-bite transmission of rabies virus infection. *Br Vet J.* 1979;135:142–148.

48. Soave OA. Transmission of rabies to mice by ingestion of infected tissue. *Am J Vet Res.* 1966;27:44–46.

49. Barnard B, Hassel R, Geyer H, et al. Nonbite transmission of rabies in kudu (*Tragelaphus strepsiceros*). *Onderstepoort J Vet Res.* 1982;49:191–192.

50. Howard DR. Transplacental transmission of rabies virus from a naturally infected skunk. *Am J Vet Res.* 1981;42:691–692.

51. Podberscek AL. An appetite for dogs: consuming and loving them in Vietnam. In: Pręgowski M, ed. *Companion Animals in Everyday Life.* New York: Palgrave Macmillan; 2016.

52. Ajoke E, Solomon A, Ikhide S. The role of dog trading and slaughter for meat in rabies epidemiology with special reference to Nigeria - a review. *J Exp Biol Agric Sci.* 2014;2(2):131–136.

53. Garba A, Dzikwi A, Okewole P, et al. Evaluation of dog slaughter and consumption practices related to the control of rabies in Nigeria. *J Exp Biol Agric Sci.* 2013;1:125–130.

54. Wertheim H, Nguyen T, Nguyen K, et al. Furious rabies after an atypical exposure. *PLoS Med.* 2009;6(3):e1000044. https://doi.org/10.1371/journal.pmed.1000044.

55. Dato V, Campagnolo E, Long J, et al. A systematic review of human bat rabies virus variant cases: evaluating unprotected physical contact with claws and teeth in support of accurate risk assessments. *PloS One.* 2016;11(7):e0159443.

56. Ugolini G, Hemachudha T. Rabies: changing prophylaxis and new insights in pathophysiology. *Curr Opin Infect Dis.* 2018;31(1):93–101.

57. Manning S, Rupprecht C, Fishbein D, et al. Human rabies prevention--United States, 2008: recommendations of the Advisory Committee on Immunization Practices. *MMWR Recomm Rep (Morb Mortal Wkly Rep).* 2008;57(RR-3):1–28.

58. Wandeler A, Bauder W, Prochaska S, et al. Small mammal studies in a SAD baiting area. *Comp Immunol Microbiol Infect Dis.* 1982;5(1–3):173–176.

59. Tomori O. Wild life rabies in Nigeria: experimental infection and transmission studies with the shrew (*Crocidura* sp.). *Ann Trop Med Parasitol.* 1980;74(2):151–156.

60. Sipahioglu U, Alpaut S. Transplacental rabies in humans. *Mikrobiyoloji Bulteni.* 1985;19(2):95–99.

61. Gautret P, Blanton J, Dacheux L, et al. Rabies in nonhuman primates and potential for transmission to humans: a literature review and examination of selected French national data. *PLoS Neglected Trop Dis.* 2014;8(5):e2863.

62. Centers for Disease Control and Prevention, Human rabies - Kentucky/Indiana, 2009. *Morb Mortal Wkly Rep.* 2010;59(13):393–396.

63. VMA. Rabies and Your Pet. https://www.avma.org/public/Health/Pages/rabies.aspx.

64. Centers for Disease Control and Prevention. Prevention in Animals. https://www.cdc.gov/rabies/prevention/animals.html.

65. Texas Department of State Health Services, Zoonosis Control. Rabies. In: *Animal Control Officer Training Manual.* ; 2014:1–16. http://dshs.texas.gov/idcu/health/zoonosis/education/training/aco/manual/information/basChapters.asp.

66. U. of Saskatchewan. Clinical Signs of Rabies. http://homepage.usask.ca/~sjd220/virology/clinsigns.html.

67. Leslie M, Messenger S, Rohde R, et al. Bat-associated rabies virus in skunks. *Emerg Infect Dis.* 2006;12(8). www.cdc.gov/eid.

68. Eidson M, Matthews S, Wilset A, et al. Rabies Virus Infection in a pet guinea pig and seven pet rabbits. *JAVMA.* 2005;227:932–935.

69. Hampson K, Coudeville L, Lembo T, et al. Estimating the global burden of endemic canine rabies. *PLoS Neglected Trop Dis.* 2015;9(4):e0003709.

70. Moro P, Woo E, Paul W, et al. Post-marketing surveillance of human rabies diploid cell vaccine (Imovax) in the vaccine adverse event reporting system (VAERS) in the United States, 1990–2015. *PLoS Neglected Trop Dis.* 2016;10(7):e0004846.

71. Reveneau E, Cottin P, Rasuli A. Two decades of pharmacovigilance and clinical experience with highly purified rabies immunoglobulin F(ab')2 fragments. *Expert Rev Vaccines.* 2017;16(3):273–287.

72. World Health Organization. WHO Expert consultation on rabies. First report. *World Health Organ Tech Rep Ser.* 2004;(931):1–121.

73. Bharti O, Madhusudana S, Gaunta P, et al. Local infiltration of rabies immunoglobulins without systemic intramuscular administration: an alternative cost effective approach for passive immunization against rabies. *Hum Vaccines Immunother.* 2015;13(4):762–765.

74. R.E. Willoughby Jr., Rabies Treatment Protocol and Registry. 2018(5). Available from: www.mcw.edu/rabies.

75. Willoughby Jr RE. "Early death" and the contraindication of vaccine during treatment of rabies. *Vaccine.* 2009;27(51):7173–7177.

76. Lebrun A, Portocarrero C, Kean R, et al. T-bet is required for the rapid clearance of attenuated rabies virus from central nervous system tissue. *J Immunol.* 2015;195(9):4358–4368.

77. Iowa State University Center for Food Security and Public Health. *Rabies and Rabies-related Lyssaviruses.* Center for Food Security and Public Health Technical Factsheets; 2012:106. https://lib.dr.iastate.edu/cfsph_factsheets/106.

78. Rupprecht C, Briggs D, Brown C, et al. Use of a reduced (4-dose) vaccine schedule for postexposure prophylaxis to prevent human rabies: recommendations of the Advisory Committee on Immunization Practices. *MMWR Recomm Rep (Morb Mortal Wkly Rep).* 2010;59(RR-2):1–9.

79. Rupprecht C, Briggs D, Brown C, et al. Evidence for a 4-dose vaccine schedule for human rabies post-exposure prophylaxis in previously non-vaccinated individuals. *Vaccine.* 2009;27(51):7141–7148.

80. Albuquerque E, Barnard E, Porter C, et al. The density of acetylcholine receptors and their sensitivity in the postsynaptic membrane of muscle endplates. *Proc Natl Acad Sci USA.* 1974;71(7):2818–2822.

81. Madhusudana S, Ashwin B, Sudarshan S. Feasibility of reducing rabies immunoglobulin dosage for passive immunization against rabies: results of in vitro and in vivo studies. *Hum Vaccines Immunother.* 2013;9(9):1914–1917.

82. Van C, Molenaers G. Localization of the motor endplate zone in human skeletal muscles of the lower limb: anatomical guidelines for injection with botulinum toxin. *Dev Med Child Neurol.* 2011;53(2):108–119.

83. Kessels J, Recuenco S, Navarro-Vela A, et al. Pre-exposure rabies prophylaxis: a systematic review. *Bull World Health Organ.* 2017;95(3):210–219C.

84. Vashishtha V, Choudhury P, Kalra A, et al. Indian Academy of Pediatrics (IAP) recommended immunization schedule for children aged 0 through 18 years--India, 2014 and updates on immunization. *Indian Pediatr.* 2014;51(10):785–800.

85. Global Alliance for Rabies Control. *Partners for Rabies Prevention. Blueprint and Stepwise Approach to Rabies Elimination;* 2012. https://rabiesalliance.org/capacity-building/blueprint-sare.

86. Dyer J, Yager P, Orciari L, et al. Rabies surveillance in the United States during 2013. *JAVMA.* 2014;245(10):1111–1123.

87. *The Vaccine Alliance. Report to the Board: Vaccine Investment Strategy: Short List.* Geneva: Gavi; June 7, 2018. Report No. 07.

88. McLaughlin K. Infectious disease. Scandal clouds China's global vaccine ambitions. *Science.* 2016;352(6285):506.

89. Rabies vaccine–update. *Wkly Epidemiol Rec.* 2007;82(8):62–68.

90. Centers for Disease Control and Prevention Human Rabies Prevention – United States; 2008. Morb Mortal Wkly Rep. https://www.cdc.gov/mmwr/preview/mmwrhtml/rr57e507a1.htm.

91. Hanlon C, Niezgoda M, Morrill P, et al. The incurable wound revisited: progress in human rabies prevention? *Vaccine.* 2001;19(17–19):2273–2279.

92. Legal Help. Home Rule and Legal Definition. https://definitions.uslegal.com/h/home-rule.

93. National League of Cities. https://www.nlc.org.

94. Centers for Disease Control and Prevention. *Veterinarians: Rabies Vaccination - Rabies;* 2011. https://www.cdc.gov/rabies/specific_groups/veterinarians/vaccination.html.

95. Canadian Council of Chief Veterinary Officers. Recommendations of the Canadian Council of Chief Veterinary Officers Subcommittee for the Management of Potential Domestic Animal Exposures to Rabies. http://www1.agric.gov.ab.ca/$Department/deptdocs.nsf/all/cpv16353/$FILE/CCVO-Recommendations-Rabies-Exposure.pdf.

96. Texas Department of State Health Services. Zoonosis Control. Rabies Prevention in Texas. Stock No. 6-108. Revised January 2016. http://www.oie.int/en/conferences-events/other-oie-key-events/2014/.

97. Darkaoui S, Fihri O, Schereffer J, et al. Immunogenicity and efficacy of Rabivac vaccine for animal rabies control in Morocco. *Clin Exp Vaccine Res.* 2016;5(1):60–69.

98. Moore S. Humoral Immune Response Ad Rabies Virus Concentration Timelines. Kansas State Veterinary Diagnostic Laboratory.

99. Smith T, Millien M, Franso A, et al. Evaluation of immune responses in dogs to oral rabies vaccine under field conditions. *Vaccine*. 2017.

100. Shimazaki Y, Inoue S, Takahashi C, et al. Immune response to Japanese rabies vaccine in domestic dogs. *Zoonoses Public Health*. February 2003;50(2):95–98.

101. Moore M, Davis R, Kang Q, et al. Comparison of anamnestic responses to rabies vaccination in dogs and cats with current and out-of-date vaccination status. *JAVMA*. 2015;246(2):205–211.

102. Brown C, Slavinski S, Ettestad P, et al. Compendium of animal rabies prevention and control. *JAVMA*. 2016; 248(5):505–517.

103. OIE. *World Organization for Animal Health*; 2014.

104. Wilson P, Clark K. Postexposure rabies prophylaxis protocol for domestic animals and epidemiologic characteristics of rabies vaccination failures in Texas: 1995-1999. *JAVMA*. 2001;218(4):522–525.

105. Wilson P, Oertli E, Hunt P, et al. Evaluation of a postexposure rabies prophylaxis protocol for domestic animals in Texas: 2000-2009. *JAVMA*. 2010;237(12):1395–1401.

106. Clark KA, Wilson PJ. Postexposure rabies prophylaxis and preexposure rabies vaccination failure in domestic animals. *JAVMA*. 1996;208(11):1827–1830.

107. Texas Administrative Code 169.30. http://txrules.elaws.us/rule/title25_chapter169.

108. Colorado Disease Control and Environmental Epidemiology Division. Algorithm for Management of Domestic Animals Exposed to Wildlife. Colorado Resource Guide: Rabies. Colorado State U. Fort Collins, CO.

109. New York Department of Health. Rabies Post Exposure Prophylaxis (RPEP) Algorithm. www.health.NY.gov/publications/3028.pdf.

110. Indiana State Department of Health. Rabies Education Website: https://www.in.gov/isdh/files/rabies_treatment_algorithm.pdf.

111. North Dakota Enforcement Authority 23-36-03 (Paragraph 5). https://www.legis.nd.gov/cencode/t23c36.pdf.

112. Moore D, Sischo W, Hunter A, et al. Animal bite epidemiology and surveillance for rabies postexposure prophylaxis. *JAVMA*. 2000;217:190–194.

CHAPTER 7

Assessment of Potential Exposure Scenarios

PAMELA J. WILSON, MEd, LVT, MCHES • RODNEY E. ROHDE, PhD, MS, SM(ASCP)[CM], SV[CM], MB[CM], FACSc

INTRODUCTION AND BACKGROUND OF REAL-LIFE SCENARIOS

Hey this is a great article and very helpful one but I have a question. I got bit by a stray cat July 4. The cat seemed very healthy but she was hungry so I was feeding her but stupid me I had it in my hand and she bit me. I did not get the vaccine for rabies and my doctor told me that I was fine but the day after I got bit I had a sore throat and a headache is it possible that I could have contracted rabies? Is it too late to get the vaccine? We saw the cat 7ish days after the bite and she was healthy too. I overthink too much so please help me before I overthink to death.

Answer: Having a sore throat and headache the day after a bite is not typically characteristic of rabies. However, there is always a potential for getting an infection from a bite wound. Your doctor would need to evaluate it to determine if antibiotics are needed; he/she can also determine if you should get a tetanus shot. The standard is that if a cat is alive and healthy at least 10 days after it has bitten someone, it could not have transmitted rabies through that particular bite scenario. If you have any doubts, you should consult your physician again and ask him/her to reevaluate your bite scenario to determine if there is a need for any type of treatment. Wishing you well.—Pam and Rodney

This chapter presents real-life rabies concerns that were submitted by readers worldwide in response to two articles that were published in Elsevier Connect.[1,2] Inquiries and concerns submitted by readers of the aforementioned articles are followed by responses provided by the authors (Wilson and Rohde), who worked in collaboration with Alison Bert, an Executive Editor for Elsevier. Some were questions posed on the basic nature and fundamentals of rabies. The majority of these inquires, however, pertained to what constitutes a rabies exposure and whether rabies

postexposure prophylaxis (PEP) was warranted in a wide variety of scenarios. The description of the variable incubation period for rabies, including that it could potentially be years, was one of the most unsettling concepts for readers, as was the mention that, although rabies is typically transmitted through the bite of a rabid animal, transmission could potentially occur through infected saliva from a rabid animal contacting mucous membranes or an opening in the skin. These submissions are being shared because they reflect the type of inquiries health professionals actually receive.

In their responses to the inquiries that were submitted, the authors consistently provided the disclaimer that they are not physicians and that anyone suspecting that they were exposed to rabies should contact a physician immediately and not wait for a response to a question posted on the Internet. Additionally, the following disclaimer was posted on the website with each article: "While we welcome your comments, anyone who thinks they might have been exposed to rabies should contact a physician immediately and not wait for a response to an Internet inquiry."

SUBMITTED RABIES INQUIRIES AND RESPONSES

The following are the questions submitted by readers of the Elsevier Connect rabies articles[1,2] and the authors' subsequent responses as described previously. They were divided into categories by species depending on the extent of exposure probability or general rabies inquiries. Timeframes for receiving comments and providing responses on the Internet are not reflected in the following section. Therefore, to assure accuracy of the statements, the term "and well" or its equivalent has been added pertaining to the 10-day

Rabies. https://doi.org/10.1016/B978-0-323-63979-8.00007-6
Copyright © 2019 Elsevier Inc. All rights reserved.

observation period for dogs, cats, and domestic ferrets (i.e., if the animal is alive [and well] 10 days after a bite incident, it could not have transmitted rabies at the time of that particular bite). To save the reader too much repetitiveness in the compiled responses, disclaimers pertaining to not being medical doctors and recommendations to contact a physician pertaining to PEP needs were removed from multiple responses. **Please note that the questions from readers are being presented verbatim with no modifications by the authors unless it was to remove any identifying information.**

Definite/Probable or Contemplative Exposures

Dog

1. Following sad incident happened with my 3-year-old son in India:
   a. Rabies infected dog bites on his right ear on June 13, 2017 at ~8:30 p.m.
   b. The wound was washed with soap water then dettol and victim receives tetanus vaccine approximately after 30 min after the bite incident.
   c. The rabies-infected dog died on June 14, 2017.
   d. Victim receives first dose of Rabipur antirabies vaccine on June 14, 2017, at ~3 p.m.
   e. Victim receives human rabies immune globulin (HRIG) vaccine with help of body anesthesia on June 14, 2017, at ~10 p.m.
   f. Victim receives second dose of antirabies vaccine on June 17, 2017 (3rd day).
   g. Remaining doses of antirabies vaccine will be given on following days:
      June 21, 2017 (7th day)
      June 28, 2017 (14th day)
      July 12, 2017 (28th day)
      September 15, 2017 (62nd day)

      All vaccinations mentioned above are done by medical professionals.

      I understand that we have to cure this during initial period as there is no treatment after infection spreads into his nervous system; we are doing whatever has been advised by doctors to prevent him from getting infected. Please advise me if there is anything else we can do to save our kid. Thanks!

      Is there any tests possible to detect the following:
   1. Rabies virus is not active in his body.
   2. HRIG given to him is effective and it is really working.

      I don't know what else to ask I really need urgent help!

   Answer: Hi, We are sorry that you are going through this issue. However, it appears that your medical professionals are following all postexposure protocols for rabies virus infection. To answer your final two questions, there is no reliable test to determine if rabies virus is active in the body. There are some antemortem (before death) molecular testing that is occasionally done if the case merits its use. However, these tests can present a "false-negative" result because of the pathogenesis of the rabies virus. To my knowledge, there are not tests to determine if HRIG is effective in "real time." We are not medical doctors; we always recommend that you contact/consult a physician as soon as possible pertaining to concerns about a possible exposure to rabies if you have major concerns. You have done that! Thanks for the question!—Dr. Rohde and Pam

2. Hello, Thanks for the informative article :) Everyone seems to have had an encounter that has brought them to this page, and here is mine:

   Earlier today, I found a dog outside on my porch. I tried to coax it into eating and drinking water, and while it certainly ate, it only did so when I had returned indoors—I'm not sure if it drank the water. It appeared to have injured legs and was shivering, so I decided to bring it in from the cold against my better judgment. I picked it up with a giant bag and placed it in a bin and noticed that the pup was extremely docile the entire time. Although a call to the state health department initially left me less worried about the dog having rabies because of it not being aggressive, the more I searched the disease on the Google, the more I saw traits the dog exhibited. Finally, my father called and told me that the dog I had brought in had tried to bite him yesterday after staggering around, and I was then 99% positive the animal was rabid. Although I wasn't bitten, I'm fairly sure I moved the bowl the dog drank out of before placing him in the bin. My question, I guess, is how worried should I be about the chances of the disease being transmitted this way because the bowl may have had saliva around it? I'm doubtful that I touched my face or any areas that would've allowed the disease to travel into my bloodstream, but should I consider a shot to be on the safe side nonetheless? Thank you in advance. *Answer:* Hello, you did not mention if you still had the dog. If so, you should take it to a veterinarian. A veterinarian will be able to better evaluate the animal's health status. Additionally, the dog can be observed for rabies; if the dog is alive (and well) 10 days after any possible exposure you might have had, it could not have transmitted rabies in its saliva during that particular exposure. The dog can also be tested for rabies if the veterinarian determines that is the necessary route to take; the dog must be euthanized to test it for rabies, so it is not a step to take without due consideration.

Your physician would be the one who would ultimately decide whether or not to prescribe post-exposure treatment for you. Rabies is primarily transmitted via a bite from an infected animal, but it could potentially be transmitted if saliva containing the rabies virus contacted a break in the skin or a mucous membrane. Hope all goes as well as possible.—Pam and Rodney

Cat

1. Hello, I am in dire need of advice. Recently, two stray kittens (about 4 months old) showed up to my door. I fed them once and now they keep coming (it's been 3 days). They basically live on my porch now. They're quite friendly, they like to be pet, and they lick me sometimes. But they are strays and so I'm scared that they have rabies. I've been licked quite a few times, and the cats also bite (but not an aggressive bite—it's the kind of bite my old pet cats would give me, like they put their teeth on you but don't break skin). I don't have enough money to take them to the vet and I don't know what to do. How do I know if they have rabies or not? Thanks in advance!

   Answer: Hi, you cannot tell if an animal has rabies or not just by looking at it or having a veterinarian examine it. The only way to confirm if an animal has rabies is to euthanize it and submit its head for testing, which you surely want to avoid doing.

   If a cat is alive (and well) 10 days after it has been suspected of exposing a person to rabies via a bite (or its saliva contacting a mucous membrane or open cut on the skin of the person), it could not have transmitted rabies in its saliva during that particular suspected exposure scenario. It could be incubating rabies, but it would not have been passing the virus in its saliva at that time. A good recommendation would be for you to take these two strays to a veterinarian to have them vaccinated against rabies. Good luck.—Pam and Rodney

Possible Exposures
Dog

1. Hi Sir, I got bitten by a small dog 7 years ago and I don't know whether it was dead or not. Is there any possibility of rabies? Can I take vaccine now?

   Answer: Because of the varying range of the incubation period for rabies, treatment should be started even if there was a delay in recognizing a rabies exposure. However, the sooner the treatment has begun after exposure, the better the chance of effectiveness. The PEP combination of rabies immune globulin and rabies vaccine is recommended, regardless of the interval between exposure and treatment. Thank you for your interest.—Pam and Dr. Rohde

2. My two puppies, "K" and "D," were recently attacked by a rabid dog (July 8, 2016) at around 1:30 a.m. I woke up and rushed to my doorstep and found "K" badly wounded. Unfortunately, he died the following morning by 10:00 a.m. "D" was traumatized and he decided to come back home at around 12:00 noon. So far, he seems fine and doesn't have any symptoms or bite marks. He has no wounds and I therefore assume that he wasn't infected. However, he seems scared and he is not as confident and playful as he used to be. Should I be worried that he might be infected or is this change of behavior as a result of the trauma? *The darker one is "K" and the lighter one is "D"*

   Answer: Hello, sorry to hear about the death of "K." It's such a significant loss to have a pet pass away. Plus, that was certainly a tragic scenario. It could have had enough impact on "D" to cause him to act differently, so could the loss of his playmate.

   Was the attacking dog actually tested and laboratory confirmed to be rabid?

   You did not mention the age of "D," his vaccination status, or in what state you reside. If there was, indeed, an attack by a rabid dog in which "D" may have gotten even a small wound or had saliva from the attacking dog contact a mucous membrane (i.e., eyes, nose, or mouth), it would be better to err on the side of caution and get rabies postexposure prophylaxis (PEP) for him. Because PEP protocols can vary by state, I am going to include as an example information from the Texas Administrative Code, Rabies Control and Eradication, which covers PEP for domestic animals; during various decades of data analyses on Texas' PEP protocol, it has been, at a minimum, 99.5% effective. In Texas, if the animal was not currently vaccinated when it was exposed to rabies, it would be immediately vaccinated against rabies, placed in confinement for 90 days, and given booster vaccinations during the third and eighth weeks of confinement. For young animals, additional vaccinations may be necessary to ensure that the animal receives at least two vaccinations at or after the age prescribed by the US Department of Agriculture (USDA) for the vaccine administered. If the animal was currently vaccinated when it was exposed, it would be immediately given a booster rabies vaccination and placed in confinement for 45 days. Confinement can be conducted at home with one primary caregiver to keep the number of people exposed to a minimum if the animal did develop rabies.

As mentioned in our article, although rabies incubation periods can range from days to years, the average is 3–8 weeks. Dogs, cats, and domestic ferrets with rabies may shed the rabies virus 3–6 days before they show clinical signs of rabies and only live for a few days after the clinical signs appear. Even after having PEP administered, if "D" becomes ill, remind your veterinarian of this incident so he/she can determine if rabies needs to be considered as a differential diagnosis. Again, with sincere sympathy on your loss.—Pam and Dr. Rohde

3. Hi, my child had dog bite on the day before yesterday. Now the dog is died. I have already vaccinated my child on the same day. Is it dangerous to my child because the dog is died?

Answer: Hello, if the dog which recently bit your child just died, the dog should be tested for rabies. Contact your local animal control agency or a veterinarian about the testing process. If the dog is confirmed to be negative, that can relieve your worries about rabies. If it tests positive, you will know to be diligent about getting the full rabies postexposure prophylaxis for your child. Hope all goes well.—Pam and Dr. Rohde

4. I was bitten by a dog but it is only a scrape and not bleeding. Do I need to take a vaccine? Thank you.

Answer: Thank you for your question. There are many elements to consider when determining whether or not a person should get rabies postexposure prophylaxis (PEP). Rabies is primarily transmitted by warm-blooded mammals via a bite or scrape, as well as other minor routes like contact with mucous membranes. Any small scrape, even without bleeding, is a potential route for rabies to be transmitted from an animal to a person (or other animal). There are many questions for you to consider such as do you know the dog and its location so that it can be observed (and, determine if the dog is currently vaccinated for rabies.). However, the most important thing for you to do is to visit your physician/doctor as soon as possible to determine whether or not you should receive rabies PEP.—Dr. Rohde and Pam

Cat

1. Hi Doc R. I have a question. I got bitten by our cat 3 days ago. Is it okay if wouldn't take the antirabies shot? Before the incident, we visit a veterinarian to do rabies vaccine on our cat. During his vaccination, my cat escaped and we tried to capture it. I was bitten two times in the process before my cat had the vaccine. Now, I'm worried if my cat has rabies. My cat is healthy, eating, and drinking. There is no change of behavior since the day of vaccination up to now. If my cat survives after 10 days, does it mean I am safe? Do I need to be concerned because he got his vaccine and does the 10-day process still apply?

Answer: Hi, thank you for your inquiry. Although incubation periods can vary, typically it is within 10 days that the animal would (show clinical signs or) die from rabies. As a reminder, it is always important to consult with your physician after any animal bite (pet or wildlife) to consider not only a rabies risk but also any type of bacterial infection that might occur from the animal's mouth flora. So, the good news is that there has been no change in the cat's behavior but because it is still within the 10 days, we recommend you always consult with your physician. Thanks for your interest in our article.—Dr. Rohde and Pam

Unlikely Exposures
Dog

1. I took four puppies to my home before 1 week because their mother was killed by a truck. Those puppies were of a street bitch, which were unvaccinated. When the puppies were playing with me 2 days before, then I found their scratches in my hand. But I've no wounds there. Will it be a problem?

Answer: Thank you for your question. The primary route of exposure to rabies is via the bite of a rabid animal. Other possible routes of exposure could be infected saliva contacting a break in the skin or a mucous membrane. If the puppies were still alive (and well) 10 days after the scenario you described, they could not have been transmitting rabies at that time.

It was kind of you to rescue the puppies. Please note that they can be vaccinated against rabies as early as when they are 12 weeks of age. Hope all is going well for them and for you.—Pam and Rodney

2. I have a question. My unvaccinated puppy had a possible encounter with a possum (I say possible because a dead possum was found on our deck and I don't know if one of our three dogs killed it or it randomly died). I checked over my puppy and couldn't find any clear bite marks but his back foot seems to be bothering him so the situation is ambiguous. I immediately got my puppy vaccinated for rabies but I am still concerned that if he did develop rabies that he could infect my young 8-year-old son who plays with him/kisses/receives licks from him often. Should I ask my son's pediatrician for the rabies vaccine to be on the safe side or am I overreacting?

Answer: Thank you for your question. There are many elements to consider when determining whether or not a person should get rabies postexposure prophylaxis (PEP). Your doctor would be the person who would ultimately decide whether or not to prescribe PEP for your son.

Although any warm-blooded animal could develop rabies, opossums are considered to be low risk for this disease. Plus, as you mentioned, it is nebulous as to whether any of your animals even had direct contact with this opossum.

If on the very rare chance that this opossum was rabid, PEP protocols for domestic animals are generally very effective. You did not mention the age of your puppy, the vaccination status of your other dogs, or in what state you reside. Because PEP protocols can vary by state, I am going to include as an example information from the Texas Administrative Code, Rabies Control and Eradication, which covers PEP for domestic animals; during various decades of data analyses on Texas' PEP protocol, it has been, at a minimum, 99.5% effective. In Texas, if the animal was not currently vaccinated when it was exposed to rabies, it would be immediately vaccinated against rabies, placed in confinement for 90 days, and given booster vaccinations during the third and eighth weeks of confinement. For young animals, additional vaccinations may be necessary to ensure that the animal receives at least two vaccinations at or after the age prescribed by the US Department of Agriculture (USDA) for the vaccine administered. If the animal was currently vaccinated when it was exposed, it would be immediately given a booster rabies vaccination and placed in confinement for 45 days. Confinement can be conducted at home with one primary caregiver to keep the number of people exposed to a minimum if the animal did develop rabies.

When you find a dead animal in your yard and you don't know if your pets or child had contact with it, you can request that animal control or a veterinarian submit its head, or whole body for bats or small rodents, for rabies testing; a person trained in head-removal techniques should remove the head to ensure that all the required portions of the brain are submitted for testing. Do not handle the body with bare hands (wear gloves, use a shovel, etc.) when you place it in a plastic bag. For improved testing success, keep the body cool in a refrigerator or a cooler; do not freeze it. If this is not possible or the body already looks decomposed, still request submission for testing. The laboratory will then determine if it is testable or not.

As mentioned in our article, although rabies incubation periods can range from days to years, the average is 3–8 weeks. Dogs, cats, and domestic ferrets with rabies may shed the rabies virus 3–6 days before they show clinical signs of rabies and only live for a few days after the clinical signs appear. If one of your dogs becomes ill, remind your veterinarian of this incident so he/she can determine if rabies needs to be considered as a differential diagnosis.

Again, you have described a very low-risk scenario, plus you have done well to get the puppy immediately vaccinated against rabies. I hope this has provided you with the information you were seeking and also helps to relieve your concern.—Pam

3. Dear Sir, I have tasted 1 teaspoon of cooked slice pork with little mayonnaise today at 11 a.m., but I didn't know that my pet dog ate some of it. My dog had vaccine antirabies more than a year now. My dog eats clean foods and is healthy, but now she got one ear problem because of water and just stays in the house. Would I get PEP?

   Answer: Hi, a dog licking food before she ate it actually presents an incredibly low-risk situation. However, it is always important to consult with your physician after any animal exposure to consider not only a rabies risk, but also any type of other exposure (bacterial infection) that might occur from the animal's mouth flora. Thanks for your interest in our article.—Pam and Dr. Rohde

4. Hello. I would just like to ask. 9–10 years ago I tried to pet our neighbor's dog and it suddenly flinched, maybe it thought I was gonna hit her. Then, I noticed a small wound, maybe a size of a half rice grain, on my finger. I am really worried about the possibility of rabies occurring after 9–10 years. Is that possible? Thank you.

   Answer: Hi, it is not clear as to why you think you may have been exposed to rabies by this dog as you do not describe any type of physical contact with it. If your concern is that you petted it while you had a wound on your hand, just touching the dog would not constitute an exposure unless it had fresh saliva on its coat that happened to contain the rabies virus and that saliva came into contact with your wound. You mentioned that the dog flinched, but did not state that it bit you. Do you think that it did bite you and created the small wound on your hand? If so, rabies incubation periods can range from days to years; however, the average is 3–8 weeks. However, if you are able to remember that your neighbor's dog was still alive (and well) 10 days after this incident, then it could not have transmitted rabies to you at that time; even if the dog had been incubating rabies virus when it created a wound or your wound contacted fresh saliva on its coat, by the time the virus was in the dog's saliva and actually transmissible, the dog would have (showed clinical signs or) died from the disease within 10 days (probably even sooner than that). Thanks for reading our article.—Pam and Dr. Rohde

5. If a dog is shedding the virus and receives a normal vaccine after it begins shedding, is there any chance of the dog surviving the rabies? I ask because my dog had a limp a few months ago (didn't check it for bites), and there have been some visits from a raccoon at the very edge of our yard who was attacking our chickens. So I don't know if they had contact. The point being, today I took the dog for her first rabies shot. She was acting fine, but the article says she can shed even before symptoms. Anyway, I went to scratch her back and got her saliva on my hand (she had been biting herself because of fleas). I don't have any open wounds on my hands, but two recently healed wounds. I have two questions. (1) Is there a possibility of exposure, if she did have rabies? And (2) can I still use the 10-day rule, even though she just got her shot today? This brings me back to the original question, once a dog starts shedding the virus, can a vaccine stop death? If it can't, and she's doomed, then I can watch for 10 days, but if there's a chance she can survive, then I guess I'll go to the doctors. This sort of information isn't really clear over the Internet. Thanks for any reply.

Answer: Hi, I know we've answered your questions already via other means. However, I wanted to post this answer for the benefit of other readers. (Answers are in brackets.)

My question is simple. Once a dog starts shedding the rabies virus, is there any way to provide treatment, such as a normal rabies vaccine, that can help save the animal from death? (No)

It is to my understanding that once the rabies virus enters the brain/nervous system and the virus starts shedding through the saliva, nothing can be done to save the animal and it will most certainly die. So a rabies vaccine, administered after shedding begins, would have no effect, and the animal should die within 10 days, correct? (Yes)

Here's my dilemma, and I apologize if this isn't the correct medium in contacting you. There has been a racoon that has been visiting our yard in the past, and a few months back, my dog (which was unvaccinated at the time) had a slight limp. It is unsure if the limp was a result from a bite, or even if the two had any sort of contact with each other. The problem lies in that I read an article by you and another expert, suggesting that rabies can be secreted from an animal even before symptoms arrive. Just yesterday, the day that I finally took my dog to be vaccinated, I scratched my dogs back that was covered in her saliva (she had been apparently biting it because of fleas) and this probably would have not bothered me, but I have two recently healed wounds on my hands, and I've read, albeit rare, that the virus can penetrate microabrasions in the skin. (In the Rabies Prevention in Texas postexposure prophylaxis guide, an exposure is defined as (1) an animal bite [or scratch] that breaks the skin or (2) exposure of broken skin [bled or had serous drainage within the past 24 h] or mucous membranes to saliva or cerebrospinal fluid.)

This all leads up to now. I know there's an incredibly low risk of my dog actually having the virus, and the "exposure" would be an incredibly low risk because she didn't bite or break skin, and that my wounds are technically healed, but considering how rabies exposure is an urgent matter, I want to be sure. Ordinarily, I would just wait and see if the animal dies within 10 days to see if I need postexposure treatment; however, the day I had contact with her saliva was the day she received her first vaccination. This brings me back to my original question, if the dog received a rabies vaccine "after" it had already began shedding the virus, is there any way of the dog surviving the disease? (No, it's highly unlikely.)

Or am I correct in my understanding that once the dog begins shedding, there is nothing medically to be done to save the dogs life, that it will, without a doubt, die. (One can never say without a doubt; however, it's very unlikely.)

If the later is true, then I can wait 10 days to verify exposure. (Although I believe your risk is very low and would be prone to tell you to wait 10 days, I am not a medical doctor. My colleagues and I always recommend you consult with your physician to make the ultimate decision.)

Thanks for any reply, and my apologies for any inconvenience, or if this isn't the right method in asking the question. (Thanks for reading our article and good luck.—Dr. Rohde and Pam)

6. Sir, there's anything to worry about, because last week the dog of my friend attacked my feet and there is no wound or scratches caused by bite; it left saliva but at that moment I felt pain. Still will I pursue to receive PEP?

Answer: If the animal is not available for observation/quarantine or if it was not submitted for rabies testing, then it's impossible to rule out a rabid animal. Anytime, if you think you may have been exposed to rabies, you should always consult with a physician even if a long period of time has passed.—Dr. Rohde and Pam (Note: Saliva contacting intact skin does not constitute an exposure.)

7. Hello Sir, I have been in great worry for 1 month. I have also searched a lot about rabies, but I couldn't get any answer. So, please help me. I lived in a village that is a backward area in India. When I was studying 10th standard (2010), I took a small new born puppy to my home and that new born puppy was of a street bitch. Now (2016) the puppy is 6-year-old. I never tie up my dog at home and he plays and fights with other street dogs also, comes to my home when he likes, and wanders here and there outside my home. On June 18, 2016, I was playing with my dog. After 3–4 days, I found a small wound on my leg. I didn't know, either the wound was made by dog's teeth or with its paw during playing. After 4 days, I went to a local doctor and he gave me a tetanus shot. Still now, that is, after 1 month, my dog is healthy and okay. One more thing I want to tell you is that I vaccinated my dog only three times—firstly, when it was 1 year old, secondly, in October 2015, and thirdly in March 2016. Now please tell me whether I am infected with rabies virus by my dog's bite by taking into consideration the following points: (1) the date March 2016 when I vaccinated my dog last time; (2) the date June 18, 2016, when my dog bit me; (3) the date June 22, 2016, when the local doctor gave me a tetanus shot; (4) I never tie up my dog, and he plays and fights with other streets dogs also till now; (5) at present, the date is July 22, 2016, and my dog is okay. Please reply me as soon as possible; otherwise, I will be depressed by thinking about it.

Answer: Although the animal could be incubating rabies, if a dog, cat, or domestic ferret is alive (and well) 10 days after an exposure, such as a bite, it could not have transmitted rabies via that particular exposure. Because your dog was alive (and well) 10 days after the bite you described, he could not have transmitted rabies to you at that time.

To lower the chances of your dog being exposed to and developing rabies, you should keep him currently vaccinated against rabies and not allow him to run loose where he encounters and fights with other dogs. Hope this information aids you in preventing the spread of this disease.—Pam and Rodney

8. Nicely written article. I have a query, recently my friend got bitten by a dog with rabies symptoms, and he started PEP and took AR vaccine on the same day and immunoglobulin on the next day. After an hour from taking immunoglobulin while conversing, a particle of his saliva fell on my mouth. Is his saliva contagious at that time? This happened a week back, my friend is healthy and taking his PEP shots regularly. Should I be worried about myself and undergo PEP treatment. What is the scope of rabies transmission between humans? Thank you.

Answer: We are glad that you enjoyed our article. Thank you.

Was the dog that bit your friend tested for rabies? If not, was it available for the 10-day observation period? If the dog was alive (and well) 10 days after the bite incident, it could not have transmitted rabies via that bite.

Rabies is elusive in that it has a varying incubation period of days to years, with an average of 3–8 weeks, plus it can be spread in a variety of ways, including when infected saliva contacts mucous membranes. Therefore, it's difficult to give absolutes. That said, it is highly improbable given the time frames that you presented that your friend could have had rabies virus in his saliva so quickly. Additionally, the immunoglobulin would not cause his saliva to be contagious. Hope all is well.—Pam and Rodney

9. Hello Dr. Rohde, I recently had a small bite from a friend's dog (9 years old, female, shiz tzu) about 7 days ago. It was my first time encountering a dog bite and I am kind of worried. I have read your wonderful article and I now have pretty good idea but I would like to ask couple of questions to make sure the dog and I do not need to seek medical attention. The dog, I believe, had vaccine regularly and most recent vaccine paper dates 8/3/2016, "killed" as vaccine type, and Zoetis as manufacturer. The dog is a house dog and lives in an apartment. I have few questions and I would really appreciate if you could please answer for me. (1) Should I be concerned with possible rabies? (2) Ultimately, if the dog is fine after three more days, I do not need to see doctor, right? (3) Would there be failure of this protocol? (4) Can dog have rabies and live perfectly fine? I guess what I am trying to ask is do I need a PEP for this incident. Thank you!

Answer: Hi Steve, thanks for the questions (and photo). I love Shiz tzu dogs! I'm so sorry you had that type of encounter. First, it's very unlikely that an apartment-dwelling dog which is vaccinated for rabies poses any risk to you. However,

Question 1: Although I do not believe you have much to worry about, it's always our recommendation to seek the opinion of your doctor/physician to have a medical opinion.

Question 2: As mentioned in other comments, if the dog was alive (and well) 10 days after the bite incident, she could not have transmitted rabies to you through that bite.

Question 3: Your doctor would be the person who would ultimately decide whether or not to prescribe PEP for you.

Thanks. Dr. Rohde

10. Hello Dr. Rohde, 1 month ago I went to a park. There was a couple with their small dog, we chatted a little bit. Then the dog jumped on the rock I was sitting on. I used my hand to keep him at a distance. His nose touched my palm, and I could feel center of my palm was wet a little bit. We continued chatting about 5 more minutes. I went back to my car and washed my hands with liquid hand sanitizer (I can't remember when I washed my hands, the dog's sweat had been dried or not). However, after I used the sanitizer, I remembered that there was a paper cut I had got 2 days before on my finger. The sanitizer may have come into the wound. I am very worried if this whole thing will give rabies and maybe the liquid sanitizer may bring alive virus into the paper cut wound? And is it still working if I go to get my PEP now, after a month? The dog was stranger's pet, so I couldn't know if he is healthy now. Thanks.

Answer: Hello, thank you for your inquiry. The sooner that rabies postexposure prophylaxis (PEP) is started, the better the chances are of it being effective; however, even if time has passed since the possible exposure, it is worthwhile to have PEP administered in hopes that it was timely enough (rabies has a varying incubation period). Rabies is transmitted via infected saliva, usually through the bite from a rabid animal; although rare, it's possible that infected saliva contacting a mucous membrane or a break in the skin could be a means of exposure. Exposure to body fluids/excretions other than saliva and possibly tears (i.e., urine, blood, stool…) from a rabid animal or human generally is not considered to constitute an exposure. Using a hand sanitizer also would not constitute an exposure. Wishing you good health.—Pam and Dr. Rohde

11. I was staying at a friend's home for a bit and he has two dogs. One has the vaccine and is a year old; the other is a puppy about 4 months old and is not vaccinated. Around the third day, I found out the puppy is not vaccinated and remember a time when the pup licked my hands and I ate pizza

right after. I know it might sound odd to ask, but I gotta ask. Is it possible I can get rabies this way? I am very hydrophobic and can't seem to get the thought out of my head that it's a possibility. I was absolutely scared to even stay another night. You assume things like vaccines should be covered, but people are people. It's been a week since it happened, someone please give me an answer that pup was way too friendly (a husky) and it scares me.

Answer: Hi, it is true that, with rabies, a change in behavior is a clinical sign of rabies and the behavior of an individual puppy can range from extroverted to introverted. That said, a puppy that's really playful and licks people sounds like it is exhibiting typical puppy behavior.

Rabies is transmitted via infected saliva, usually through the bite from a rabid animal; although rare, it's possible that infected saliva contacting a mucous membrane (i.e., in the eye, mouth, or nose) or a break in the skin could be a means of exposure. That said, this sounds like an incredibly low-risk scenario. Additionally, if a dog, cat, or domestic ferret is alive (and well) 10 days after an exposure incident, they could not have transmitted rabies virus in their saliva at the time of that particular incident. It appears from your description that this time interval has passed. Wishing you well.—Pam and Dr. Rohde

12. Hello, Yesterday morning, my little doggie was sniffing around the trails near my home and she sniffed up something that stayed on her nose. I reached down to pluck it off of her and dropped it to the ground. Then I noticed it was a tiny tuft of fur (possibly from a squirrel) with tiny flecks of skin attached. It was not bloody or wet that I could tell, but I always have rough, dry, scratched hands, so I'm sort of worried now. Is this something I should be concerned about or will my doctor throw me out of his office? I'm serious, please help. Thank you.

Answer: Hi Christine, thank you for your question. There are many elements to consider when determining whether or not a person should get rabies postexposure prophylaxis (PEP). Although any warm-blooded animal could develop rabies, squirrels, opossums, etc. are considered to be low risk for this disease. As always, it's also critical that your dog(s) and other domestic animals have been vaccinated against rabies. The first line of protection for humans is the vaccination of their animals.

As mentioned in our article, although rabies incubation periods can range from days to years, the average is 3–8 weeks. Dogs, cats, and domestic ferrets with rabies may shed the rabies virus 3–6 days before they show clinical signs of rabies and only live for a few days after the clinical signs appear. If your dog becomes ill, remind your veterinarian of this incident so he/she can determine if rabies needs to be considered as a differential diagnosis.

I hope this has provided you with the information you were seeking and also helps to relieve your concern.—Dr. Rohde and Pam

13. Hi I have a question. As a person with anxiety, you could only imagine the suffering I'm going through. I had a cut that was under my fingernails that came out just slightly to the outer skin on May 6. The dog we have is confined to the backyard, she never leaves it, and unfortunately we have not been vaccinating her and she did get all her shots when she was little but we fell off track. But she has killed mice and a bird. But that was 2 or 3 months ago and she's still fine. No fighting with other animals or at least from what I saw watching her all these years. Two days later after the cut, on May 7, my dog somehow got into the house. She was very friendly, tail wagging, and everything; not foaming at the mouth, and she didn't bite or scratch me. But I can't figure out if she licked it or it was her nose that brushed against my cut and that left the wet feeling. I talked to the doctor and he said it's not necessary for the vaccines as I wasn't bitten or scratched and the dog didn't show rabid behavior. But I totally forgot to tell him I had a cut where she licked or her nose could have come into contact with. It's been 7 days so far from May 7 and she's not showing any of the symptoms. My family said I shouldn't worry because a rabid dog would never lick someone. So should I not worry or go ahead and take action immediately?

Answer: Hello, the observation period following a possible exposure to rabies is 10 days for dogs; if the dog is alive (and well) after 10 days, it could not have transmitted rabies through that particular possible exposure. Saliva containing rabies virus contacting an open area of the skin can constitute a possible exposure, but you have your pet available for the observation period, so that should ease your worries. Generally, if a dog was at the point of transmitting virus in its saliva, it probably would be dead in a shorter period of time than 10 days, but the observation period is extended to 10 days as an extra precaution.

You mentioned actions that you should take. When 10 days have passed, get your dog vaccinated against rabies. It's one of the best ways that you can

prevent the spread of this disease, plus it's usually required by law. It also sounds like your dog would enjoy spending time with you in the house! Hope this helps to ease your anxiety.—Pam and Rodney

14. Hi, I am glad you put up this article but I'm really worried about something. I volunteer at this dog day care, and about 5 weeks ago, one of the small dogs there bit my finger. My finger shook for a few minutes and then stopped and I think that happened because of shock. It bled and at the time I don't think I washed it but what I did do was cleaned it with alcohol wipes. I think an hour later when the wound was healing, the veterinarian who works there applied betadine to clean it (the wound was already closing up when he was cleaning it up). The place I volunteer at is basically a place where the dog's owners drop them off when they're busy/have no one to have them taken care of or when they're traveling and can't take their pets along with them. Even dogs that are up for adoption stay there (animal shelter). It's logical to say that all the dogs are healthy there and that they wouldn't be allowed to play with the other dogs if they were sick/rabid, but even with that, I am still paranoid and scared. I can't recall having felt any of the early symptoms of rabies, that is, fever/muscle pain. I don't know if I had those over the course of 5 weeks. I cannot remember but I do get body pain after a long day of school, especially when my bag is heavy. Other days I'm fine. I do get headaches every now and then but that's normal to me so I cannot tell if it's because of rabies. The dog that bit me is most probably alive right now but I'm not too sure. I know the dog is not rabid but I still can't get this fear out of my head that I'm too late on treatment and that I might die. The bite is small by the way, but it still bled. Is it when I start experiencing symptoms such as hallucinations, agitation, sleep paralysis, etc., when I'm too late or am I too late when I start experiencing the early symptoms like fever or head ache? It is now, after 5 weeks, that I am getting vaccinated. I got the first dose 3 days ago and I got the second one today. I will be getting five injections. Am I too late? Also, will a rabid animal still die even if its bite was really minimal like my case? Why do rabid animals die after biting someone? By the way, the veterinarian there told me that most of their dogs are vaccinated and that the one that bit me was probably vaccinated too. I am familiar with that dog too. It only bites or gets aggressive when it's being held by someone and someone else tries to pet or touch it. Like if I were

holding it and my friend tried to pet or touch it, it would growl and try to bite. Otherwise, it's usually friendly and wants to be pet when it's not being held by anyone.

Answer: The straightforward solution to addressing concerns about rabies transmission from this dog bite is to contact the owner and get confirmation that the dog was alive (and well) after 10 days from the time of the bite, which should be possible to do for a dog that had spent time at a day care center. As mentioned in our article, dogs with rabies may shed the rabies virus 3–6 days before they show clinical signs of rabies and only live for a few days after the clinical signs appear (whether or not they have bitten someone). If the dog was alive (and well) 10 days after the bite, it could not have been at the point of passing rabies virus in its saliva at the time of that specific bite and, therefore, could not have exposed you to rabies; the dog still could possibly be incubating rabies, but it could not have been at the point of transmitting the virus in its saliva. Thank you for your inquiry.—Pam

15. Hi I am gonna ask but I have been bitten by my puppy 2–3 months ago I think? Is it possible for me to have rabies?

   Answer: Thank you for your question. The primary route of exposure to rabies is via the bite of a rabid animal. Other possible routes of exposure could be infected saliva contacting a break in the skin or a mucous membrane. If the puppy is still alive (and well) 10 days after the scenario you described, they could not have been transmitting rabies at that time.

   Thank you for your question.—Dr. Rohde and Pam

Cat

1. Hi, I have a question. My daughter was bitten by our cat on her nose. She was given a vaccine after more than 48 h and 5 days after she was bitten, she was given another dose and another that's called Berirab. Although the cat seems fine and my daughter is okay too, is there something else that I need to be worried? She was bitten last July 24.

   Answer: Hello, it would be best for you to check with the doctor who administered your daughter's vaccinations. We are not familiar with Berirab as it is not a vaccine licensed by the USDA.

   It's good to hear, though, that the cat is fine and you seem to understand that some cats do nip, even when playing.

   Although you did not mention the vaccination status of your cat, one of the best preventive measures against rabies is to keep your cat currently vaccinated

against the disease. Wishing the best for you, your daughter, and your cat.—Pam and Rodney

2. Wonderful article! I was curious to see if you could comment on my situation. I was walking with my dog and a stray cat jumped out of a tree and scratched me on two locations on my shoulder. The "wounds" are pretty superficial … I didn't even notice them until my wife pointed out that one was bleeding a little. I went to the doctor and standard procedure is to perform the PEP treatment. The immunoglobin shot was administered in and around the two scratch sites with the rest being administered into my thighs (two on left, one on right). When I got home, I noticed that there is a third scratch site on my side right above my hip. I am not 100% confident that this was from the encounter with the stray but I can't remember any other time that I would have scratched myself. This scratch is also superficial as indicated that I hadn't noticed it before. My question is this… Should I be concerned that this potential site was missed in the application of the immunoglobin? Thanks!

   Answer: Hello, thank you for the positive comment on our article. We are very pleased that you found it helpful.

   Sorry to hear about your cat encounter; PEP was certainly warranted in this potential exposure scenario. It's always best to consult directly with your physician on concerns such as yours. However, there are times when it's not even anatomically possible to inject all of the human rabies immune globulin (HRIG) into and around the potential exposure wound(s). Additionally, you should not give more than the recommended dose of HRIG.

   From Rabies Prevention in Texas pertaining to HRIG:

   If anatomically feasible, the full dose should be infiltrated around and into the wound(s), and any remaining volume should be administered at an anatomical site (intramuscular [IM]) distant from vaccine administration.

   and

   As much as possible of the full dose of HRIG should be thoroughly infiltrated into and around the wound(s). Any remaining volume of HRIG should be administered IM in the closest muscle mass of suitable size to accommodate the remaining volume, with the caveat that it should not be administered in the same site as the first vaccine dose. Anterior lateral thigh muscles are frequently used as HRIG injection sites when the complete amount, because of anatomic limitations, cannot be administered around the wound(s). The HRIG should be injected into muscle, not adipose tissue. Particular care should be taken when administering HRIG in the gluteal area because of the increased risk of injection into adipose tissue. The HRIG may partially suppress the active production of antibodies; therefore, no more than the recommended dose of HRIG should be given.

Wishing you the best.—Pam and Rodney

3. Hi! I saw two stray cats eating on my dog's food that's sitting on the counter top. I tried to scare them away. I picked up food and realized that there was a trace of saliva at the container. I did wash my hands after. I touched the container again just so I could transfer its content. This time, I touched the parts of the container which I think was safe from the saliva. And then I accidentally touched the inside of my nose. What is the possibility of getting rabies from this? What if some saliva slipped from that side of the container that I touched?

Answer: Hi, the type of exposure you describe (hands to saliva and touching your nose) is relatively unlikely to have allowed transmission of rabies virus. As in other scenarios described in the comments of this article, there are many elements to consider when determining whether or not a person should get rabies postexposure prophylaxis (PEP). Because you do not know the health status of the cats after the "exposure," you may also want to follow up with your physician (doctor) about it to see if you need the PEP. Thanks.—Dr. Rohde and Pam

4. I am really happy to have found this post. I think I know the answer to my question but I want to make sure. My mom has been in the hospital recently (hopefully coming home Friday-yay!), and my family and I have been taking turns staying with her. I live in a pretty urban area. On Sunday May 14, 2017, I noticed a friendly cat in the parking deck of the hospital so I stopped and petted him. I noticed he wasn't fixed, but he looked well taken care of so I assumed he probably was just wondering looking for food. The next morning when I left he was still hanging out there, and a woman was talking about calling animal control. I thought he was a perfectly nice cat and I couldn't let that happen so I petted him, carefully picked him up (which he allowed, no problems), and put him in my car (I know, approaching strange animals is bed!!!). I started posting online looking for owners immediately. If I can't find one, I plan on keeping him. He seems to have a very nice temperament. I do have other pets which are vaccinated but because I do not know if this cat is vaccinated, I have been keeping him in my guest bedroom.

On May 16, 2017, I went in to feed him and pet him some (I feel bad he's all quarantined by himself).

As cats do, he nipped me ever so lightly when he was done with me petting him. It wasn't aggressive, and he did not bite to hurt me. It didn't draw blood, and although it left an indention for a moment, it was gone quickly and it did not break the skin (I have one grumpy cat who does like to bite to hurt and play to rough so I feel I know the difference). I tend to worry a lot so I immediately began thinking how dumb it was to pick up a stray animal and that I probably have rabies now. The cat is acting normal, I had even taken him to the vet earlier that day to see if he had a microchip (he didn't), and they commented how he looked like he was in good shape and may have owners. I called the vet to see what they thought and they suggested just bringing him in to get the vaccine to protect myself and the other pets at my house which I am planning on doing. I also called urgent care and asked if this was something I should come in for and was told they weren't really sure what they would do because there was no "bite" per se and that if it didn't break the skin it was a slim to none chance of contracting rabies if the cat even has it. I feel silly because there is no bite mark, it didn't draw blood, but I kept seeing how saliva is, what transmits rabies. I expect I will have the cat at my house for a while. If everything is good after 10 days, is it safe to say that I am okay? Should I go to an urgent care anyways and have them look at it? I just want to cover all my bases. I am attaching a picture of the cat because he is pretty cute. How could I leave him for animal control to get?

Answer: Hello, if saliva containing the rabies virus contacts intact skin (such as you described), it is not considered to be an exposure.

Just to answer your question, if a cat is at the point of being able to transmit the rabies virus in its saliva, it will not be alive (and well) after 10 days (usually within even fewer days, but 10 days if used as a precaution), which is why there is a 10-day observation period for a cat that has potentially exposed a person to rabies.

It is good that you sought advice from a physician/urgent care and a veterinarian. It's advisable to get a pet vaccinated against rabies to help prevent the spread of this disease.

Hope this cat experiences a well-deserved happy, full life in a good home.—Pam and Rodney

5. Hello. Thank you for the informative advice! I was wondering though, what about scratches specifically, not just bites? 3–4 years ago, I was scratched by a stray kitten, and I remember there being some blood drawn. I phoned my doctor about cat scratch

fever, and he said not to worry, but I never thought to ask about rabies. I know it's been many years, but because there have been a few rare cases, I am thinking that I should just go and get the set of PEP shots, just in case. Are cat scratches just as high-risk as bites?

Answer: Hi and thanks for your questions. Although bites are the primary route of exposure to the rabies virus, scratches "can be" a route for the virus. Because it's been 3–4 years since the scratch, it's unlikely that you have rabies. However, because of the varying range of the incubation period for rabies, treatment should be started even if there was a delay in recognizing a rabies exposure. The sooner the treatment is begun after exposure, the better the chance of effectiveness. The PEP combination of rabies immune globulin and rabies vaccine is recommended, regardless of the interval between exposure and treatment. Domestic cats and dogs are not as likely to be rabid as wildlife or feral animals. Thanks.—Doc R

Other animals

1. Hello, a few hours ago, our family came to a cabin in Canada for fishing, and we noticed a chipmunk acting very tame to us, would feeding it by hand but then wash your hands be dangerous without the vaccine? A chipmunk that seemed very tame toward humans from the wild tried to come up to my hand for food scratched my leg left no openings but just redness, should I be concerned?

Answer: Hi, rabies is usually spread by the bite of a rabid animal. It can also be transmitted when saliva from a rabid animal contacts a break in the skin or mucous membranes, such as found in the eyes, nose, and mouth. It is not uncommon for chipmunks to appear tame because of people feeding them, so that could be considered typical behavior. They become trusting of people and get positive reinforcement for doing so via the reward of food. It's best not to feed wildlife because it modifies their diet, which could be detrimental to their health; encourages them to trust people, which could also be detrimental to their health; and increases the chances for an unfortunate encounter, such as the person accidentally being bitten while hand-feeding the animal. Even though chipmunks are considered to be low-risk animals for rabies, such an exposure then opens the door for speculation on possible rabies exposure, which would need to be discussed with a physician.

Enjoy the wonderful wildlife surrounding your cabin, but please resist trying to hand-feed the chipmunks even though they are irresistibly adorable.—Pam and Rodney

2. Hello, my son was bitten by mongoose at the petting zoo in Russia. Zoo officials told us that the animals are vaccinated with Nobivac vaccine. But we started with rabies shots vaccine for my son. We observe the animal and they seem okay. We also learn that mongooses have immunity to rabies. My question is, should we complete full course of vaccine which is of 90 days and six doses here in Russia? Or can we stop if animal is not sick?

Answer: Thank you for the question. I don't have experience with that vaccine in Russia. However, you are correct that it would be very unlikely for a zoo animal to have rabies. Likewise, if the animal (mongoose) is still healthy, that also is in your favor. However, ultimately, your doctor would be the person who would ultimately decide whether or not to continue PEP for your son. We are so sorry you were bitten at a zoo, a place that we all go to admire wildlife and other animals. Good luck! Thanks.—Dr. Rohde (Note: A mongoose does not have immunity to rabies.)

3. Hello, after taking trash out, I noticed the trash bags had been torn into by some unknown animal. I picked up the bag(s) and placed them inside bin and touched the areas of the bag, which were ripped/torn into. The bags were wet from rain as well. Could this constitute an exposure? There are groundhogs and raccoons in area but no recent reported instances of rabies.

Answer: Hi, thank you for your inquiry. Rabies is transmitted via infected saliva, usually through the bite from a rabid animal; although rare, it's possible that infected saliva contacting a mucous membrane or a break in the skin could be a means of exposure. Exposure to body fluids/excretions other than saliva and possibly tears (i.e., urine, blood, and stool) from a rabid animal or human is not considered to constitute a rabies exposure. Wishing you good health.—Pam and Dr. Rohde

4. Hello, I had a potential exposure from a bat, and I did go get PEP 7–8 days after this incident. It has been over 90 days since the potential exposure, I had my titer level checked and it came back at 5.5 UL/mL. Should I consider myself safe from developing rabies?

Answer: Bat exposures are certainly a growing concern with respect to rabies transmission. Because bat "bites and/or scratches" can be very difficult to document, one should always check with their physician regarding rabies vaccination and postexposure prophylaxis. Because you got PEP so soon after the incident and your rabies titer has been determined to be 5.5 UL/mL, it appears you are in the clear but please seek a physician's opinion if you have any further questions.—Doc R

5. Thank you for the wonderful information. We had rescued a baby mongoose, which lived with us for few months as we were deciding where to send her for proper rehabilitation. Many times she licked us. Also I couldn't give her bath so she was covered with her urine. She used to climb on me and she was extremely playful, she even used to play with water, she used to do some strange action with her hand before drinking water. Can she be infected with rabies, or carrier of rabies?

Answer: Hello, any warm-blooded animal can become infected with rabies, including mongooses, which can be a notable animal pertaining to rabies in certain areas of the world (for example, Puerto Rico).

Transmission of rabies is through contact with infected saliva, typically through a bite, but potentially through infected saliva contacting an open wound in the skin or mucous membranes. Licks to intact skin or contact with urine are not modes of transmission for rabies.

It sounds like she was exerting her playfulness with the water. On a side note, if you decide to become involved with rehabilitating wildlife, it would be advisable for you to get preexposure rabies vaccinations. Best wishes.—Pam and Rodney

Not Exposures

Dog

1. Dear Sir, I had a dog bite long back in 1996 then I was 15 years old and I was not vaccinated. It is 20 years now. Is there still a possibility of infection? That dog was a pet and during feeding by mistake I had a bite by the dog. The dog was young but died in within 1–2 months of that bite, we did not understand the reason that time but he seemed to healthy.

Answer: Thank you for your inquiry. Because you stated that the dog was alive 1–2 months after the bite incident, it could not have transmitted rabies to you via that particular bite. Although incubation periods can vary and the dog could have been incubating rabies virus when it bit you, by the time the virus was in the dog's saliva and actually transmissible via a bite, the dog would have died (or been ill) from the disease within 10 days (probably even sooner than that). Again, thank you for your interest.—Pam and Rodney

2. Hi, I recently visited my parents' house where I got a small wound (nearly 15 days back). There was a pet dog nearly 1 year old which might have licked me on the sight of the wound. My parents are saying that the dog had received a rabies vaccine 3–4 months back, so there is nothing to worry about but they didn't retain the prescription for the shot. So I'm worried that I should take rabies vaccine or not.

I would also like to add up that dog is completely healthy right now and has shown no sign of any disease since. Please advise. Thanks!

Answer: Hi, thank you for your inquiry. Because you stated that the dog was alive (and well) 15 days after the incident you described, it could not have transmitted rabies to you via licking that wound. Although incubation periods can vary and the dog could have been incubating rabies virus when it licked you, by the time the virus was in the dog's saliva and actually transmissible via a bite, the dog would have died (or been ill) from the disease within 10 days (probably even sooner than that). Additionally, it sounds very likely that the dog had been vaccinated; that lowers the risk even further. As a reminder, it's always important to consult with your physician after any animal bite (pet or wildlife) to consider not only a rabies risk, but also any type of bacterial infection that might occur from the animal's mouth flora. Thanks for your interest in our article.—Dr. Rohde and Pam

3. Hi Sir, I got dog bite 20 years before, not a very severe bite but it bled. I had not taken any vaccination or medication after the bite. What shall I do now? Can any vaccination help me? Please suggest. I am now 35 years old and I got the bite when I was 13–15 years old. Recently, I heard a news in which a man got rabies after 25 years of dog bite. Can anything be done now?

Answer: Hi, as mentioned in our article, although rabies incubation periods can range from days to years, the average is 3–8 weeks. Dogs, cats, and domestic ferrets with rabies may shed the rabies virus 3–6 days before they show clinical signs of rabies and only live for a few days after the clinical signs appear. It is very unlikely that you have anything to worry about after such a long period of time.—Dr. Rohde and Pam

4. Dear Sir, I was bitten by a dog 24 years ago and I wasn't vaccinated. Are there any chances of getting infected after such a long period. Also I don't know what happened to that dog.

Answer: Hi, I'm the editor of Elsevier Connect. Dr. Rohde and Pam Wilson just answered a similar question. Here is their previous response: "As mentioned in our article, although rabies incubation periods can range from days to years, the average is 3–8 weeks. Dogs, cats, and domestic ferrets with rabies may shed the rabies virus 3–6 days before they show clinical signs of rabies and only live for a few days after the clinical signs appear. It is very unlikely that you have anything to worry about after such a long period of time."—Dr. Rohde and Pam

5. Hello doctor, a month back my dog was ill and she bit on my right-hand finger; the wound was very small and I washed it with water and soap and applied dettol. My dog at that time was vaccinated 2 months back even though as a precaution sake I took two Rabipur injections but doctor gave me those injections on my back. However, dog is fine.
   Answer: Thank you for your inquiry. If the dog was alive (and well) 10 days after the bite incident, she could not have transmitted rabies to you through that bite. We are not familiar with Rabipur as it is not licensed by the USDA, so any questions on the administration of that vaccine should be directed to the doctor or other health professionals who administered the vaccine. Unfortunately, people sometimes get bitten by their own dog when the animal is ill either because they are trying to administer oral medications or because the dog is not feeling well and might be more sensitive to being disturbed. It is commendable that your dog was vaccinated against rabies as that's one of the best ways to prevent exposure to and spread of the disease.

6. Two months ago I encountered a neighbor dog, which barked a lot and seem to have aggression issues. It got off its leash and ran straight toward me and circled me. I felt its mouth and teeth on my leg but didn't seem to have any scratches of bites. It has been 2 month and the dog is still alive. Is it possible that I could be infected?
   Answer: Thank you for your question. Because you stated that the dog was alive 2 months after the incident, it could not have transmitted rabies to you via that particular bite. Although incubation periods can vary and the dog could have been incubating rabies virus when it "touched your leg," by the time the virus was in the dog's saliva and actually transmissible via a bite, the dog would have (been ill or) died from the disease within 10 days (probably even sooner than that). As always, a physician would determine whether or not to prescribe PEP based on various factors surrounding the possible exposure incident. Again, thank you for your interest.—Pam and Rodney

7. I was bitten by my pup by accident and I am observing her right now, if after 10 days or so she is still alive, it means that I don't have rabies? Do I still need to get vaccine for rabies? I am getting paranoid.
   Answer: Hi Adrian, thank you for your inquiry. If the dog is alive (and well) more than 10 days after the bite incident, it could not have transmitted rabies to you via that particular bite. Although incubation periods can vary and the dog could have been incubating rabies virus when it bit you, by the time the virus was in the dog's saliva and actually transmissible via a bite, the dog would have (been ill or) died from the disease within 10 days (probably even sooner than that). As a reminder, it's always important to consult with your physician after any animal bite (pet or wildlife) to consider not only a rabies risk, but also any type of bacterial infection that might occur from the animal's mouth flora. Likewise, it's important that you always vaccinate your pets! Again, thank you for your interest.—Doc R

Cat

1. Thank you for this article. It is the most helpful article I've read all day searching on the Internet. I was bitten by a kitten living under my neighbor's porch. I wasn't thinking about rabies until it was mentioned that there is also a skunk living under this porch. The kittens were taken to the SPCA and euthanized before we realized we should tell them about the bite. The SPCA released the kittens to my neighbor who then took the three kittens to the Department of Agriculture where they will send out for testing (because I do not know which bit me). We live in Pennsylvania. We are waiting for the results. Is it possible that the kittens could test negative but still have been had rabies? Could the rabies virus be in her saliva but not in her brain? I went to the ER. They recommended waiting for the results before starting the vaccines.
   Answer: We were pleased to hear that you found our article helpful. By now, you should have received the results from the laboratory. If they confirmed that the kitten was negative for rabies, it could not have transmitted rabies to you. Hope that the results were negative and that this relieves your worries.—Pam and Dr. Rohde

2. Good day Mr. Rodney Rohde. I received the complete (five shots) of PCEC last 2015. I was bitten again by my cat last 2016 and received two more shots. Then I was bitten again by our new kitten last month (March 2017) on my nose. I received the first shot but traveled to a new country and I was not

able to get the second one. My cat is still alive after 15 days and not acting weird. Can I get another set of booster after I return to our country (1 year from now) or the previous shots are not sufficient and should get the boosters ASAP? Thank you very much.

Answer: The good news is that, because your new kitten is alive past the 10-day rabies observation period since the time of the bite, it could not have transmitted rabies to you at the time of that particular bite. All good wishes.—Pam and Rodney

3. My cat doesn't exhibit any signs of rabies but lately she's become extremely violent for no reason. If I hold her, she starts hissing and scratching. Is that normal? Does the rabies virus transmit through scratches or just saliva?

Answer: Hello, you did not mention how long your cat has been displaying this change of behavior. Technically, a change in behavior is one of the classic clinical signs of rabies; however, once a cat is at the point of passing the virus in its saliva, it will not (be well and) alive past 10 days (probably shorter than that, but 10 is cited to cover possible outliers). With cats, though, you need to keep in mind that various changes in their environment or routines can cause them to have notable changes in their behavior. It's also a good idea to have your cat evaluated by a veterinarian to ensure that there isn't a health issue that might be causing these changes as well. Of course, the best way to reduce concern about your cat having rabies is to make sure it is currently vaccinated against this disease.

The disease is spread by infected saliva entering the body, usually via the bite of a rabid animal, but it could possibly enter through contact with a mucous membrane or an opening in the skin (possibly created by a scratch). Thank you.—Pam

Other animals

1. Hello, about 6 days ago, I hit a racoon that was under my deck with a broom and it hissed at me and I don't know if it was rabid and this was in the middle of the day. Could I have gotten rabies without even being bitten.

Answer: When you encounter a wild (or feral/unknown) animal in your yard or other locations, one should always avoid contact with it and contact your local animal control to handle the situation. In your description, the encounter sounds like you would not have been exposed (i.e., if there was no bite or scratch). The most direct type of exposure is a bite.—Dr. Rohde and Pam

2. Hello! Is it possible that a human transmits rabies to me through the air? 5 months ago I went by a stranger who was rabid and had dripping saliva all around his mouth. He was inadequate and clearly not fine emotionally. He walked by less than 1 m away from me with a speedy walk. I had an open wound on my lip at that time. Is it possible that a very small amount of the virus entered my body? Today, it's been 2 days in a roll that I have 38°C fever, indescribable headache, very sore throat, overall unwellness and body pain, as well as intense pain behind the eyes and an aphtha in my mouth that lasts for 2 weeks. Is it all just the winter flu? I never ever get so sick.

Answer: Offhand, for you to have been exposed to rabies in the scenario you described, saliva containing the rabies virus would have had to actually contact your open wound or a mucous membrane. It would be questionable that this stranger actually had rabies unless it was confirmed by a laboratory. It is true that rabies can have a varying incubation period of days to years, but the average length is 3–8 weeks. Hope you are feeling much better.—Pam and Dr. Rohde

3. What are the chances of infected saliva getting onto a piece of metal and infecting someone? I ask this because in November last year (about 5 months ago) I caught raccoons and moved them off my land. On one particular incident, I let the raccoon go and went to pick up the cage and scratched myself. I went to my doctor. He told me I probably have nothing to worry about and didn't talk about the incident further. I talked to the rabies hotline in my state and he stated that he doesn't recommend PEP after such a long time with no guaranteed exposure. I was wondering your thoughts on the situation.

Answer: Hello, the rabies virus survives for only a short period of time outside the body; it is sensitive to light and air. How long it will subsist depends on the surrounding environment and how quickly the saliva dries, which is contingent upon the amount of saliva, the surrounding temperature, etc. Once the saliva has dried, the virus is not viable within minutes. Although transmission could conceivably occur in the situation you describe, it is not the typical way in which rabies is transmitted. Plus, there are many unknowns in your particular situation, such as whether or not the raccoon had rabies; whether or not there was any infected saliva present on the cage; and whether or not your cut contacted any infected saliva. Wishing you well.—Pam and Rodney

4. Hi, I have a question about contracting rabies from a dead bat. I found a dead bat at the park about

6 weeks ago. I crouched down to look at it, probably about 2 ft away. Is it possible to contract aerosolized rabies if it was rabid? Or could a flea have gone from it to me without me realizing it? I did not touch it, but rabies is such a horrible disease I keep thinking what if. Thank you for your help.

Answer: Hi, Kelly, rabies is not transmitted by fleas. In the scenario you described, aerosolized virus as a source of exposure would not be a concern. Take care.—Pam and Rodney

General Questions on Rabies

1. Can someone still pursue PEP years after exposure? Will there be any side effects if the person actually didn't get infected but still receive PEP?

Answer: Hello, thank you for your inquiry. Anytime a person (or animal) is administered a drug (for example, antibiotics, vaccinations, etc.), that individual has the possibility of developing negative side effects. However, there wouldn't be side effects specifically because of a person receiving rabies postexposure prophylaxis (PEP) just because they weren't really exposed to rabies.

Because of the varying range of the incubation period for rabies, treatment should be started even if there was a delay in recognizing a rabies exposure. However, the sooner the treatment is begun after exposure, the better the chance of effectiveness. The PEP combination of rabies immune globulin and rabies vaccine is recommended, regardless of the interval between exposure and treatment. A physician would determine whether or not to prescribe PEP based on various factors surrounding the possible exposure incident. Thank you for your interest.—Pam

2. I have a question. Can a dead coyote with rabies still transfer rabies to other animals?

Answer: Hi, we appreciate the question. As stated in many of the other posts on this thread, rabies is transmitted via infected saliva, usually through the bite from a rabid animal; although rare, it's possible that infected saliva contacting a mucous membrane or a break in the skin could be a means of exposure. Exposure to body fluids/excretions other than saliva and possibly tears (i.e., urine, blood, stool…) from a rabid animal or human generally is not considered to constitute an exposure. So, your question is a valid one. If another animal were to "feed" or "lick" on a rabid, dead coyote with respect to rabid material (brain matter, spinal cord, nerve tissue), then that animal went and bit another animal or human (when it was to the point of being able to transmit virus in the saliva after the incubation period), it's

"possible" but is still likely a lower risk. Thanks for the question!—Doc R

3. Hello, thanks for this article. I have one question? If I have had antirabid vaccine but another animal bites me, what can I do?

Answer: Hi, the main thing that you should do is contact a physician and discuss whether the biting animal is available or not for observation (or testing), the potential need for postexposure treatment, the treatment/biologicals you actually received previously, etc. The following are recommendations for certain scenarios:

When an immunized person who was vaccinated according to the recommended preexposure or postexposure regimen with human diploid-cell vaccine (HDCV) or purified chick embryo cell vaccine (PCECV), or who has previously demonstrated rabies antibody, is exposed to rabies, that person should receive two IM doses (1.0 mL each) of HDCV or PCECV, one immediately and one 3 days later. The human rabies immune globulin (HRIG) should not be given in these cases. If the immune status of a previously vaccinated person who did not receive the recommended HDCV or PCECV regimen is not known, full primary PEP (HRIG plus five doses of HDCV or PCECV) may be necessary.

Hope this helps. Thanks.—Pam

4. I was fishing and there was a dead animal in the water. I pushed it away with a stick and then went in the water with waders on. It is possible that the river water got in my mouth, nose, and eyes. I did not physically touch the carcass. The water was very cold and fast flowing.

Answer: Hello, as mentioned in our article, rabies is spread by saliva infected with the rabies virus entering the body, most commonly through a bite from a rabid animal; it can also be spread by infected saliva contacting a cut in the skin or a mucous membrane. The scenario you described in which river water contacted mucous membranes and a dead animal was in the rushing water does not suggest an exposure scenario because the volume of river water would create a significant dilution effect and the rushing water would have removed the virus from the site. Hope you are doing well.—Pam and Rodney

5. Does rabies occur naturally or does it have to be spread by biting, clawing, etc.?

Answer: Thank you for your question. Rabies is spread by saliva infected with the rabies virus entering the body, most commonly through a bite from a rabid animal; it can also be spread by infected saliva contacting a cut in the skin or a mucous membrane.

The virus can only live briefly outside the body in moist saliva (once the saliva has dried, the virus will die within minutes and it cannot be revived by remoistening it), so there is a potential for fresh, infected saliva on an inanimate object to contact a cut in the skin or mucous membranes, but this would be considered a rare route for exposure. Best regards.—Pam and Rodney

6. Thanks for the great article! Because rabies might be transmitted through broken skin, I was wondering if dry/rough skin is considered broken and a possible entrance for the virus?

    Answer: Hello, as stated in many of the other posts on this thread, rabies is transmitted via infected saliva, usually through the bite from a rabid animal; although rare, it's possible that infected saliva contacting a mucous membrane or a break in the skin could be a means of exposure. Exposure to body fluids/excretions other than saliva and possibly tears (i.e., urine, blood, stool …) from a rabid animal or human generally is not considered to constitute an exposure. The exposure you describe is very unlikely to transmit rabies. Thanks for the question!—Dr. Rohde and Pam

7. If a man is infected with rabies and if he kisses a lady, then how much chance of spreading rabies in the lady?

    Answer: If the infection were to the point that the virus was in the saliva of the person infected with rabies, then there would be a possibility that rabies could be spread by that saliva contacting the mucous membrane in the mouth of the other person during a kiss. Thank you for your inquiry.—Pam and Rodney

8. Sorry I got a question. Can a 9-week-old puppy get rabies from drinking hot water? I was told that someone's dog drank hot water and got rabies so they had to put the dog down to sleep and everyone in contact had to get a bunch of shots into the stomach.

    Answer: Thank you for your inquiry. No, a puppy (or any other animal for that matter) does not get rabies from drinking hot water. Maybe there was some other factor involved, like the puppy was sharing a bowl of water with an animal that was subsequently confirmed to have rabies and there was a concern about the rabid animal's saliva being in the bowl and contacting the mucous membranes in the mouth of the puppy when it drank from the bowl. Additionally, rabies vaccinations are no longer given in the stomach. It also doesn't sound appropriate that the puppy was given hot water to drink. Thanks.—Pam and Rodney

9. Recently, I visited a home of person who died few days before because of rabies. Is there any chance of infection? Should I go for antirabies injection?

    Answer: Hello, transmission of rabies occurs when saliva containing the rabies virus is introduced into an opening in the skin, usually via the bite of a rabid animal. Although rare, transmission could occur through infected saliva contacting mucous membranes or a scratch or other break in the skin.

    The rabies virus is very sensitive to light and air. How long the virus remains active depends on how long the saliva remains moist (many variables affect this, such as a cool temperature, shady environment, volume of saliva …). Once the saliva dries, the virus will not be revived by remoistening it. Therefore, in the scenario you describe, it sounds very unlikely that there would be any moist saliva with viable rabies virus in that house. Thank you for your question.—Pam

10. Here's what I don't get about vaccinating pets for rabies: my cats, age 14 and 10 years, are indoor cats. The very few times they've been outside, which has been like on the porch under close supervision. I suppose it's possible we might not notice a mouse run up and bite them really quickly and run away, but the odds are so slim. And if a pet is strictly an indoor pet, is it something you need to worry about at all? A rabid mouse or bat that somehow got into your house could just bite you and not your pets.

    Answer: Indoor animals are, indeed, less likely to be exposed to rabies. However, there is always a chance that an exposure could occur. A rabid bat can gain entrance to a house fairly readily. We even have had scenarios in which larger animals, such as a rabid skunk, have entered a household through a pet door. Therefore, laws pertaining to vaccinating animals against rabies tend to be all inclusive. It also would be difficult to delineate specific exceptions in the law and determine if somebody, for example, truly kept their pet indoors and totally isolated (if that's possible) from any rabid animals or if they let them outside occasionally and may or may not be diligent (as you mentioned you are) about supervising the animal the entire time that it is outside. It only takes a moment for a cat (or dog) to pick up a downed rabid bat or get in a scuffle with any rabid animal. Thanks for your interest.—Pam and Rodney

REVIEW

Real-life scenarios provide a learning ground for addressing possible rabies exposures and evaluating the need for PEP. Not only do they provide opportunities to contemplate rationales for handling different situations, but they also provide a memorable format on which to reflect when faced with similar inquiries from future patients or clients.

REFERENCES FOR RABIES CONCEPTS COMMONLY FEATURED IN RESPONSES

Within the replies to the Internet inquiries, there are reoccurring themes based on some key rabies concepts. Given that many of the answers focus on the recommendation to contact a physician, the lead author (Wilson) compiled the following referenced statements to support the responses for physicians and to provide veterinarians and other health professionals with readily available key points. Many variables need to be considered when evaluating a patient for administration of PEP; see Chapter 6 for detailed guidelines.

- Rabies is a medical urgency, not an emergency.[3]
- If a bite does occur, wash the bite wound immediately with soap and water, plus a virucidal agent, such as povidine-iodine solution (if available and not allergic). Washing the wound thoroughly with soap and water is one of the most effective ways to avoid infection with the rabies virus.[3-6] Promptly seek medical attention and guidance from a physician on the possible need for PEP; PEP must be prescribed by a physician (for humans) or a veterinarian (for animals if in a locale that allows it). The physician may decide to prescribe antibiotics and tetanus prophylaxis[7] depending on the nature of the bite and the circumstances of the bitten person.
- No cases of rabies have been reported in association with transmission by fomites or environmental surfaces.[8]
- The PEP regimen no longer features the much-feared extensive series of vaccinations in the abdomen, but in the United States consists of a dose of human rabies immune globulin (HRIG) administered as much as possible near the bite site and a series of four vaccinations (five vaccinations for immunocompromised individuals) in the deltoid area over a 2- to 4-week period (days 0, 3, 7, and 14, plus day 28 if immunocompromised).[9] The dose of HRIG is administered at the beginning of PEP; the amount of HRIG is based on the weight of the patient.[5]
- Rabies postexposure treatment is highly effective if administered correctly and before the virus enters the nervous system.[10] Failure rates of PEP have been estimated from 1 in 80,000 in developed countries to 1 in 12,000 in underdeveloped countries. Failure

is typically associated with a delay in administration or a breach in protocol.[11]

- Although rabies incubation periods can range from days to years,[12] it rarely exceeds 6 months[13] and typically is cited in the literature as 3–8 weeks[14] or 3 weeks to 3 months.[13] This range is why it is important to promptly receive PEP in case the incubation period is on the short side and also why a person should still pursue PEP even if time has lapsed since the bite or other potential exposure (possibly because they didn't initially consider the possibility of rabies). In the latter case, if the incubation period is on the protracted end, the PEP may still be effective (as long as the virus has not yet entered the nervous system and clinical signs and symptoms have not developed).
- Dogs, cats, and domestic ferrets have a special grouping in the world of rabies. If they bite or otherwise expose someone to rabies, they can be observed for 10 days. If they are healthy and alive 10 days after the bite incident, they could not have transmitted rabies in their saliva at the time of the bite.[13,15,16] That does not mean that they could not be incubating rabies; it just means that the disease would not have progressed to where the virus was being shed in the saliva at the time of that particular potential exposure.
- The incubation period is not the same as the 10-day observation period (during which the animal is typically quarantined or confined) for a dog, cat, or domestic ferret that has bitten a person. After an animal is exposed to rabies and the virus has spread to its salivary glands, the animal may be able to shed the rabies virus in its saliva; this means that the animal is infectious. Clinical signs generally appear within days of salivary shedding before death ensues. Dogs, cats, and domestic ferrets with rabies typically shed the rabies virus a few days[13,17-19] before they show clinical signs of rabies and only live for a few days after the clinical signs appear. This is why it is so important to observe animals that have bitten or otherwise potentially exposed a person to rabies. If a dog, cat, or domestic ferret is alive and healthy 10 days after the incident, it can be concluded that the rabies virus could not have been in the animal's saliva at the time of the incident and it could not have exposed the person to rabies.[13,15,16] Again, the animal still could possibly be incubating rabies, but it could not have been at the point of transmitting the virus in its saliva.
- When rescuing or adopting a stray animal, it is important to get it examined by a veterinarian and vaccinated against rabies; rabies preexposure vaccination will help to protect the animal from acquiring

rabies, and, by doing so, reduce the potential for it to subsequently be a source of disease exposure for people or other domestic animals.[13]

- When considering the need for PEP, it is significant to know the geographical location of the person who is submitting an inquiry about a possible exposure. For instance, the bite of a mongoose would not typically be correlated with rabies concerns in the 50 states, but would be in Puerto Rico.[4,20,21] Even different states have variations in species in which rabies has been documented.

- If the biting animal dies or is euthanatized, a suitable specimen should be kept appropriately cooled and submitted for testing in a timely fashion to avoid decomposition to the point of being untestable. However, if this does not happen, it is never too late to submit a specimen and let the laboratorians determine if it is testable.[22]

- Bat bites are so small that they can be undetected, so the recommendation is that in a situation in which a bat is physically present and the person(s) cannot exclude the possibility of a bite (for instance, a bat found in a room with a young child, a person who had been sleeping, a sensory or mentally challenged person, or an intoxicated person), PEP should be considered unless prompt testing of the bat rules out the possibility of rabies.[22,23]

REFERENCES

1. Wilson PJ, Rohde RE. *8 Things You May Not Know about Rabies - But Should*. Elsevier Connect; September 2015. htpps://www.elsevier.com/connect/8-things-you-may-not-know-about-rabies-but-should.
2. Wilson PJ, Rohde RE. *The Many Faces of Rabies*. Elsevier Connect; September 2016. htpps://www.elsevier.com/connect/the-many-faces-of-rabies.
3. Centers for Disease Control and Prevention. When Should I Seek Medical Attention? http://www.cdc.gov/rabies/exposure/index.html.
4. Birhane MG, Cleaton JM, Monroe BP, et al. Rabies surveillance in the United States during 2015. *JAVMA*. 2017;250(10):1117–1130.
5. Centers for Disease Control and Prevention. Human rabies prevention – United States, 2008: recommendations of the Advisory Committee on Immunization Practices. *MMWR*. 2008;57(RR-3):1–28.
6. World Health Organization. Rabies. http://www.who.int/meidacentre/factsheets/fs099/en/.
7. Willoughby RE. Rabies: rare human infection – common questions. *Infect Dis Clin*. 2015;29:637–650.
8. Centers for Disease Control and Prevention. Investigation of rabies infections in organ donor and transplant recipients – Alabama, Arkansas, Oklahoma, and Texas, 2004. *MMWR*. 2004;53(Dispatch):1–3.
9. Rupprecht CE, Briggs D, Brown CM, et al. Use of a reduced (4-dose) vaccine schedule for postexposure prophylaxis to prevent human rabies: recommendations of the Advisory Committee on Immunization Practices. *MMWR Recomm Rep*. 2010;59(RR-2):1–9.
10. Susilawathi NM, Darwinata AE, Dwija IB, et al. Epidemiological and clinical features of human rabies cases in Bali 2008-2010. *BMC Infect Dis*. 2012;12(81):1–8.
11. De Serres G, Dallaire F, Cote M, et al. Bat rabies in the United States and Canada from 1950 through 2007: human cases with and without bat contact. *Clin Infect Dis*. 2008;46:1329–1337.
12. Pan American Health Organization. Rabies. In: *Zoonoses and Communicable Diseases Common to Man and Animals*. PAHO; 2003:246–275.
13. Brown CM, Slavinski S, Ettestad P, et al. Compendium of animal rabies prevention and control, 2016. *JAVMA*. 2016;248(5):505–517.
14. Centers for Disease Control and Prevention. Human rabies-Missouri, 2014. *MMWR*. 2016;65(10):253–256.
15. Niezgoda M, Hanlon CA, Rupprecht CE. Animal rabies. In: Jackson AC, Wunner WH, eds. *Rabies*. San Diego: Academic Press, An Elsevier Science Imprint; 2002:163–218.
16. Hanlon CA. Rabies in terrestrial animals. In: Jackson AC, ed. *Rabies: Scientific Basis of the Disease and Its Management*. San Diego: Academic Press, An Elsevier Science Imprint; 2013:179–213.
17. Fekadu M. Canine rabies. In: Baer GM, ed. *The Natural History of Rabies*. 2nd ed. Boca Raton: CRC Press, Inc; 1991:367–387.
18. Vaughn JB, Gerhardt P, Paterson JCS. Excretion of street rabies virus in the saliva of cats. *JAMA*. 1963;184:705–708.
19. Vaughn JB, Gerhardt P, Newell KW. Excretion of street rabies virus in the saliva of dogs. *JAMA*. 1965;193(5):113–118.
20. Centers for Disease Control and Prevention. Human rabies – Puerto Rico, 2015. *MMWR*. 2017;65(52):1474–1476.
21. Krebs JW, Williams SM, Smith JS, et al. Rabies among infrequently reported mammalian carnivores in the United States, 1960-2000. *J Wildl Dis*. 2003;39(2):253–261.
22. Centers for Disease Control and Prevention. Human rabies – Washington, 1995. *MMWR*. 1995;44(34):625–627.
23. Mayes BC, Wilson PJ, Oertli EH, et al. Epidemiology of rabies in bats in Texas (2001-2010). *JAVMA*. 2013;243(8):1129–1137.

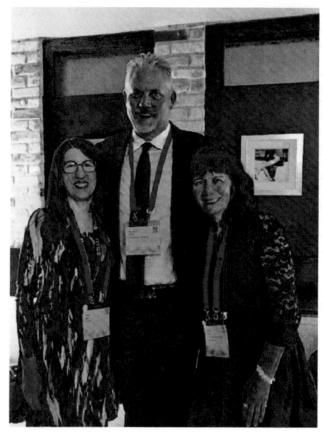

Dr. Alison Bert, Dr. Rodney E. Rohde, and Pamela Wilson (left to right) developed the concept for this book based on questions submitted by readers worldwide on two rabies articles published in Elsevier Connect and the authors' responses. (Photo taken at an Elsevier gathering in Austin, TX.)

CHAPTER 8

Education and Prevention Tips

PAMELA J. WILSON, MEd, LVT, MCHES

SCENARIO

From an actual rabies case investigation: an owner took a pregnant dog to an emergency clinic because it was acting strange. The clinic was advised by the owner that the dog was current on its vaccinations; however, she was not. The owner then took the dog to her regular veterinarian, who suspected rabies (the dog also smelled of skunk) and submitted the dog's brain for testing; the dog was laboratory-confirmed positive with the south central skunk rabies virus variant. Four veterinary clinic personnel and four members of the family who owned the dog had been exposed. The owners had rescued the dog some time previously; it had a leg and an abdominal injury (the injuries were not characteristic of being caused by an animal and were not believed to be the source of exposure), plus the dog had a fever at the time of the exam, so vaccinations were not administered. The owners thought the dog was vaccinated on subsequent appointments with their veterinarian. The cost for rabies biologics to administer postexposure prophylaxis came to $20,000 ($9000 for veterinary personnel and almost $11,000 for family members); additionally, the dog had lost her life as well as those of her unborn puppies. All were costs that could have been avoided with an inexpensive rabies preexposure vaccination for the dog.[a,b]

INTRODUCTION

"Don't go near that dog. Do you understand? He's just as dangerous dead as alive." Atticus Finch in the 1962 movie *To Kill a Mockingbird* warning his young children not to touch a rabid dog that he just shot.[1]

Providing information on rabies prevention can have lifesaving consequences. Educational efforts, including those directed toward children, should be included in the goals of public health programs. One of the challenges in providing communications on rabies prevention is to present the reality of the severity of the disease and the elusiveness of what can constitute an exposure, plus the intricacies of the variable incubation period, without creating a panic. The goal is not to make people fear having contact with animals or engender a desire to destroy every bat they see. Rather, the goal is to make them aware of the potential for exposure to this disease and how to approach animal-related situations with an educated caution and informed respect.

Note: In the example of Atticus Finch's warning to his children, the still moist saliva on the rabid dog contacting a mucous membrane or break in their skin would constitute a possible exposure.

CONCEPTS OF PREVENTION—HEALTH BELIEF MODEL

The premise of the Health Belief Model (HBM) is that a person's belief in a threat to his/her personal health or potential to acquire a disease combined with his/her belief that a particular behavior or action will deter that threat will predict whether or not the person adopts that particular behavior. Some of the elements of the HBM include the following:

- perceived susceptibility—the person's perception of how likely they are to acquire a disease;
- perceived severity—the person's perception of the seriousness of a disease;
- perceived benefits—the person's perception as to how effective certain behaviors or actions will be toward circumventing a disease; and
- perceived barriers—the person's perception of the affordability and obtainability of an action to prevent disease.[2]

One goal in prevention techniques would be to reach the target population and address these perceptions in real life. For example, there was a case investigation conducted on a rabid dog in South Texas during an epizootic (an epidemic in animals) of rabies involving the domestic dog/coyote rabies virus variant in the 1990s.[c] The dog had not been vaccinated against rabies. During the course of the investigation, the owner of the rabid dog inquired as to whether or not he would need to receive rabies postexposure prophylaxis (PEP) again since he had received PEP a year before that when his other

Rabies. https://doi.org/10.1016/B978-0-323-63979-8.00008-8
Copyright © 2019 Elsevier Inc. All rights reserved.

unvaccinated dog died of rabies. One would think that there would be nothing more effective than a first-hand experience with a disease such as this to make a person aware of being susceptible, and pets being susceptible, to rabies; that rabies is an extremely serious disease to the point of being nearly 100% fatal; and that preexposure rabies vaccinations for pets would be beneficial and effective in preventing rabies. In retrospect, was the missing factor in this case addressing perceived barriers, like the availability and affordability of rabies vaccinations for his pets? Or was he left with the misguided assumption that he was now invincible to rabies because he had received PEP? Plus, after having a dog die from rabies, why was the importance of getting rabies preexposure vaccinations for his future dogs not evident to him? Evaluating exposure scenarios and reviewing case investigations are all opportunities for benefitting from lessons learned and lending insights on the development of educational techniques pertaining to disease prevention.

Note: The answer to the question posed by the owner of the rabid dogs is that two booster vaccinations (one on day 0 and one on day 3) are recommended for previously vaccinated persons who are exposed to a rabid animal.[3]

RABIES PREEXPOSURE VACCINATIONS FOR ANIMALS

For disease control efforts in a given population, those who don't vaccinate depend on those who do.—William D. Wilson, Science Department, Spoon River College, Canton, Illinois

From Wilson PJ. *Caring for your puppy pal.* In: *Puppy Pal Pointers: From the True Tails of Ripple and Jessie.* Bloomington: AuthorHouse; 2004:1–66.[4]

Parenteral Vaccine for Domestic Animals

Rabies preexposure vaccination of domestic animals is a fundamental component of rabies control and prevention. By preventing animals from developing rabies, vaccination will also serve to help protect the people who own them or have contact with them from potential exposure to rabies. Before the 1960s, the majority of reported cases of rabies in animals occurred in domestic animals.[5] With the advent of rabies vaccination campaigns and animal control programs for domestic animals in the 1940s and 1950s, that is no longer the case.[6-8] Although wildlife now accounts for more than 90% of yearly rabies cases in the United States,[9,10] pets can be exposed via rabid wildlife. Those exposed pets can bring the disease into the home either because they are infected and shedding the virus or by transporting

the rabid animal into the home, such as a cat carrying a downed rabid bat and depositing it in the house.[11]

Most, if not all, states require that dogs be vaccinated against rabies.[12] Although state laws may vary on the requirement for vaccinating cats, all cats should be vaccinated against rabies. Domestic ferrets should also be vaccinated against rabies.[13,14] State laws and local ordinances cover vaccination requirements for a specific location; this information can be obtained through state and local health departments, plus city and county animal control agencies.

> Rabies preexposure vaccination of domestic animals is a fundamental component of rabies control and prevention; it serves to not only protect the animals against rabies, but also helps prevent people who have contact with them from being exposed to the disease.

The majority of rabies vaccines for animals licensed by the US Department of Agriculture (USDA) have a schedule of an initial vaccination at 3 months of age followed by a booster in 1 year.[13] There are some vaccines for cats that allow vaccination at 8 weeks of age followed by boosters every 3–4 weeks until 3 months of age and then annually thereafter.[13] If a stray animal of unknown age and vaccination status receives a vaccination, it would be considered an initial vaccination because of the fact that there is no known vaccination history, so that animal would also have a booster administered in 1 year. Subsequent boosters would then be given according to the duration of immunity of the specific vaccine used (which is typically annually or triennially). A list of licensed vaccines and their vaccination schedules is available through the most current publication of the *Compendium of Animal Rabies Prevention and Control*,[13] which is compiled by the National Association of State Public Health Veterinarians (NASPHV). If an animal is overdue for a rabies booster vaccination, it is recommended that the animal be considered currently vaccinated immediately after receiving the booster.[13] However, state laws and local ordinances may have more restrictive requirements.

The NASPHV recommends that all horses be vaccinated against rabies.[13] The American Association of Equine Practitioners considers rabies to be a core vaccine for all equids.[15] Manufacturers of vaccines licensed for horses by the USDA typically recommend vaccination at 3 or 4 months of age and annually thereafter.[13,15,16] Again, refer to the most recent version of the *Compendium of Animal Rabies Prevention and Control* for a list of licensed vaccines and their vaccination schedules.[13]

In addition to the recommendation to vaccinate all equids against rabies, other livestock that are in frequent contact with humans should be vaccinated against rabies.[14] Exhibition animals and livestock "pets" are examples of such animals.[17] The recommendation for vaccination includes domestic animals for which there is a USDA-licensed vaccine, such as sheep and cattle (especially dairy cattle from which unpasteurized milk is used for direct human consumption),[17] plus animals for which a licensed vaccine is not available, such as goats, pigs, and animals in petting zoos, fairs, and public exhibitions.[13,17] Although there is no approved parenteral vaccine for wild animals or their hybrids,[13] vaccination of wolf-dog hybrids should be considered.[14] When a rabies vaccine is used in a species for which it is not licensed, the animal is not considered to be officially vaccinated against rabies in the event of an exposure situation (whether the animal bit or otherwise potentially exposed a person or was potentially exposed by another animal to rabies)[14]; however, the hope is that the animal will get some level of response to the vaccine and be protected against rabies. When extra-label use of a vaccine is implemented, it would behoove the veterinary practitioner to explain these caveats to the client, plus document the conversation in the patient's file and/or have the client sign a statement acknowledging the conversation.

It can be confusing to the owner of a vaccinated animal that has bitten or otherwise potentially exposed a person that the animal must still be observed for rabies.[13] The rationale behind this is that, although very uncommon, there is the possibility that the vaccine was not effective in that animal.[18-20] Vaccine failures may occur possibly because the animal was immunocompromised and did not get a good response to the vaccine or the cold-chain storage of the vaccine was not effectively maintained. However, health-care providers should feel confident in observing the animal for rabies rather than testing it if the animal has been previously vaccinated and the animal is not exhibiting any signs compatible with rabies. The decision to test an animal for rabies instead of observing it warrants serious consideration because the testing procedure requires euthanatizing and decapitating the animal to submit its brain to a laboratory for testing. Of course, if the animal starts displaying clinical signs of rabies or dies during the observation period, testing is necessitated.

Although vaccines are very effective, a rabies case in a leukemia-positive cat provides an example of why biting animals are to be observed for rabies even if they have been vaccinated. This cat would have been immunocompromised because of leukemia and was presenting with weakness and posterior paresis, which are clinical signs

that can be exhibited in leukemia and in rabies. The cat had been vaccinated with a rabies vaccine approved for a 1-year duration of immunity and was 4 months overdue on the annual booster. During an office visit, the attending veterinarian noticed that the owner had been bitten on the hand by the cat and recommended that the client seek medical attention. The client followed this recommendation; the physician who examined the wound subsequently reported the bite, resulting in the cat being quarantined for a 10-day observation period. The animal's condition deteriorated, so it was euthanatized and tested for rabies; test results determined that the cat was positive for rabies.[21,22] This case exemplifies the importance of reporting animal bites and the fact that, as successful as they usually are, no vaccine is 100% effective, particularly in immunocompromised animals. Rabies should still be considered as a differential diagnosis even if the animal has been previously vaccinated. Although in most cases involving vaccinated animals, rabies is a remote possibility, it is better to err on the side of caution from a public health perspective.

Oral Rabies Vaccine for Wildlife and Herd Immunity

In addition to rabies vaccination requirements or recommendations for domestic animals being prevalent throughout the United States, there are also vaccination programs for wildlife, including raccoons, foxes, and coyotes[23]; field studies for skunks are ongoing.[24,25] In these programs,[23,26,27] the vaccine/baits consist of vaccinia- or adeno-rabies glycoprotein recombinant rabies vaccine inside a sachet (plastic packet) surrounded with flavorings and attractants to make them appealing to the target animals to eat (see Fig. 8.1). The vaccine/baits are distributed in designated areas primarily from aircraft with supplemental distribution by hand. When an animal bites into the sachet, the sachet ruptures, vaccine covers the oral cavity and throat, and the virus enters the animal's system through lymphatic tissue of the pharynx, thereby vaccinating the animal against rabies.

The vaccine/baits are nontoxic and do not become established in the environment. Studies have indicated their safety in many different species of animals. The vaccine cannot cause the animal to develop rabies.[23,26,27] Although the vaccine/baits are harmless if eaten by a domestic animal (and the vaccine possibly could provide some protection from the disease), that animal would still need to be inoculated with a parenteral rabies vaccine to be properly vaccinated; vaccinating an animal with a parenteral vaccine would be safe to do even if the animal ingested oral rabies vaccine the same day. The vaccine/baits are distributed through

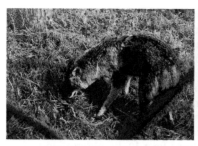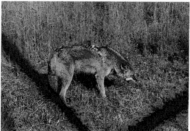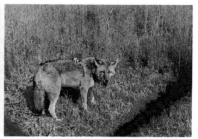

FIG. 8.1 Coyote locating and consuming a bait containing oral rabies vaccine. (Courtesy of Dr. M. Gayne Fearneyhough, former Director, Oral Rabies Vaccination Program, Austin, TX.)

government programs and not available for individual use.

The principle behind oral rabies vaccination is to produce herd immunity. Herd immunity can be described as the resistance of a group to infection and spread of the rabies virus as a result of immunity in a high proportion of individuals in the group. Transmission of rabies is a product of the number of susceptible animals and the probability that a susceptible animal will come into contact with an infected animal.[26,27] The higher the level of herd immunity, the lower the number of susceptible animals and the lower the probability that an infected animal will come into contact with a susceptible animal. The concept of herd immunity can also be applied to the aforementioned success of parenteral vaccination campaigns and mandatory vaccination requirements in effectively reducing rabies cases in dogs in the United States.[7] However, all owners should take responsibility to ensure that their domestic animals are properly vaccinated against rabies and not depend on those who do to provide herd immunity.[4]

RABIES PREEXPOSURE VACCINATIONS FOR HUMANS

As with certain domestic animals, rabies preexposure vaccinations are also available for humans. Preexposure vaccinations are given for several reasons. First, they may provide protection to people with unapparent exposures to rabies. Second, they may protect people whose postexposure therapy is delayed. This is particularly important for people at risk of being exposed while traveling or working in countries where the rabies biologics are difficult to obtain. Although these vaccinations do not totally eliminate the need for additional vaccinations after a rabies exposure, the preexposure vaccinations reduce the amount of treatment needed compared with PEP for a person who has not received the preexposure vaccinations.

The rabies preexposure vaccination regimen consists of three vaccinations given over a period of 3–4 weeks: one on day 0 and boosters on days 7 and 21 or 28 (see Table 8.1).[3] Periodic serologic testing should be conducted per recommendations for the level of risk the person has for exposure to rabies (see Table 8.2). The minimum acceptable antibody level is complete virus neutralization at a 1:5 serum dilution by a rapid fluorescent foci inhibition test (RFFIT) (or minimum neutralizing antibodies of 0.5 IU/mL[3,28]); a booster dose should be administered if the titer falls below the acceptable level (see Tables 8.1 and 8.2).[3]

Even if a person has received rabies preexposure vaccinations, if an exposure occurs, administer two booster vaccinations, one immediately and one 3 days later. The reason for this practice is that there have been cases in which individuals who had preexposure vaccinations still developed rabies after an exposure[3] as no vaccine is 100% effective or there was a natural decrease in the level of protection over time. Another factor is that the person may have been immunocompromised by pregnancy, disease (for example, cancer or viral infections), or certain medical procedures or treatments (such as chemotherapy, organ transplantations, or use of anti-inflammatory drugs) when preexposure vaccinations were administered and was unable to achieve a good response to the vaccine.

> Rabies preexposure vaccination is available for people and recommended for individuals involved in occupations or activities with a high risk of exposure to rabies.

Nonetheless, the intent of rabies preexposure vaccinations is that they are anticipated to be effective in protecting people in high-risk occupations or activities for rabies exposure who might have an unapparent exposure (see Table 8.2).[3,29] Examples of people at higher risk for being exposed to rabies who should consider getting the preexposure vaccinations include rabies research and

TABLE 8.1		
Rabies Preexposure Vaccination Schedule		
Type of Vaccination	**Route**	**Regimen**
Primary	IM	Human diploid cell vaccine (HDCV) or purified chick embryo cell vaccine (PCECV); 1.0 mL (deltoid area), one each on days 0, 7, and 21 or 28
Booster[a]	IM	HDCV or PCECV; 1.0 mL (deltoid area), day 0 only

[a]Administration of a booster dose of vaccine depends on exposure risk category and serologic testing results as noted in Table 8.2. HDCV or PCECV can be used for booster vaccinations or PEP even if another vaccine was used for the initial preexposure vaccination.
(From Centers for Disease Control and Prevention. Human rabies prevention—United States, 2008: Recommendations of the Advisory Committee on Immunization Practices. *MMWR.* 2008;57(RR-3):1–283.[3])

TABLE 8.2			
Rabies Preexposure Vaccination Guide			
Risk Category	**Nature of Risk**	**Typical Populations**	**Preexposure Recommendations**
Continuous	Virus present continuously, often in high concentrations. Aerosol, mucous membrane, bite, or nonbite exposure. Specific exposures may go unrecognized.	Rabies research lab worker, rabies biologics production workers.	Primary course. Serologic testing every 6 months; booster vaccination if antibody titer falls below acceptable level.[a]
Frequent	Exposure usually episodic, with source recognized, but exposure may also be unrecognized. Aerosol, mucous membrane, bite, or nonbite exposure.	Rabies diagnostic lab workers, cavers (spelunkers), veterinarians, veterinary staff and students, and animal control and wildlife workers in rabies-enzootic areas; all persons who frequently handle bats.	Primary course. Serologic testing every 2 years; booster vaccination if antibody titer falls below acceptable level.[a]
Infrequent (greater than population at large)	Exposure nearly always episodic with source recognized. Mucous membrane, bite, or nonbite exposure.	Veterinarians, veterinary staff and students, and animal control and wildlife workers in areas of low-rabies occurrence. Travelers visiting foreign areas where rabies is enzootic and access to medical care including biologics is limited.	Primary course; no serologic testing or booster vaccination.
Rare (population at large)	Exposures always episodic. Mucous membrane or bite with source recognized.	US population at large, including persons in rabies-enzootic areas.	No vaccination necessary.

[a]Minimum acceptable antibody level is complete virus neutralization at a 1:5 serum dilution (or titer is >/= 0.5 IU/mL) by RFFIT. Booster dose should be administered if the titer falls below this level.
From Centers for Disease Control and Prevention. Human rabies prevention—United States, 2008: Recommendations of the Advisory Committee on Immunization Practices. *MMWR.* 2008;57(RR-3):1–28[3]; Texas Department of State Health Services. Rabies Prevention in Texas.[29]
https://dshs.texas.gov/idcu/disease/rabies/information/prevention/pamphlet/.

laboratory workers, rabies biologics production workers, veterinarians, veterinary technicians and assistants, veterinary students, animal control personnel/animal shelter employees, wildlife workers (including pest management professionals and wildlife rehabilitators), and students working with wildlife for classes or research projects. Since the 1960s, rabies preexposure vaccination has been advised for cavers (spelunkers).[30] Travelers visiting foreign areas with enzootic rabies should also consider getting preexposure vaccinations,[7] particularly if they plan to be in locations or participate in activities that might enhance their exposure to animals and/or they will be in areas with limited access to medical care and rabies biologics. Routine rabies vaccinations are not recommended for the general population in the United States or for travelers to areas where rabies is not endemic.[3,29]

USE OF PERSONAL PROTECTIVE EQUIPMENT

With the implementation of standard precautions, the risk of transmission of rabies from an infected patient to a health-care provider is low; there have been no documented rabies cases because of this type of exposure.[31] The use of appropriate personal protective equipment (PPE), however, continues to be crucial to prevent medical staff from being exposed to rabies while caring for patients with suspected or confirmed rabies. Plus, because rabies in humans is rare in the United States and the clinical signs and symptoms of rabies mimic those of other diseases, cases may not be recognized until days after medical care has been initiated. Examples of PPE to use include mask and goggles or face shields to protect mucous membranes and gloves and gowns to cover any breaks in the skin from having contact with any potentially infectious substances, most notably saliva and neural tissue (and conceivably tears).[32,33] The clinical sign of hypersalivation could lead to increased potential for exposure to infected saliva. Dysphagia, a clinical sign that makes it difficult for a patient with rabies to swallow saliva,[34–36] results in copious amounts of saliva being available as a possible source of exposure. Additionally, there is documentation of cases of patients who succumbed to undiagnosed rabies that were only discovered because of rabies developing in recipients of organs donated by those individuals.[3,33] Use of standard precautions at all times when working with patients will help provide protection against an unapparent exposure from such a patient.

> Use personal protective equipment, such as mask and goggles or face shields to protect mucous membranes and gloves and gowns to cover any breaks in the skin, to prevent possible exposure to rabies.

Standard precautions should also be taken to prevent aerosol transmission during medical procedures.[37] Percutaneous injuries, such as needle sticks, are considered to be exposures because of potential contact with nervous tissue.[33] Contact with a nuchal biopsy would also be a potential source of exposure.[31] Personnel conducting autopsies should implement, in addition to standard PPE, the use of N95 masks to provide protection from aerosolized brain matter that may occur when an oscillating saw is used during the procedure.[32]

It is imperative for laboratorians to implement the use of PPE to prevent being exposed to rabies while conducting rabies research or handling and testing submitted specimens that may be positive for rabies. There was a 1972 US case of rabies involving a laboratory worker who had received four preexposure doses of experimental (never licensed) rabies vaccine, but he did not develop a positive serum antibody response when tested a year later. He did not receive any additional vaccinations during the 13 years between vaccination and onset of illness.[38] Hypotheses are that he inhaled substantial amounts of rabies virus while pipetting homogenized rabid goat brains from a blender jar to other containers or, although he was wearing PPE (gown, gloves, and mask), he apparently removed his mask for a few minutes during the process supposedly to perform mouth pipetting, which may have made exposure to mucous membrane possible.[39] Although this is a dated story, it still serves to emphasize the importance of properly utilizing PPE, plus being vaccinated against rabies and demonstrating an adequate serum antibody titer, if working in a rabies-oriented laboratory.

> For individuals at higher risk of exposure to rabies, remember the three Ps of rabies prevention: **p**reexposure vaccination, **p**ersonal protective equipment, and **p**ostexposure prophylaxis.

Even though they already should have rabies preexposure vaccinations, veterinarians, veterinary technicians, and veterinary assistants also need to implement precautions when handling patients. A realistic scenario is to treat a patient, send it home, and never hear that it subsequently died of undiagnosed rabies. Veterinary staff may have had their hands in the animal's mouth checking for possible dental problems, obstructions, or other complications unbeknownst that the animal actually was exhibiting clinical signs of rabies, such as hypersalivation, dysphagia, and choking sounds. There was a case of rabies in a veterinarian in Brazil who had not received rabies preexposure vaccination and did not implement PPE when handling rabies-suspect herbivores that were subsequently confirmed to be positive for rabies; after laboratory confirmation of rabies in these animals, the veterinarian refused PEP as well. There was no record of him being bitten by any bovines or caprines, so exposure was considered to be through coming in contact with infected saliva when he was handling the rabid animals.[40] Use of the three Ps of rabies prevention for those at high risk for exposure—preexposure vaccination, personal protective equipment, and postexposure prophylaxis (if an exposure occurs)—were not utilized in this case scenario, leading to the veterinarian developing rabies and dying.

Transmission could possibly occur during contact with infected materials, such as neural tissue, during the process of butchering or skinning an infected carcass.[7,41] Therefore, persons handling animal tissues or carcasses, including meat processors, butchers, and hunters, should utilize PPE (for example, gloves, eye protection, and face shield).[17] Depending on the extent of their exposure risk, they may even consider getting rabies preexposure vaccination.[17]

WOUND WASHING

One of the most crucial prevention measures to take if bitten by an animal (or otherwise potentially exposed to rabies) is to reduce the viral load if the animal was, indeed, rabid by washing the wound thoroughly with soap and water as promptly as possible.[9,42] Additionally, apply a virucidal agent, such as povidine-iodine solution (if available and not allergic to it). This also is essential advice to provide to patients or clients.

> Promptly and thoroughly washing a bite wound with soap and water, plus applying a virucidal agent, is one of the most effective ways to reduce viral load and help reduce chances of a productive rabies infection.

Similarly, washing the wound(s) of an animal that has been bitten using copious amounts of soap and water will help to reduce the possibility of a productive rabies infection.[43] Wear gloves in case fresh saliva from the biting animal is present; if the biting animal was rabid, rabies virus may be viable if the saliva is still moist.

SPECIAL CONSIDERATIONS FOR POTENTIAL RABIES EXPOSURE SCENARIOS INVOLVING BATS

I love bats more than ever. It's the disease, not the animal's fault. I never associated the bat with rabies. The bat was just a carrier.—Jeanna Giese, rare survivor of rabies after acquiring the virus via a bat bite.[44]

From Finley D. *Unvaccinated rabies survivor lives to tell her tale. San Antonio Express News.* 22.06.12.[45]

Most bats do not have rabies and serve an important role in agriculture and the environment via insect control (including insects that can damage crops or spread disease), seed dispersal, and pollination of plants. They fill a vital ecologic niche and care should be directed toward their continued conservation, especially when their survival is being challenged with monumental obstacles, such as white-nose syndrome (a fungal disease that has killed millions of bats).[46] When considering their role in rabies, remember that the battle is with the disease, not the animals that are devastatingly affected by it. Still, bats with rabies are more likely to be handled by people or pets than healthy bats. A clinical sign of rabies in bats is difficulty flying, so a rabid bat might be downed and fluttering on the ground.[47,48] Unfortunately, people are often tempted to pick them up and handle them with bare hands, leading to potential exposure (a bite mark from a bat may be too small to detect) and the need for PEP.[48] For instance, in one scenario, two people were playing catch with a downed bat they found while waiting at a bus stop. An astute observer reported the incident, which led to the bat that was abandoned by these individuals after they boarded the bus being recovered and tested for rabies. After the bat was laboratory-confirmed positive for rabies, a media campaign had to be initiated to find the two persons who had ill-advisedly chosen to play a game of catch with a sick animal.[49] A bat, like any animal, should be treated humanely.

Another example of unfortunate improper handling of a bat was a teacher who passed a downed bat in a bucket around the classroom while encouraging all of the students to touch it. Subsequently, the bat tested positive for rabies, with the aftermath including interviews with all the students to determine if they had any contact with the bat that could be considered a potential exposure. Just touching a rabid animal does not constitute an exposure to rabies, but infected saliva contacting a break in the skin or a mucous membrane does.[49] Bat bites are very small, leaving a mark about the size of a hypodermic needle injection, and can be easily overlooked.

Lack of knowledge about rabies or fear related to either the possibility of having PEP administered or getting in trouble, especially in children or adolescents, could prevent sharing a possible exposure history.[50] Concern by adolescents that they might be in trouble for their actions and conflicting statements by individuals and associated peers about a possible exposure incident, coupled with uncooperative attitudes, can make risk assessment difficult.[11] This makes it all the more critical to counsel young people on rabies prevention tips, especially on the importance of reporting bites from animals and the possible exposure scenarios related to bats.

> Conservation of bats is a desirable mission. However, education about the unique rabies exposure scenarios associated with bats and how to assess them for the need of PEP is of vital importance.

Given the fact that bat bites are not always visible, in situations in which a bat is physically present and there is a possibility of an unapparent exposure, the bat should be captured and submitted to a rabies laboratory for testing. Such situations could include finding a bat in a room during a time while someone had been sleeping there or in a room with an unattended child, a sensory or mentally challenged person, or an intoxicated person.[11,51,52] If rabies cannot be ruled out by laboratory testing, people with a reasonable probability of an exposure are recommended to receive PEP, and potentially exposed domestic animals may be recommended for rabies vaccinations and confinement or euthanasia (depending on state and local requirements). Scenarios that indicate a reasonable probability of exposure involving bats are provided in a client education sheet at the end of this chapter.

REVIEW

One of the most critical components of rabies prevention is to vaccinate dogs, cats, and other animals in close association with humans against rabies. People with high-risk occupations or activities for exposure to rabies should receive rabies preexposure vaccinations. Personal protective equipment should be consistently implemented.

There are materials available to provide patients or clients with information on how to recognize possible clinical signs of rabies and how to avoid being exposed to rabies, including special concerns related to exposure to bats. Educating children on these topics is imperative.

Through the course of rabies case investigations, missed opportunities have been revealed pertaining to rabies education, including what could have been life-saving information about bats being high-risk animals for transmitting rabies and the caveats of what constitutes an exposure to bats. It is of fundamental importance for health professionals to learn from these

unfortunate scenarios and, in doing so, protect the lives that are entrusted to their care and depend on them for disease-prevention guidance.

EXAMPLES OF CASES AND CASE INVESTIGATIONS

1. In Florida where raccoon rabies is endemic, a teenage boy found an ill-appearing raccoon in a wooded area on his way to school and put the animal in his backpack. While still on his way to school, the boy realized he better call for assistance, so he set the backpack in a garbage can in a residential area with permission by the home owner and called Animal Care and Control (ACC). The boy was gone by the time ACC arrived, and no contact information for him was available. The homeowner denied having been exposed to the raccoon.

   The ACC notified the Florida Department of Health (DOH) of the incident and that the raccoon was being processed for rabies testing (euthanatized and decapitated); the DOH then transported the head to the rabies laboratory. The DOH soon was able to make contact with the exposed child and his parent after he presented to a hospital in another county for a raccoon bite to the hand. The parent was given education on rabies and the necessity of continuing PEP. The parent stated no one else had contact with the raccoon.

   The raccoon tested positive for rabies the next day, and the parent was updated with the test results. Upon medical-record review by the DOH for the day 0 treatment, it was discovered that the exposed child was not given enough human rabies immune globulin (HRIG) at the hospital according to his body weight. The child returned to the hospital for the day 3 vaccination and was not given the outstanding HRIG. He received the rest of the HRIG on day 7 and finished out the rest of his series at the DOH clinic.[d,e]

   Note: HRIG provides passive immunity as protection in case of a short incubation period. By day 8 of administering the vaccine, which produces active immunity, HRIG should not be administered. This scenario is another reminder of the importance of teaching children about rabies, to avoid physical contact with wild animals, and to alert a responsible adult (parent, teacher, policeman, animal control officer...) when they have encountered an apparently sick animal.

2. At an animal shelter's weekend adoption event, a man deposited a young dog that was a stray his family had been feeding for about 6 weeks, but they could no longer afford to care for it. The receptionist took the man's name and street address before he left. Although policy typically was to hold a relinquished animal for observation, staff violated protocol and carried the puppy throughout the facility so that people could pet it. One family took an interest in the puppy and adopted it on Sunday. Shortly after they took it home, the puppy's health started to decline and it started snapping at people. The family returned the puppy to the shelter Monday where it was euthanized and a specimen was submitted for rabies testing; the puppy was laboratory-confirmed positive with the south central skunk rabies virus variant. The family had to be evaluated for potential exposure to infected saliva, plus the public had to be notified about the incident to discern about possible exposures depending on the type of contact they might have had with the puppy at the animal shelter during the period when it was being circulated at the adoption event. Various media were utilized for this purpose and phone lines were created to receive the calls. Additionally, there were complications locating the man who originally brought the puppy to the shelter because he was actually from a neighboring community, not the city where the adoption event was being held. When he was located, he and his family were evaluated for the possible need for PEP. By the end of the case investigation, 22 people received PEP.[a]

   Note: This case scenario is provided for educational purposes pertaining to rabies awareness; it in no way is intended to deter anyone from adopting a shelter animal that needs a good home nor is its intent to shed a negative light on the positive work accomplished at shelters for the benefit of deserving animals. Adoption of animals from shelters should be supported at all levels, including by local communities, dedicated shelter staff, and those seeking a new pet to enrich their lives.

3. A rancher and his son both had to receive PEP after their prize bull was confirmed to have rabies. They had both stuck their hands in the bull's mouth because it appeared to be choking on something (a clinical sign of rabies).[f]

   Note: A rabies vaccination would have been a small price to pay to keep a prize bull from succumbing to rabies and prevent the expense of PEP for two people; rabies vaccinations are recommended for livestock that are in close association with humans or are expensive.

4. A man was using an emergency toilet near a barn when he felt something rub on his legs like a cat; when he looked down, he discovered it was actually a skunk that proceeded to climb onto his lap. The man slowly pushed the skunk away and, after it dropped to the ground, he was able to distance himself from the animal and observe it. He subsequently shot the skunk and used various garden tools (hedge clippers, spade, shovel, ax, and machete) to remove its head. The specimen tested positive for rabies. Because of the amount of body fluids and tissue being spattered during the decapitation attempts, the possibility of virus-laden matter having contact with the man's mucous membranes or a break in his skin could not be ruled out and, therefore, PEP was administered to him.[g,h,i]

   Note: Although the man was astute to consider rabies in a situation in which a wild animal was acting abnormally by exhibiting no fear of him and was a nocturnal animal active during the day, he should have taken the skunk's body (without touching it with his bare hands) to a qualified person, such as a veterinarian or an animal control officer, to have the head removed properly as they would be aware of the need to use precautions and wear personal protective equipment.

5. A woman was strolling along a river walk when she discovered a downed bat and picked it up with her bare hands. She planned to take it to someone who could render aid to the animal, but in the journey to her destination, she decided to drape the bat from her shirt and it contacted her bare chest. The bat subsequently tested positive for rabies and its rescuer needed PEP.[j]

   Note: This is a meaningful example of the need for continued education on rabies and what to do if one encounters a downed bat.

CLIENT EDUCATION: FACT SHEETS ON RABIES, BITE PREVENTION, AND EXPOSURE TO BATS

The rabies and bite prevention tips, which can be found on the following pages, are easy to reproduce and post in an office or distribute to clients.

Client Education: Awareness of Clinical Signs of Rabies in Animals

Consider rabies if you see a/an:
- wild animal acting friendly, tame, and as if it has no fear of people or other animals;
- nocturnal animal, such as a skunk, raccoon, or bat, being active during the daytime;
- normally calm domestic animal acting aggressive or a normally friendly one being withdrawn;
- animal having difficulty walking or flying (bats);
- animal having trouble swallowing, eating, and drinking and/or appearing to be choking;
- animal displaying a thick, rope-like drool; and/or
- animal chewing too much at a bite wound (be aware, though, that a healthy animal can chew an area of its body to the point of creating a hot spot due to allergies).

Client Education: Recommendations for Bite Avoidance

There are many tips, including those listed below, that you can follow to avoid being bitten.
- Avoid interactions with wildlife or unfamiliar domestic animals.
- Do not handle downed bats.
- Report bites to the proper officials (such as the local rabies control authority, animal control officer, game warden, or local health department employee; for children, a teacher or parent is a good reporting resource).
- Do not feed wildlife. Leaving pet food out at night often attracts wildlife and also serves to condition them not to fear humans.
- Do not handle sick, injured, or dead animals. Contact an animal control officer or park ranger for assistance.
- Teach children how to correctly behave around an animal to avoid being bitten. For example, in addition to the above tips, teach them to not pull the animal's ears or tail, tease the animal, bother the animal while it is sleeping or eating, run past the animal, move toward an unfamiliar animal, or bother a mother while she is tending to her young.
- Have dogs and cats sterilized to reduce overpopulation; this aids in decreasing the number of stray animals, plus it lowers the risk of being bitten and potentially being exposed to rabies.

Client Education: Avoiding Interactions With Wildlife

There have been reports of rabid skunks gaining access to a house through a dog or cat door. Therefore, precautions should be taken when installing a pet door. Some are designed to prevent unwelcome intruders, such as styles that are triggered to open upon recognizing a specific tag provided by the door manufacturer for a pet to wear on its collar.

This leads to another recommendation. Keep cats indoors so they do not accidentally associate with skunks and raccoons (both high-risk animals for transmitting rabies) or pick up a downed bat (downed bats are more likely to be rabid than bats capable of flying). Cats will readily prey on downed bats and have a tendency to carry their victims into the home. Dogs, too, like to play with downed or dead bats, all which serves as another reason to have your pets vaccinated against rabies. As a side note, with urban spread destroying the habitat of wild animals, some species, such as coyotes, are more frequently seen in urban areas. It is very unfortunate for the animals, but cats, and also small dogs, have become meal sources for these animals in search of food.

Do not feed wildlife by hand because it

- modifies their diet, which could be detrimental to their health;
- encourages them to trust people, which could also be detrimental to their health (they could mistakenly trust someone who might harm them or someone may incorrectly interpret the learned tame behavior to be a clinical sign of rabies); and

- increases the chances for an unfortunate encounter, such as a person being bitten during the hand-feeding process.

Even though chipmunks and squirrels are considered to be low-risk animals for rabies, any animal bite opens the door for speculation on possible rabies exposure that should be discussed with a physician as well as a public health rabies expert.

Keep garbage in covered trash cans to prevent enticing wildlife to your yard. Do not leave any food, including bowls of pet food, outside where it could attract wild animals.

Do not try to make pets out of wildlife. This is especially tempting to do if you happen to find an adorable baby animal. It is best to let an experienced wildlife rehabilitator assist with rescue efforts of wildlife so they can raise and care for the animal with the intent of preparing it to be released back to its natural habitat. Plus, wildlife rehabilitators should have received rabies preexposure vaccinations because they are in frequent contact with wild animals (you do not know if the animal had been potentially exposed to rabies). In making a wild animal a pet, it has an increased opportunity for nipping or scratching someone, even if in play. If it is a high-risk animal for transmitting rabies, it will then most likely have to be euthanized and tested for rabies; the end result is the unfortunate demise of the animal. Additionally, there are laws prohibiting possession of certain wildlife.

Client Education: Tip List for How to Handle Finding a Bat

What to Do if You Find a Bat

If you find an injured, sick, or dead bat, do not touch it. If you need assistance, contact your local animal control agency or local health department. Your local animal control agency should be able to send a trained officer to capture the bat.

If you are unable to reach anyone for assistance, recommendations for bat capture are as follows:

- Remove any children or pets from the room.
- Wear gloves, preferably made of pliable, thick leather (never handle a bat with bare hands).
- Do not let the bat touch bare skin.
- Confine the bat to one room by closing the windows and doors.
- Turn on the lights if the room is dark.
- Wait for the bat to land.
- Cover the bat with a coffee can, cardboard box, Tupperware, or similar container.
- Slide a piece of cardboard (or the lid to the Tupperware) under the container that has the bat trapped.
- Tape the cardboard directly to the container (or snap close the Tupperware lid).
- Punch small holes in the container to allow air flow so the bat can breathe.

If any possible contact between the bat and a person or domestic animal has occurred, including the bat-specific exposure scenarios* listed at the end:

- Do *not* release the bat.
- Contact your local animal control agency or law enforcement agency to arrange for immediate submission of the bat for rabies testing. If none of these entities are available, a veterinarian can assist with the specimen submission.

If you are certain *no* contact between the bat and a person or domestic animal has occurred:

- Take the container outside.
- Release the bat, preferably at night and away from populated areas.

When capturing a bat, avoid striking it if at all possible. Physical trauma can damage the brain and make it impossible to conduct rabies laboratory tests. Do not release the bat if any of the following potential scenarios* occurred:

- A child touches a live or dead bat.
- An adult touches a bat without seeing the part of the body that was touched.
- A bat flies into a person and touches bare skin.
- A bare-footed person steps on a bat.
- A person awakens to find a bat in the same room.
- A bat is found near an infant, toddler, a person who is sensory or mentally challenged, or a person who is intoxicated (i.e., any person who cannot reliably explain what happened).
- A person puts their hand in firewood, brush, a crevice, or a dark space (e.g., a closet), then sees a bat close to that hand.

Client Education: Advice on Submitting a Specimen for Rabies Testing

Even though the animal is dead, do not handle it with bare hands. Place it in a plastic bag without touching it; use a shovel or pick it up with a gloved hand. If the animal needs to be submitted for testing because of concerns about rabies exposure and there will be a delay in getting it to an animal control officer or a veterinarian for specimen preparation and submission or a delay in taking a bat (whole bodies of bats can be submitted) to a rabies laboratory, keep the body cool in a refrigerator or an ice cooler; do not use dry ice and do not freeze. Decomposition of the specimen can result in the inability to get a confirmatory positive or negative report.

If you do happen to freeze it or do not keep it cool enough and decomposition has started, still submit it to the laboratory for testing. The laboratorians are sometimes able to salvage enough of the specimen to effectively perform testing. An example of this occurred in a case of rabies in a human in which the family of a child hospitalized with a yet undetermined diagnosis recollected that a bat had been found in the child's bedroom. Upon examination, the family saw no evidence of a bite, so they destroyed the bat and buried it. Based on this report, the child was tested and confirmed to have rabies. The local health department exhumed the bat and, even though it was partially decomposed, submitted it for testing; enough tissue was available to determine that the bat had the same rabies virus variant as the child.

Client Education: Bat Exclusion Tips

In dealing with problematic bats in a building, seal them out by using materials such as expanding foam, insulation, and wire mesh (knitted copper mesh does not deteriorate or corrode like steel wool eventually can) to fill in any openings with a diameter larger than 3/8 inch. A one-way exit tube should be provided where the bats are roosting for 7–10 days before the roost area is completely sealed. A tube or check valve with polypropylene netting that is open at the bottom will allow bats to exit the building but not enter. For larger areas, use not more than ¼-inch polypropylene mesh or hardware cloth; apply sealant at night after the bats have exited for their nightly journey in search of food. Another possible material is backer rod, which does not absorb water and caulk can be applied over it. However, and very importantly, avoid sealing openings if there is a potential that baby bats were left behind while the adults went to feed. One female bat usually has just one pup annually and needs to be in continual care of her young to enable its survival. May through August is generally the time of year to avoid bat proofing, while fall and winter are preferable; however, some warmer climates might dictate a longer period (i.e. into the fall) to avoid implementing exclusion techniques. Check with a professional bat excluder, bat conservation facility, or a local parks and wildlife office for the bat-proofing times in your area to avoid sealing babies inside and sealing adults outside.

Some environments may be conducive for bat houses to be erected as alternative roosts. If you install bat houses, cats will be attracted to chasing and hunting the bats, so for the health and safety of the cats and bats, it is advisable to keep cats indoors. Dogs also have been reported as playing with downed or dead bats that subsequently test positive for rabies. Therefore, as always, keep your pets currently vaccinated against rabies.

Bats fill a valuable ecologic niche, such as performing insect control (including insects that can damage crops or spread disease), seed dispersal, and plant pollination, so make a concerted effort to deal with them in a humane and protective manner. Additionally, in some areas, bats are protected by law.

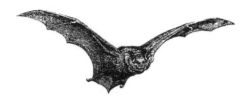

Whether it's on the ground or flying around, If it's a bat, don't touch that!

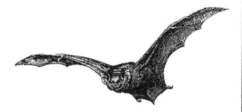

It is tempting to pick up a bat because they look so unusual. Don't do it! Leave bats alone.

Bats are helpful in nature. However, they also can spread rabies.

Rabies is a deadly disease caused by a virus. You can get rabies if an animal that has rabies bites you. Bat teeth are so small you might not even know you were bitten!

You can also get rabies if the saliva from an animal with rabies gets in your eyes, nose, or mouth. This can happen if you get the saliva on your fingers and then touch your face. Another way you can get rabies is by touching an animal with rabies and getting its saliva in open cuts on your skin.

Tell an adult, such as a teacher, nurse, parent, school guard, or police officer, right away if you have touched a bat or a bat has touched you. There is medicine that can keep you from getting rabies. For the medicine to work well, it must be given soon after contact with a bat.

Remember, if you find any bat, even if it is dead, __do not touch it__. Tell an adult right away about the bat and where you found it.

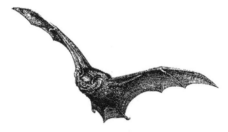

TEXAS
Department of
State Health Services

1/07 Zoonosis Control Stock No. 7-39

Both of these raccoons are cute and fuzzy. Can you tell which one has rabies?*

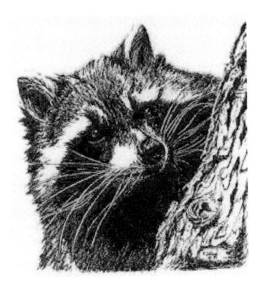 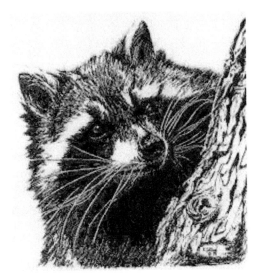

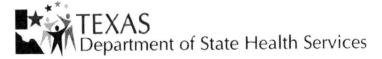

*You cannot tell if an animal has rabies by looking at it.

You can be exposed to rabies anywhere you encounter wildlife. It is good to enjoy nature, but you need to respect and understand it. Leave wild animals alone. Do not try to hand-feed them. Teach children to do the same.

Do not touch sick, injured, or dead animals. If you need help, call a local animal control officer, health department official, game warden, law enforcement officer, park employee, or rabies control authority.

TEXAS
Department of State Health Services

Zoonosis Control
Stock No. 7-25 8/05

REFERENCES

1. Universal Pictures. *To Kill a Mockingbird*; 1962. https://en.wikipedia.org/wiki/To_Kill_a_Mockingbird.
2. Green WH, Simons-Morton BG. Internal determinants of behavior. In: *Introduction to Health Education*. Prospect Heights: Waveland Press; 1984:148–178.
3. Centers for Disease Control and Prevention. Human rabies prevention – United States, 2008: recommendations of the Advisory Committee on Immunization Practices. *MMWR*. 2008;57(RR-3):1–28.
4. Wilson PJ. *Caring for your puppy pal*. In: *Puppy Pal Pointers: From the True Tails of Ripple and Jessie*. Bloomington: AuthorHouse; 2004:1–66.
5. Centers for Disease Control and Prevention. Cost of Rabies Prevention. https://www.cdc.gov/rabies/location/usa/cost.html.
6. Hanlon CA, Childs JE. Epidemiology. In: Jackson AC, ed. *Rabies: Scientific Basis of the Disease and its Management*. San Diego: Academic Press, An Elsevier Science Imprint; 2013:61–121.
7. Childs JE. Epidemiology. In: Jackson AC, Wunner WH, eds. *Rabies*. San Diego: Academic Press, An Elsevier Science Imprint; 2002:113–162.
8. Petersen BW, Rupprecht CE. *Human Rabies Epidemiology and Diagnosis. Intechopen*; 2011; November 16. https://www.intechopen.com/books/non-flavivirus-encephalitis/human-rabies-epidemiology-and-diagnosis.
9. Birhane MG, Cleaton JM, Monroe BP, et al. Rabies surveillance in the United States during 2015. *JAVMA*. 2017;250(10):1117–1130.
10. Ma X, Monroe BP, Cleaton JM, et al. Rabies surveillance in the United States during 2016. *JAVMA*. 2018;252(8):945–957.
11. Mayes BC, Wilson PJ, Oertli EH, et al. Epidemiology of rabies in bats in Texas (2001-2010). *JAVMA*. 2013;243(8):1129–1137.
12. Centers for Disease Control and Prevention. Issuance and Enforcement Guidance for Dog Confinement Agreements: Rabies Vaccine Requirements. https://www.cdc.gov/importation/laws-and-regulations/faq.html.
13. Brown CM, Slavinski S, Ettestad P, et al. Compendium of animal rabies prevention and control, 2016. *JAVMA*. 2016;248(5):505–517.
14. Texas Administrative Code. *Rabies Control and Eradication*; 2013. Sections 169.21-169.34 http://texreg.sos.state.tx.us/public/readtac$ext.ViewTAC?tac_view=5&ti=25&pt.=1&ch=169&sch=A&rl=Y.
15. American Association of Equine Practitioners. Rabies. https://aaep.org/guidelines/vaccination-guidelines/core-vaccination-guidelines/rabies.
16. Wilson PJ. Rabies. In: Sprayberry KA, Robinson NE, eds. *Robinson's Current Therapy in Equine Medicine*. 7th ed. St. Louis: Elsevier-Saunders; 2015:171–172.
17. Roach J. Rabies Management in Livestock and Horses. Animal Industry Services Division, Oklahoma Department of Agriculture.

18. Clark KA, Wilson PJ. Postexposure rabies prophylaxis and preexposure rabies vaccination failure in domestic animals. *JAVMA*. 1996;208(11):1827–1830.
19. Wilson PJ, Clark KA. Postexposure rabies prophylaxis protocol for domestic animals and epidemiologic characteristics of rabies vaccination failures in Texas: 1995-1999. *JAVMA*. 2001;218(4):522–525.
20. Murray KO, Holmes KC, Hanlon CA. Rabies in vaccinated dogs and cats in the United States, 1997-2001. *JAVMA*. 2009;235(6):691–696.
21. Murnane TG. Importance of observing animal bite reporting procedures. *TX Prev Dis News*. 1990;50:5.
22. Mahlow J, Wilson P. *Healthy Texans: The Veterinary Perspective*. Texas Department of Health Report. TVMA: *TX Vet*; 1996.
23. United States Department of Agriculture – Animal and Plant Health Inspection Service. National Rabies Management Program. https://www.aphis.usda.gov/aphis/ourfocus/wildlifedamage/programs/nrmp/ct_rabies.
24. Fehlner-Gardiner C, Rudd R, Donovan D, et al. Comparing ONRAB and RABORAL V-RG oral rabies vaccine field performance in raccoons and striped skunks, New Brunswick, Canada, and Maine, USA. *J Wildl Dis*. 2012;48(1):157–167.
25. Wohlers A, Lankau EW, Oertli EH, et al. Challenges to controlling rabies in skunk populations using oral rabies vaccination: a review. *Zoo Pub Hlth*. 2018;65(4):373–385.
26. Fearneyhough MG, Wilson PJ, Clark KA, et al. Results of an oral rabies vaccination program for coyotes. *JAVMA*. 1998;212(4):498–502.
27. Sidwa TJ, Wilson PJ, Moore GM, et al. Evaluation of oral rabies vaccination programs for control of rabies epizootics in coyotes and gray foxes: 1995-2003. *JAVMA*. 2005;227(5):785–792.
28. World Health Organization. WHO Expert Consultation of Rabies –Third Report. *WHO Technical Report Series*. 2018;1012:1–183.
29. Texas Department of State Health Services. Rabies Prevention in Texas. Zoonosis Control. https://dshs.texas.gov/idcu/disease/rabies/information/prevention/pamphlet/.
30. Miller ET, Marsh RH, Harris NS. Rabies exposure-implications for wilderness travelers. *Wilderness Environ Med*. 2009;20:290–296.
31. Centers for Disease Control and Prevention. Human rabies – Wyoming and Utah, 2015. *MMWR*. 2016;65(21):529–533.
32. Wallace RM, Bhavnani D, Russell J, et al. Rabies death attributed to exposure in Central America with symptom onset in a US detention facility-Texas, 2013. *MMWR*. 2014;63(20):446–449.
33. Centers for Disease Control and Prevention. Investigation of rabies infections in organ donor and transplant recipients – Alabama, Arkansas, Oklahoma, and Texas, 2004. *MMWR*. 2004;53(Dispatch):1–3.
34. Jackson AC. Human disease. In: Jackson AC, Wunner WH, eds. *Rabies*. San Diego: Academic Press, An Elsevier Science Imprint; 2002:219–244.

35. Fooks AR, Banyard AC, Horton DL, et al. Current status of rabies and prospects for elimination. *Lancet.* 2014;384:1389–1399.

36. Warrell MJ, Warrell DA. Rabies: the clinical features, management, and prevention of the classic zoonosis. *Clin Med.* 2015;15(1):78–81.

37. Centers for Disease Control and Prevention. Human rabies–South Carolina, 2011. *MMWR.* 2013;62(32):642–644.

38. Winkler WG, Fashinell TR, Leffingwell L, et al. Airborne rabies transmission in a laboratory worker. *JAMA.* 1973;226(10):1219–1221.

39. Gibbons RV. Cryptogenic rabies, bats, and the question of aerosol transmission. *Ann Emerg Med.* 2002;39(5):528–536.

40. de Brito MG, Chamone TL, da Silva FJ, et al. Antemortem diagnosis of human rabies in a veterinarian infected when handling a herbivore in Minas Gerais, Brazil. *Rev Inst Med Trop.* 2011;53(1):39–44.

41. Niezgoda M, Hanlon CA, Rupprecht CE. Animal rabies. In: Jackson AC, Wunner WH, eds. *Rabies.* San Diego: Academic Press, An Elsevier Science Imprint; 2002:163–218.

42. Rupprecht CE, Hanlon CA, Hemachudha T. Rabies re-examined. *Lancet Infect Dis.* 2002;2:327–343.

43. Hanlon CA. Rabies in terrestrial animals. In: Jackson AC, ed. *Rabies: Scientific Basis of the Disease and its Management.* San Diego: Academic Press, An Elsevier Science Imprint; 2013:179–213.

44. Willoughby RE, Tieves KS, Hoffman GM, et al. Survival after treatment of rabies with induction of coma. *N Engl J Med.* 2005;352:2508–2514.

45. Finley D. Unvaccinated rabies survivor lives to tell her tale. San Antonio Express News. 22.06.12.

46. National Park Service. What is White-Nose Syndrome? https://www.nps.gov/articles/what-is-white-nose-syndrome.htm.

47. De Serres G, Dallaire F, Cote M, et al. Bat rabies in the United States and Canada from 1950 through 2007: human cases with and without bat contact. *Clin Infect Dis.* 2008;46:1329–1337.

48. Baer GM, Smith JS. Rabies in nonhematophagus bats. In: Baer GM, ed. *The Natural History of Rabies.* 2nd ed. Boca Raton: CRC Press, Inc; 1991:341–366.

49. Wilson PJ, Rohde RE. *The Many Faces of Rabies.* Elsevier Connect; September 2016. htpps://www.elsevier.com/connect/the-many-faces-of-rabies.

50. Smith JS, Fishbein DB, Rupprecht CE, et al. Unexplained rabies in three immigrants in the United States. *NEJM.* 1991;324(4):205–211.

51. Centers for Disease Control and Prevention. Human rabies – Washington, 1995. *MMWR.* 1995;44(34):625–627.

52. Rohde RE, Wilson PJ, Mayes BC, et al. Rabies methods and guidelines for assessing a clinical rarity. Microbiology No MB-4; Tech Sample. *Am Soc Clin Path.* 2004:21–29. https://www.researchgate.net/publication/256816514.

53. Wilson PJ. Understanding your puppy pal. In: *Puppy Pal Pointers: From the True Tails of Ripple and Jessie.* Bloomington: AuthorHouse; 2004:103–155.

54. Oertli EH, Wilson PJ, Hunt PR, et al. Epidemiology of rabies in skunks in Texas. *JAVMA.* 2009;234(5):616–620.

55. New York State Department of Health. *Guidelines for Managing Bats and Risk of Rabies Transmission. Rabies Policies And Procedures;* 2004.

56. Cornell University. *The Facts about Bats: Exploring Conflicts and Designing Solutions.* Cornell Cooperative Extension; 2002.

57. Texas Department of State Health Services. *Bats and Rabies Poster for Schools.* Zoonosis Control. Stock No. 7-39. http://dshs.texas.gov/idcu/health/zoonosis/education/pamphlets/.

58. Texas Department of State Health Services. *Rabies and Wildlife.* Zoonosis Control. Stock No. 7-25. http://dshs.texas.gov/idcu/health/zoonosis/education/pamphlets/.

Personal Communications

a. McDonald KM. Zoonosis Control Specialist, Department of State Health Services, Lubbock, TX. Communications on 15.12.17; 10.05.18.

b. Finch TG. Public Health and Prevention Specialist, Department of State Health Services, Canyon, TX. Communication on 10.05.18.

c. Pye GE. Zoonosis Control Specialist, Texas Department of Health, Harlingen, TX. Departed. Communication based on rabies case investigations: 1995–96.

d. O'Sullivan BJ. Zoonosis Control Epidemiologist, Department of State Health Services, Austin, TX. Communication on 28.09.18.

e. Hensley DS. Epidemiologist, Health Protection and Response, Florida Department of Health in Pasco County, Dade City, Florida. Communication on 28.09.18.

f. Moore GM. Zoonosis Control Program Specialist and Wildlife Biologist, Department of State Health Services, Austin, TX. Retired. Communication on 15.05.18.

g. Ferguson NW. Zoonosis Control Specialist. Department of State Health Services, Abilene, TX. Communication on 27.04.18; 08.10.18.

h. Stonecipher SD. Regional Zoonosis Control Veterinarian, Department of State Health Services, Arlington, TX. Communication on 08.10.18.

i. Hunt PR. Zoonosis Control Program Specialist, Department of State Health Services, Austin, TX. Communication on 27.04.18.

j. Phillips CR. Zoonosis Control Specialist, Department of State Health Services, El Paso, TX. Communication on 23.10.18.

REFERENCES FOR CLIENT EDUCATION MATERIALS

1. Client Education: Awareness of Clinical Signs of Rabies in Animals.
   Source: Wilson PJ, Rohde RE. *The Many Faces of Rabies*. Elsevier Connect; September 2016.[49] https://www.elsevier.com/connect/the-many-faces-of-rabies.
2. Client Education: Recommendations for Bite Avoidance.
   Source: Wilson PJ. Understanding your puppy pal. In: *Puppy Pal Pointers: From the True Tails of Ripple and Jessie*. Bloomington: AuthorHouse; 2004:103–155.[53]
3. Client Education: Avoiding Interactions With Wildlife.
   Sources: Oertli EH, Wilson PJ, Hunt PR, et al. Epidemiology of rabies in skunks in Texas. *JAVMA*. 2009;234(5):616–620.[54]
   Mayes BC, Wilson PJ, Oertli EH, et al. Epidemiology of rabies in bats in Texas (2001–2010). *JAVMA*. 2013;243(8):1129–1137.[11]
   Wilson PJ, Rohde RE. *The Many Faces of Rabies*. Elsevier Connect; September 2016.[49] https://www.elsevier.com/connect/the-many-faces-of-rabies.
4. Client Education: Tip List for How to Handle Finding a Bat.
   Sources: New York State Department of Health. Guidelines for managing bats and risk of rabies transmission. *Rabies Policies and Procedures*. 2004.[55]

Wilson PJ, Rohde RE. *The Many Faces of Rabies*. Elsevier Connect; September 2016.[49] https://www.elsevier.com/connect/the-many-faces-of-rabies.
5. Client Education: Advice on Submitting a Specimen for Rabies Testing.
   Source: Centers for Disease Control and Prevention. Human rabies—Washington, 1995. *MMWR*. 1995;44(34):625–627.[51]
6. Client Education: Bat Exclusion Tips.
   Sources: Cornell University. *The Facts About Bats: Exploring Conflicts and Designing Solutions*. Cornell Cooperative Extension; 2002.[56]
   Wilson PJ, Rohde RE. *The Many Faces of Rabies*. Elsevier Connect; September 2016.[49] https://www.elsevier.com/connect/the-many-faces-of-rabies.
7. Flier on Bats and Rabies.
   Source: Texas Department of State Health Services. *Bats and Rabies Poster for Schools*. Zoonosis Control. Stock No. 7-39.[57] http://dshs.texas.gov/idcu/health/zoonosis/education/pamphlets/.
8. Flier on Rabies and Wildlife.
   Source: Texas Department of State Health Services. *Rabies and Wildlife*. Zoonosis Control. Stock No. 7-25.[58] http://dshs.texas.gov/idcu/health/zoonosis/education/pamphlets/.

Index

Note: Page numbers followed by "f" indicate figures, "t" indicate tables, and "b" indicate boxes.

Printed and bound by CPI Group (UK) Ltd, Croydon, CR0 4YY

03/10/2024

01040373-0006